The Bishop Family
204 Holly Ln
Palatka, FL 32177
386.315.2144

上海市重点图书

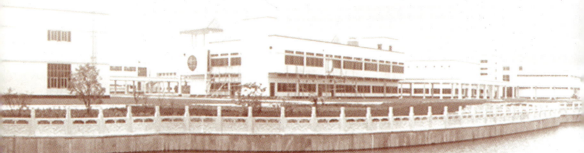

Full View Of Yangtze River Pharmacy Group ( Taizhou, Jiangsu, China )
扬子江药业集团全景（中国·江苏·泰州）

Newly Compiled
Practical English-Chinese Library
of Traditional Chinese Medicine
（英汉对照）新编实用中医文库

Compiled by Nanjing University of Traditional Chinese Medicine
Translated by Shanghai University of Traditional Chinese Medicine

General Compiler-in-Chief ZUO Yanfu
总主编 左言富

Translators-in-Chief
ZHU Zhongbao, HUANG Yuezhong, TAO Jinwen, LI Zhaoguo
主译 朱忠宝 黄月中 陶锦文 李照国（执行）

南京中医药大学 主编
上海中医药大学 主译

# DIAGNOSTICS OF TRADITIONAL CHINESE MEDICINE

## 中医诊断学

Examiner-in-Chief       LI Guoding
Compiler-in-Chief       WANG Lufen
Vice-Compilers-in-Chief YUE Peiping
                        TANG Chuanjian
Translators-in-Chief    LI Zhaoguo
                        BAO Bai
Vice-Translators-in-Chief DONG Jing
                         CAO Lijuan

主审 李国鼎芬
主编 王鲁平
副主编 岳沛俭
       唐传照
主译 李照国 白
     鲍 晶
副主译 董 丽娟
       曹

上海浦江教育出版社（原上海中医药大学出版社）
Shanghai Pujiang Education Press
Shanghai University of Traditional Chinese Medicine Press

Shanghai Pujiang Education Press (Shanghai University of Traditional Chinese Medicine Press)
1200 CaiLun Road, Shanghai, 201203, China

Diagnostics of Traditional Chinese Medicine
Compiler-in-Chief Wang Lufen   Translator-in-Chief Li Zhaoguo   Bao Bai
(A Newly Compiled Practical English-Chinese Library of TCM General Compiler-in-Chief Zuo Yanfu)

All rights reserved. No part of this book may be reproduced, stored in a retrieval system, or transmitted in any form or by any means, electronic, mechanical, photocopying, recording or otherwise, without the prior permission in writing of the Publisher.

### 图书在版编目(CIP)数据

中医诊断学／王鲁芬主编；李照国，鲍白主译．—上海：上海中医药大学出版社，2002(2011.9重印)
(英汉对照新编实用中医文库／左言富总主编)
ISBN 978-7-81010-652-8

Ⅰ.中…　Ⅱ.①王…②李…③鲍…　Ⅲ.中医诊断学-对照读物-英、汉　Ⅳ.R241

中国版本图书馆CIP数据核字(2002)第038445号

**中医诊断学**　　主编 王鲁芬　主译 李照国 鲍白

上海浦江教育出版社(原上海中医药大学出版社)出版发行　(蔡伦路1200号　邮政编码201203)
新华书店上海发行所经销　　　　　　　　　上海新华印刷有限公司印刷
开本　787mm×1092mm　1/18　　印张 17.444　　插页 4　　字数 417千字
版次 2002年10月第1版　　印次 2011年9月第5次印刷

ISBN 978-7-81010-652-8/R·618　　　　　　定价 46.00元

# Compilation Board of the Library

**Honorary Director**  Zhang Wenkang
**General Advisor**  Chen Keji
**Advisors**  (Listed in the order of the number of strokes in the Chinese names)

| | | | |
|---|---|---|---|
| Gan Zuwang | You Songxin | Liu Zaipeng | Xu Zhiyin |
| Sun Tong | Song Liren | Zhang Minqing | Jin Shi |
| Jin Miaowen | Shan Zhaowei | Zhou Fuyi | Shi Zhen |
| Xu Jingfan | Tang Shuhua | Cao Shihong | Fu Weimin |

**International Advisors**  M. S. Khan (Ireland)  Alessandra Gulí (Italy)  Secondo Scarsella (Italy)  Raymond K. Carroll (Australia)  Shulan Tang (Britain)  Giovanni Maciocia (Britain)  David Molony (America)  Tzu Kuo Shih (America)  Isigami Hiroshi (Japan)  Helmut Ziegler (Germany)

**Director**  Xiang Ping
**Executive Director**  Zuo Yanfu
**Executive Vice-Directors**  Ma Jian  Du Wendong  Li Zhaoguo
**Vice-Directors**  Huang Chenghui  Wu Kunping  Liu Shenlin  Wu Mianhua
  Chen Diping  Cai Baochang

**Members**  (Listed in the order of the number of strokes in the Chinese names)

| | | | | |
|---|---|---|---|---|
| Ding Anwei | Ding Shuhua | Yu Yong | Wan Lisheng | Wang Xu |
| Wang Xudong | Wang Lingling | Wang Lufen | Lu Zijie | Shen Junlong |
| Liu Yu | Liu Yueguang | Yan Daonan | Yang Gongfu | Min Zhongsheng |
| Wu Changguo | Wu Yongjun | Wu Jianlong | He Wenbin | |
| He Shuxun (specially invited) | | He Guixiang | Wang Yue | |
| Wang Shouchuan | | Shen Daqing | Zhang Qing | Chen Yonghui |
| Chen Tinghan (specially invited) | | Shao Jianmin | Lin Xianzeng (specially invited) | |
| Lin Duanmei (specially invited) | | Yue Peiping | Jin Hongzhu | |
| Zhou Ligao (specially invited) | | Zhao Xia | Zhao Jingsheng | Hu Lie |
| Hu Kui | Zha Wei | Yao Yingzhi | Yuan Ying | Xia Youbing |
| Xia Dengjie | Ni Yun | Xu Hengze | Guo Haiying | Tang Chuanjian |
| Tang Decai | Ling Guizhen (specially invited) | | Tan Yong | Huang Guicheng |
| Mei Xiaoyun | Cao Guizhu | Jiang Zhongqiu | Zeng Qingqi | Zhai Yachun |
| Fan Qiaoling | | | | |

# 《（英汉对照）新编实用中医文库》编纂委员会

**名誉主任** 张文康
**总 顾 问** 陈可冀
**顾   问**（按姓氏笔画为序）
　　于祖望　尤松鑫　刘再朋　许芝银　孙 桐　宋立人　张民庆　金 实
　　金妙文　单兆伟　周福贻　施 震　徐景藩　唐蜀华　曹世宏　符为民
**外籍顾问**
　　萨利姆（爱尔兰）　亚历山大·古丽（意大利）　卡塞拉·塞肯多（意大利）
　　雷蒙特·凯·卡罗（澳大利亚）　汤淑兰（英国）　马万里（英国）
　　大卫·莫罗尼（美国）　施祖谷（美国）　石上博（日本）　赫尔木特（德国）

**主　　　任** 项 平
**执 行 主 任** 左言富
**执行副主任** 马 健　杜文东　李照国
**副　主　任** 黄成惠　吴坤平　刘沈林　吴勉华　陈涤平　蔡宝昌
**编　　　委**（按姓氏笔画为序）
　　丁安伟　　　丁淑华　　　于 勇　　　万力生　　　王 旭
　　王旭东　　　王玲玲　　　王鲁芬　　　卢子杰　　　申俊龙
　　刘 玉　　　刘跃光　　　严道南　　　杨公服　　　闵仲生
　　吴昌国　　　吴拥军　　　吴建龙　　　何文彬　　　何树勋（特邀）
　　何贵翔　　　汪 悦　　　汪受传　　　沈大庆　　　张 庆
　　陈永辉　　　陈廷汉（特邀）　邵健民　　　林显增（特邀）
　　林端美（特邀）岳沛平　　　金宏柱　　　周礼杲（特邀）
　　赵 霞　　　赵京生　　　胡 烈　　　胡 葵　　　查 炜
　　姚映芷　　　袁 颖　　　夏有兵　　　夏登杰　　　倪 云
　　徐恒泽　　　郭海英　　　唐传俭　　　唐德才　　　凌桂珍（特邀）
　　谈 勇　　　黄桂成　　　梅晓芸　　　曹贵珠　　　蒋中秋
　　曾庆琪　　　翟亚春　　　樊巧玲

# Translation Committee of the Library

**Advisors**  Shao Xundao   Ou Ming
**Translators-in-Chief**  Zhu Zhongbao   Huang Yuezhong   Tao Jinwen
**Executive Translator-in-Chief**  Li Zhaoguo
**Vice-Translators-in-Chief**  (Listed in the order of the number of strokes in the Chinese names)

Xun Jianying   Li Yong'an   Zhang Qingrong   Zhang Dengfeng   Yang Hongying
Huang Guoqi   Xie Jinhua

**Translators**  (Listed in the order of the number of strokes in the Chinese names)

| | | | |
|---|---|---|---|
| Yu Xin | Wang Ruihui | Tian Kaiyu | Shen Guang |
| Lan Fengli | Cheng Peili | Zhu Wenxiao | Zhu Yuqin |
| Zhu Jinjiang | Zhu Guixiang | Le Yimin | Liu Shengpeng |
| Li Jingyun | Yang Ying | Yang Mingshan | He Yingchun |
| Zhang Jie | Zhang Haixia | Zhang Wei | Chen Renying |
| Zhou Yongming | Zhou Suzhen | Qu Yusheng | Zhao Junqing |
| Jing Zhen | Hu Kewu | Xu Qilong | Xu Yao |
| Guo Xiaomin | Huang Xixuan | Cao Lijuan | Kang Qin |
| Dong Jing | Qin Baichang | Zeng Haiping | Lou Jianhua |
| Lai Yuezhen | Bao Bai | Pei Huihua | Xue Junmei |
| Dai Wenjun | Wei Min | | |

**Office of the Translation Committee**
**Director**  Yang Mingshan
**Secretaries**  Xu Lindi   Chen Li

## 《(英汉对照)新编实用中医文库》编译委员会

| | | | | | | |
|---|---|---|---|---|---|---|
|顾　　问|邵循道|欧　明| | | | |
|总 编 译|朱忠宝|黄月中|陶锦文| | | |
|执行总编译|李照国| | | | | |

副 总 编 译　（按姓氏笔画为序）

　　寻建英　李永安　张庆荣　张登峰　杨洪英　黄国琪　谢金华

编 译 者　（按姓氏笔画为序）

　　于　新　王瑞辉　田开宇　申　光　兰凤利　成培莉　朱文晓
　　朱玉琴　朱金江　朱桂香　乐毅敏　刘升鹏　李经蕴　杨　莹
　　杨明山　何迎春　张　杰　张海峡　张　维　陈仁英　周永明
　　周素贞　屈榆生　赵俊卿　荆　蓁　胡克武　徐启龙　徐　瑶
　　郭小民　黄熙璇　曹丽娟　康　勤　董　晶　覃百长　曾海苹
　　楼建华　赖月珍　鲍　白　裴慧华　薛俊梅　戴文军　魏　敏

编译委员会办公室
主　任　杨明山
秘　书　徐林娣　陈　力

# Approval Committee of the Library

**Director**  Li Zhenji
**Vice-Directors**  Shen Zhixiang   Chen Xiaogu   Zhou Zhongying   Wang Canhui
　　　　　　　 Gan Zuwang   Jiang Yuren
**Members** (Listed in the order of the number of strokes in the Chinese names)

| | | | |
|---|---|---|---|
| Ding Renqiang | Ding Xiaohong | Wang Xinhua | You Benlin |
| Shi Yanhua | Qiao Wenlei | Yi Sumei | Li Fei |
| Li Guoding | Yang Zhaomin | Lu Mianmian | Chen Songyu |
| Shao Mingxi | Shi Bingbing | Yao Xin | Xia Guicheng |
| Gu Yuehua | Xu Fusong | Gao Yuanhang | Zhu Fangshou |
| Tao Jinwen | Huang Yage | Fu Zhiwen | Cai Li |

**General Compiler-in-Chief**  Zuo Yanfu
**Executive Vice-General-Compilers-in-Chief**  Ma Jian   Du Wendong
**Vice-General-Compilers-in-Chief**  (Listed in the order of the number of strokes in the Chinese names)

| | | | |
|---|---|---|---|
| Ding Shuhua | Wang Xudong | Wang Lufen | Yan Daonan |
| Wu Changguo | Wang Shouchuan | Wang Yue | Chen Yonghui |
| Jin Hongzhu | Zhao Jingsheng | Tang Decai | Tan Yong |
| Huang Guicheng | Zhai Yachun | Fan Qiaoling | |

**Office of the Compilation Board Committee**
**Directors**  Ma Jian   Du Wendong
**Vice-Directors**  Wu Jianlong   Zhu Changren

**Publisher**  Zhu Bangxian
**Chinese Editors**  (Listed in the order of the number of strokes in the Chinese names)

| | | | |
|---|---|---|---|
| Ma Shengying | Wang Lingli | Wang Deliang | He Qianqian |
| Shen Chunhui | Zhang Xingjie | Zhou Dunhua | Shan Baozhi |
| Jiang Shuiyin | Qin Baoping | Qian Jingzhuang | Fan Yuqi |
| Pan Zhaoxi | | | |

**English Editors**  Shan Baozhi   Jiang Shuiyin   Xiao Yuanchun
**Cover Designer**  Wang Lei
**Layout Designer**  Xu Guomin

# 《(英汉对照)新编实用中医文库》审定委员会

主　　任　李振吉
副 主 任　沈志祥　陈啸谷　周仲瑛　王灿晖　干祖望　江育仁
委　　员　(按姓氏笔画为序)
　　　　　丁仁强　丁晓红　王新华　尤本林　石燕华　乔文雷　衣素梅　李　飞
　　　　　李国鼎　杨兆民　陆绵绵　陈松育　邵明熙　施冰冰　姚　欣　夏桂成
　　　　　顾月华　徐福松　高远航　诸方受　陶锦文　黄雅各　傅志文　蔡　丽

总 主 编　左言富
执行副总主编　马　健　杜文东
副 总 主 编　(按姓氏笔画为序)
　　　　　丁淑华　王旭东　王鲁芬　严道南　吴昌国　汪　悦　汪受传　陈永辉
　　　　　金宏柱　赵京生　唐德才　谈　勇　黄桂成　翟亚春　樊巧玲

编纂委员会办公室
主　　任　马　健　杜文东
副 主 任　吴建龙　朱长仁

出 版 人　朱邦贤
中文责任编辑　(按姓氏笔画为序)
　　　　　马胜英　王玲琍　王德良　何倩倩　沈春晖　张杏洁　周敦华　单宝枝
　　　　　姜水印　秦葆平　钱静庄　樊玉琦　潘朝曦
英文责任编辑　单宝枝　姜水印　肖元春
美 术 编 辑　王　磊
技 术 编 辑　徐国民

# Foreword I   序一

As we are walking into the 21st century, "health for all" is still an important task for the World Health Organization (WHO) to accomplish in the new century. The realization of "health for all" requires mutual cooperation and concerted efforts of various medical sciences, including traditional medicine. WHO has increasingly emphasized the development of traditional medicine and has made fruitful efforts to promote its development. Currently the spectrum of diseases is changing and an increasing number of diseases are difficult to cure. The side effects of chemical drugs have become more and more evident. Furthermore, both the governments and peoples in all countries are faced with the problem of high cost of medical treatment. Traditional Chinese medicine (TCM), the complete system of traditional medicine in the world with unique theory and excellent clinical curative effects, basically meets the need to solve such problems. Therefore, bringing TCM into full play in medical treatment and healthcare will certainly become one of the hot points in the world medical business in the 21st century.

Various aspects of work need to be done to promote the course of the internationalization of TCM, especially the compilation of works and textbooks suitable for international readers. The impending new century has witnessed the compilation of such a

人类即将迈入21世纪,"人人享有卫生保健"仍然是新世纪世界卫生工作面临的重要任务。实现"人人享有卫生保健"的宏伟目标,需要包括传统医药学在内的多种医学学科的相互协作与共同努力。世界卫生组织越来越重视传统医药学的发展,并为推动其发展做出了卓有成效的工作。目前,疾病谱正在发生变化,难治疾病不断增多,化学药品的毒副作用日益显现,日趋沉重的医疗费用困扰着各国政府和民众。中医药学是世界传统医学体系中最完整的传统医学,其独到的学科理论和突出的临床疗效,较符合当代社会和人们解决上述难题的需要。因此,科学有效地发挥中医药学的医疗保健作用,必将成为21世纪世界卫生工作的特点之一。

加快中医药走向世界的步伐,还有很多的工作要做,特别是适合国外读者学习的中医药著作、教材的编写是极其重要的方面。在新千年来临之际,由南京中医药大学

series of books known as *A Newly Compiled Practical English-Chinese Library of Traditional Chinese Medicine* published by the Publishing House of Shanghai University of TCM, compiled by Nanjing University of TCM and translated by Shanghai University of TCM. Professor Zuo Yanfu, the general compiler-in-chief of this Library, is a person who sets his mind on the international dissemination of TCM. He has compiled *General Survey on TCM Abroad*, a monograph on the development and state of TCM abroad. This Library is another important works written by the experts organized by him with the support of Nanjing University of TCM and Shanghai University of TCM. The compilation of this Library is done with consummate ingenuity and according to the development of TCM abroad. The compilers, based on the premise of preserving the genuineness and gist of TCM, have tried to make the contents concise, practical and easy to understand, making great efforts to introduce the abstruse ideas of TCM in a scientific and simple way as well as expounding the prevention and treatment of diseases which are commonly encountered abroad and can be effectively treated by TCM.

This Library encompasses a systematic summarization of the teaching experience accumulated in Nanjing University of TCM and Shanghai University of TCM that run the collaborating centers of traditional medicine and the international training centers on acupuncture and moxibustion set by WHO. I am sure that the publication of this Library will further promote the development of traditional Chinese med-

主编、上海中医药大学主译、上海中医药大学出版社出版的《(英汉对照)新编实用中医文库》的即将问世,正是新世纪中医药国际传播更快发展的预示。本套文库总主编左言富教授是中医药学国际传播事业的有心人,曾主编研究国外中医药发展状况的专著《国外中医药概览》。本套文库的编撰,是他在南京中医药大学和上海中医药大学支持下,组织许多著名专家共同完成的又一重要专著。本套文库的作者们深谙国外的中医药发展现状,编写颇具匠心,在注重真实,不失精华的前提下,突出内容的简明、实用,易于掌握,力求科学而又通俗地介绍中医药学的深奥内容,重点阐述国外常见而中医药颇具疗效的疾病的防治。

本套文库蕴含了南京中医药大学和上海中医药大学作为WHO传统医学合作中心、国际针灸培训中心多年留学生教学的实践经验和系统总结,更为全面、系统、准确地向世界传播中医药学。相信本书的出版将对中医更好地走向世界,让世界更好地了解中医产生更

icine abroad and enable the whole world to have a better understanding of traditional Chinese medicine.

Professor Zhu Qingsheng
Vice-Minister of Health Ministry of the People's Republic of China
Director of the State Administrative Bureau of TCM

December 14, 2000 Beijing

为积极的影响。

朱庆生教授
中华人民共和国卫生部副部长

国家中医药管理局局长

2000年12月14日于北京

# Foreword II

Before the existence of the modern medicine, human beings depended solely on herbal medicines and other therapeutic methods to treat diseases and preserve health. Such a practice gave rise to the establishment of various kinds of traditional medicine with unique theory and practice, such as traditional Chinese medicine, Indian medicine and Arabian medicine, etc. Among these traditional systems of medicine, traditional Chinese medicine is a most extraordinary one based on which traditional Korean medicine and Japanese medicine have evolved.

Even in the 21st century, traditional medicine is still of great vitality. In spite of the fast development of modern medicine, traditional medicine is still disseminated far and wide. In many developing countries, most of the people in the rural areas still depend on traditional medicine and traditional medical practitioners to meet the need for primary healthcare. Even in the countries with advanced modern medicine, more and more people have begun to accept traditional medicine and other therapeutic methods, such as homeopathy, osteopathy and naturopathy, etc.

With the change of the economy, culture and living style in various regions as well as the aging in the world population, the disease spectrum has changed. And such a change has paved the way for the new application of traditional medicine. Besides,

# 序 二

在现代医学形成之前，人类一直依赖草药和其他一些疗法治病强身，从而发展出许多有理论、有实践的传统医学，例如中医学、印度医学、阿拉伯医学等。中医学是世界林林总总的传统医学中的一支奇葩，在它的基础上还衍生出朝鲜传统医学和日本汉方医学。在跨入21世纪的今天，古老的传统医学依然焕发着活力，非但没有因现代医学的发展而式微，其影响还有增无减，人们对传统医学的价值也有了更深刻的体会和认识。在许多贫穷国家，大多数农村人口仍然依赖传统医学疗法和传统医务工作者来满足他们对初级卫生保健的需求。在现代医学占主导地位的许多国家，传统医学及其他一些"另类疗法"，诸如顺势疗法、整骨疗法、自然疗法等，也越来越被人们所接受。

伴随着世界各地经济、文化和生活的变革以及世界人口的老龄化，世界疾病谱也发生了变化。传统医学有了新的应用，而新疾病所引起的新需求以及现代医学的成

the new requirements initiated by the new diseases and the achievements and limitations of modern medicine have also created challenges for traditional medicine.

WHO sensed the importance of traditional medicine to human health early in the 1970s and have made great efforts to develop traditional medicine. At the 29th world health congress held in 1976, the item of traditional medicine was adopted in the working plan of WHO. In the following world health congresses, a series of resolutions were passed to demand the member countries to develop, utilize and study traditional medicine according to their specific conditions so as to reduce medical expenses for the realization of "health for all".

WHO has laid great stress on the scientific content, safe and effective application of traditional medicine. It has published and distributed a series of booklets on the scientific, safe and effective use of herbs and acupuncture and moxibustion. It has also made great contributions to the international standardization of traditional medical terms. The safe and effective application of traditional medicine has much to do with the skills of traditional medical practitioners. That is why WHO has made great efforts to train them. WHO has run 27 collaborating centers in the world which have made great contributions to the training of acupuncturists and traditional medical practitioners. Nanjing University of TCM and Shanghai University of TCM run the collaborating centers with WHO. In recent years it has, with the cooperation of WHO and other countries, trained about ten thousand international students from over

就与局限又向传统医学提出了挑战,推动它进一步发展。世界卫生组织早在20世纪70年代就意识到传统医学对人类健康的重要性,并为推动传统医学的发展做了努力。1976年举行的第二十九届世界卫生大会将传统医学项目纳入世界卫生组织的工作计划。其后的各届世界卫生大会又通过了一系列决议,要求各成员国根据本国的条件发展、使用和研究传统医学,以降低医疗费用,促进"人人享有初级卫生保健"这一目标的实现。

世界卫生组织历来重视传统医学的科学、安全和有效使用。它出版和发行了一系列有关科学、安全、有效使用草药和针灸的技术指南,并在专用术语的标准化方面做了许多工作。传统医学的使用是否做到安全和有效,是与使用传统疗法的医务工作者的水平密不可分的。因此,世界卫生组织也十分重视传统医学培训工作。它在全世界有27个传统医学合作中心,这些中心对培训合格的针灸师及使用传统疗法的其他医务工作者做出了积极的贡献。南京中医药大学、上海中医药大学是世界卫生组织传统医学合作中心之一,近年来与世界卫生组织和其他国家合作,培训了近万名来自90多个国

90 countries.

In order to further promote the dissemination of traditional Chinese medicine in the world, *A Newly Compiled Practical English-Chinese Library of Traditional Chinese Medicine*, compiled by Nanjing University of TCM with Professor Zuo Yanfu as the general compiler-in-chief and published by the Publishing House of Shanghai University of TCM, aims at systematic, accurate and concise expounding of traditional Chinese medical theory and introducing clinical therapeutic methods of traditional medicine according to modern medical nomenclature of diseases. Undoubtedly, this series of books will be the practical textbooks for the beginners with certain English level and the international enthusiasts with certain level of Chinese to study traditional Chinese medicine. Besides, this series of books can also serve as reference books for WHO to internationally standardize the nomenclature of acupuncture and moxibustion.

The scientific, safe and effective use of traditional medicine will certainly further promote the development of traditional medicine and traditional medicine will undoubtedly make more and more contributions to human health in the 21st century.

Zhang Xiaorui<br>
WHO Coordination Officer<br>
December, 2000

家和地区的留学生。

在南京中医药大学左言富教授主持下编纂的、由上海中医药大学出版社出版的《(英汉对照)新编实用中医文库》，旨在全面、系统、准确、简要地阐述中医基础理论，并结合西医病名介绍中医临床治疗方法。因此，这套文库可望成为具有一定英语水平的初学中医者和具有一定中文水平的外国中医爱好者学习基础中医学的系列教材。这套文库也可供世界卫生组织在编写国际针灸标准术语时参考。

传统医学的科学、安全、有效使用必将进一步推动传统医学的发展。传统医学一定会在21世纪为人类健康做出更大的贡献。

**张小瑞**<br>
**世界卫生组织传统医学协调官员**<br>
**2000年12月**

# Preface

The Publishing House of Shanghai University of TCM published *A Practical English-Chinese Library of Traditional Chinese Medicine* in 1990. The Library has been well-known in the world ever since and has made great contributions to the dissemination of traditional Chinese medicine in the world. In view of the fact that 10 years has passed since its publication and that there are certain errors in the explanation of traditional Chinese medicine in the Library, the Publishing House has invited Nanjing University of TCM and Shanghai University of TCM to organize experts to recompile and translate the Library.

Nanjing University of TCM and Shanghai University of TCM are well-known for their advantages in higher education of traditional Chinese medicine and compilation of traditional Chinese medical textbooks. The compilation of *A Newly Compiled Practical English-Chinese Library of Traditional Chinese Medicine* has absorbed the rich experience accumulated by Nanjing University of Traditional Chinese Medicine in training international students of traditional Chinese medicine. Compared with the previous Library, the Newly Compiled Library has made great improvements in many aspects, fully demonstrating the academic system of traditional Chinese medicine. The whole series of books has systematically introduced the basic theory and thera-

# 前　言

上海中医药大学出版社于1990年出版了一套《(英汉对照)实用中医文库》,发行10年来,在海内外产生了较大影响,对推动中医学走向世界起了积极作用。考虑到该套丛书发行已久,对中医学术体系的介绍还有一些欠妥之处,因此,上海中医药大学出版社特邀南京中医药大学主编、上海中医药大学主译,组织全国有关专家编译出版《(英汉对照)新编实用中医文库》。

《(英汉对照)新编实用中医文库》的编纂,充分发挥了南京中医药大学和上海中医药大学在高等中医药教育教学和教材编写方面的优势,吸收了作为WHO传统医学合作中心之一的两校,多年来从事中医药学国际培训和留学生学历教育的经验,对原《(英汉对照)实用中医文库》整体结构作了大幅度调整,以突出中医学术主体内容。全套丛书系统介绍了中医基础理论和中医辨证论治方法,讲解了中药学和方剂学的基本理论,详细介绍了236味中药、152首常用方剂和100种常用中成药;详述

peutic methods based on syndrome differentiation, expounding traditional Chinese pharmacy and prescriptions; explaining 236 herbs, 152 prescriptions and 100 commonly-used patent drugs; elucidating 264 methods for differentiating syndromes and treating commonly-encountered and frequently-encountered diseases in internal medicine, surgery, gynecology, pediatrics, traumatology and orthopedics, ophthalmology and otorhinolaryngology; introducing the basic methods and theory of acupuncture and moxibustion, massage (tuina), life cultivation and rehabilitation, including 70 kinds of diseases suitable for acupuncture and moxibustion, 38 kinds of diseases for massage, examples of life cultivation and over 20 kinds of commonly encountered diseases treated by rehabilitation therapies in traditional Chinese medicine. For better understanding of traditional Chinese medicine, the books are neatly illustrated. There are 296 line graphs and 30 colored pictures in the Library with necessary indexes, making it more comprehensive, accurate and systematic in disseminating traditional Chinese medicine in the countries and regions where English is the official language.

This Library is characterized by following features:

1. Scientific   Based on the development of TCM in education and research in the past 10 years, efforts have been made in the compilation to highlight the gist of TCM through accurate theoretical exposition and clinical practice, aiming at introducing authentic theory and practice to the world.

2. Systematic   This Library contains 14 sepa-

264种临床内、外、妇、儿、骨伤、眼、耳鼻喉各科常见病与多发病的中医辨证论治方法；系统论述针灸、推拿、中医养生康复的基本理论和基本技能，介绍针灸治疗病种70种、推拿治疗病种38种、各类养生实例及20余种常见病证的中医康复实例。为了更加直观地介绍中医药学术，全书选用线图296幅、彩图30幅，并附有必要的索引，从而更加全面、系统、准确地向使用英语的国家和地区传播中医学术，推进中医学走向世界，造福全人类。

本丛书主要具有以下特色：
(1) 科学性：在充分吸收近10余年来中医教学和科学研究最新进展的基础上，坚持突出中医学术精华，理论阐述准确，临床切合实用，向世界各国介绍"原汁原味"的中医药学术；(2) 系统性：本套丛书包括《中医基础理论》、《中医诊断学》、《中药学》、《方剂学》、《中医内

rate fascicles, i.e. *Basic Theory of Traditional Chinese Medicine*, *Diagnostics of Traditional Chinese Medicine*, *Science of Chinese Materia Medica*, *Science of Prescriptions*, *Internal Medicine of Traditional Chinese Medicine*, *Surgery of Traditional Chinese Medicine*, *Gynecology of Traditional Chinese Medicine*, *Pediatrics of Traditional Chinese Medicine*, *Traumatology and Orthopedics of Traditional Chinese Medicine*, *Ophthalmology of Traditional Chinese Medicine*, *Otorhinolaryngology of Traditional Chinese Medicine*, *Chinese Acupuncture and Moxibustion*, *Chinese Tuina (Massage)*, and *Life Cultivation and Rehabilitation of Traditional Chinese Medicine*.

3. Practical  Compared with the previous Library, the Newly Compiled Library has made great improvements and supplements, systematically introducing therapeutic methods for treating over 200 kinds of commonly and frequently encountered diseases, focusing on training basic clinical skills in acupuncture and moxibustion, tuina therapy, life cultivation and rehabilitation with clinical case reports.

4. Standard  This Library is reasonable in structure, distinct in categorization, standard in terminology and accurate in translation with full consideration of habitual expressions used in countries and regions with English language as the mother tongue.

This series of books is not only practical for the beginners with certain competence of English to study TCM, but also can serve as authentic textbooks for international students in universities and colleges of TCM in China to study and practice TCM. For those from TCM field who are going to go

科学》、《中医外科学》、《中医妇科学》、《中医儿科学》、《中医骨伤科学》、《中医眼科学》、《中医耳鼻喉科学》、《中国针灸》、《中国推拿》、《中医养生康复学》14个分册,系统反映了中医各学科建设与发展的最新成果;(3) 实用性:临床各科由原来的上下两册,根据学科的发展进行大幅度的调整和增补,比较详细地介绍了200多种各科常见病、多发病的中医治疗方法,重点突出了针灸、推拿、养生康复等临床基本技能训练,并附有部分临证实例;(4) 规范性:全书结构合理,层次清晰,对中医各学科名词术语表述规范,对中医英语翻译执行了更为严格的标准化方案,同时又充分考虑到使用英语国家和地区人们的语言习惯和表达方式。

本丛书不仅能满足具有一定英语水平的初学中医者系统学习中医之用,而且也为中医院校外国留学生教育及国内外开展中医双语教学提供了目前最具权威的系列教材,同时也是中医出国人员进

abroad to do academic exchange, this series of books will provide them with unexpected convenience.

Professor Xiang Ping, President of Nanjing University of TCM, is the director of the Compilation Board. Professor Zuo Yanfu from Nanjing University of TCM, General Compiler-in-Chief, is in charge of the compilation. Zhang Wenkang, Minister of Health Ministry, is invited to be the honorary director of the Editorial Board. Li Zhenji, Vice-Director of the State Administrative Bureau of TCM, is invited to be the director of the Approval Committee. Chen Keji, academician of China Academy, is invited to be the General Advisor. International advisors invited are Mr. M. S. Khan, Chairman of Ireland Acupuncture and Moxibustion Fund; Miss Alessandra Gulí, Chairman of "Nanjing Association" in Rome, Italy; Doctor Secondo Scarsella, Chief Editor of YI DAO ZA ZHI; President Raymond K. Carroll from Australian Oriental Touching Therapy College; Ms. Shulan Tang, Academic Executive of ATCM in Britain; Mr. Giovanni Maciocia from Britain; Mr. David, Chairman of American Association of TCM; Mr. Tzu Kuo Shih, director of Chinese Medical Technique Center in Connecticut, America; Mr. Helmut Ziegler, director of TCM Center in Germany; and Mr. Isigami Hiroshi from Japan. Chen Ken, official of WHO responsible for the Western Pacific Region, has greatly encouraged the compilers in compiling this series of books. After the accomplishment of the compilation, Professor Zhu Qingsheng, Vice-Minister of Health Ministry and Director of the State Administrative Bureau of TCM, has set a high value on the books in his fore-

行中医药国际交流的重要工具书。

全书由南京中医药大学校长项平教授担任编委会主任、左言富教授任总主编，主持全书的编写。中华人民共和国卫生部张文康部长担任本丛书编委会名誉主任，国家中医药管理局李振吉副局长担任审定委员会主任，陈可冀院士欣然担任本丛书总顾问指导全书的编纂。爱尔兰针灸基金会主席萨利姆先生、意大利罗马"南京协会"主席亚历山大·古丽女士、意大利《医道》杂志主编卡塞拉·塞肯多博士、澳大利亚东方触觉疗法学院雷蒙特·凯·卡罗院长、英国中医药学会学术部长汤淑兰女士、英国马万里先生、美国中医师公会主席大卫先生、美国康州中华医疗技术中心主任施祖谷先生、德国中医中心主任赫尔木特先生、日本石上博先生担任本丛书特邀外籍顾问。世界卫生组织西太平洋地区官员陈恩先生对本丛书的编写给予了热情鼓励。全书完成后，卫生部副部长兼国家中医药管理局局长朱庆生教授给予了高度评价，并欣然为本书作序；WHO传统医学协调官员张小瑞对于本丛书的编写给予高度关注，百忙中也专为本书作序。我国驻外教育机构，特别是中国驻英国曼彻斯特领事张益群先生、中国驻美国休斯敦领事严美华

word for the Library. Zhang Xiaorui, an official from WHO's Traditional Medicine Program, has paid great attention to the compilation and written a foreword for the Library. The officials from the educational organizations of China in other countries have provided us with some useful materials in our compilation. They are Mr. Zhang Yiqun, China Consul to Manchester in Britain; Miss Yan Meihua, Consul to Houston in America; Mr. Wang Jiping, First Secretary in the Educational Department in the Embassy of China to France; and Mr. Gu Shengying, the Second Secretary in the Educational Department in the Embassy of China to Germany. We are grateful to them all.

The Compilers<br>December, 2000

女士、中国驻法国使馆教育处一秘王季平先生、中国驻德国使馆教育处二秘郭胜英先生在与我们工作联系中,间接提供了不少有益资料。在此一并致以衷心感谢!

编　者<br>2000年12月

# Note for Compilation

Diagnostics of TCM is a subject concentrating on diagnosis of diseases and differentiation of syndromes through examination based on the theory and methodology of TCM. It serves as a bridge to connect the basic theory of TCM with clinical specialties and is the essential course for all clinical subjects.

This book, focusing on elucidation of the theory and methods of TCM in examining pathological conditions as well as analyzing and differentiating syndromes, is composed of introduction, diagnostic methods and syndrome differentiation. It is a systematic in itself and, at the same time, keeps a close association with the clinical specialties so as to preserve the systematic and integral characteristics of TCM.

In the compilation, the authors have tried to preserve the unique features of TCM and demonstrate the profound content of TCM diagnostics on one hand, and unite theory and practice so as to guide the clinical practice on the other. In the compilation, the authors have also tried to make it concise, easy to read, fluent and accurate. For this purpose, some illustrations and colour pictures are included. We hope that this book will be beneficial to both the international students with certain level of Chinese in learning traditional Chinese medicine and the readers in China who are studying traditional Chinese medicine or going abroad.

# 编写说明

中医诊断学是研究运用中医学理论和方法诊察病情,判断疾病,辨识证候的一门学科。它在中医学科体系中起着沟通基础理论与临床各科之间的桥梁作用,为中医临床各科的基础,是学习中医的必修内容之一。

本书重点阐述中医诊察病情,分析、辨识证候的理论和方法,包括绪论、诊法、辨证三个部分,自成体系,具有本学科的独立性;同时充分注意到与《中医基础理论》及临床各科的联系,以保持中医学科体系的系统性和完整性。

本书在编写内容上既注意突出中医特色,全面展示中医诊断学的丰富内容,又坚持理论联系实际的原则,突出实用性和针对性,对中医临床起到指导作用。编写者力求论述简明扼要、深入浅出、说理清楚,文字简洁精炼、通俗易懂,译文准确流畅,并适当配以插图和彩照。竭诚希望此书能成为中医院校外国留学生和具有一定汉语水平的外国读者学习中医的良师益友,同时也为国内学习中医药学的读者及中医出国人员提供帮助。

# Contents

Introduction ............................................................................ 1
1  Diagnostic methods ............................................................ 7
  1.1 **Inspection** ................................................................... 8
    1.1.1 Inspection of the whole body .................................. 8
      1.1.1.1 Inspection of spirit ......................................... 9
      1.1.1.2 Inspection of complexion ............................. 12
      1.1.1.3 Inspection of body ....................................... 17
      1.1.1.4 Inspection of postures ................................. 19
    1.1.2 Inspection of local regions .................................... 22
      1.1.2.1 Inspection of head and hair .......................... 22
      1.1.2.2 Inspection of the five sense organs .............. 25
      1.1.2.3 Inspection of neck ....................................... 30
      1.1.2.4 Inspection of skin ......................................... 31
      1.1.2.5 Inspection of infantile index finger veins ...... 35
      1.1.2.6 Inspection of excreta ................................... 38
    1.1.3 Inspection of tongue ............................................ 42
      1.1.3.1 Methods for inspection of tongue ................ 42
      1.1.3.2 Normal states of the tongue ........................ 44
      1.1.3.3 Inspection of the tongue body .................... 44
      1.1.3.4 Inspection of tongue fur .............................. 52
      1.1.3.5 Comprehensive analysis of the body of the tongue and tongue fur ......... 58
  1.2 **Listening and olfaction** .............................................. 60
    1.2.1 Listening to sounds .............................................. 60
      1.2.1.1 Speech ........................................................ 61
      1.2.1.2 Respiration .................................................. 63
      1.2.1.3 Cough ......................................................... 65
      1.2.1.4 Hiccup and belching .................................... 66
    1.2.2 Olfaction ............................................................... 67
      1.2.2.1 Smelling body odor ..................................... 68

# 目 录

| | |
|---|---|
| 绪论 | 1 |
| 第一章 诊法 | 7 |
|   第一节 望诊 | 8 |
|     一、望全身情况 | 8 |
|       （一）望神 | 9 |
|       （二）望面色 | 12 |
|       （三）望形体 | 17 |
|       （四）望姿态 | 19 |
|     二、望局部情况 | 22 |
|       （一）望头与发 | 22 |
|       （二）望五官 | 25 |
|       （三）望颈项 | 30 |
|       （四）望皮肤 | 31 |
|       （五）望小儿食指脉络 | 35 |
|       （六）望排出物 | 38 |
|     三、望舌 | 42 |
|       （一）望舌的方法 | 42 |
|       （二）正常舌象 | 44 |
|       （三）望舌体 | 44 |
|       （四）望舌苔 | 52 |
|       （五）舌体与舌苔的综合分析 | 58 |
|   第二节 闻诊 | 60 |
|     一、听声音 | 60 |
|       （一）语言 | 61 |
|       （二）呼吸 | 63 |
|       （三）咳嗽 | 65 |
|       （四）呃逆与嗳气 | 66 |
|     二、嗅气味 | 67 |
|       （一）嗅病体之气 | 68 |

  1.2.2.2 Odor in the room ·················································· 69
**1.3 Inquiry** ························································································ 69
 1.3.1 General information ·················································· 70
 1.3.2 Inquiry of chief complaint and history of present illness ············· 71
  1.3.2.1 Inquiry of chief complaint ·········································· 71
  1.3.2.2 Inquiry of the history of present illness ························ 72
 1.3.3 Inquiry of the present symptoms ·································· 73
  1.3.3.1 Inquiry of fever and cold ··········································· 73
  1.3.3.2 Inquiry of sweating ·················································· 80
  1.3.3.3 Inquiry of pain ························································ 84
  1.3.3.4 Inquiry of sleep ······················································· 90
  1.3.3.5 Inquiry of diet and partiality ······································ 92
  1.3.3.6 Inquiry of urination and defecation ····························· 97
  1.3.3.7 Inquiry of the head and face ······································ 102
  1.3.3.8 Inquiry of chest and abdomen ···································· 106
  1.3.3.9 Inquiry of the symptoms over the loins, back and four limbs ············· 108
  1.3.3.10 Inquiry of symptoms in andropathy ·························· 109
  1.3.3.11 Inquiry of symptoms in gynecology ·························· 111
  1.3.3.12 Inquiry of symptoms in pediatrics ···························· 114
 1.3.4 Inquiry of anamnesis ·················································· 116
  1.3.4.1 Inquiry of past physique ············································ 117
  1.3.4.2 Inquiry of previous illness ········································· 117
 1.3.5 Inquiry of family history ············································· 117
**1.4 Pulse-taking and palpation** ·································································· 118
 1.4.1 Pulse-taking ······························································· 118
  1.4.1.1 Regions and methods for taking pulse ·························· 119
  1.4.1.2 Normal pulse ·························································· 123
  1.4.1.3 Morbid pulse ·························································· 125
 1.4.2 Palpation ·································································· 131
  1.4.2.1 Methods for palpation ·············································· 132
  1.4.2.2 Pressing the chest and abdomen ································· 133
  1.4.2.3 Palpation of the four limbs ········································ 136
  1.4.2.4 Palpation of acupoints ·············································· 137

(二) 嗅病室之气 ································· 69
第三节　问诊 ································· 69
　一、问一般情况 ································· 70
　二、问主诉与现病史 ································· 71
　　(一) 问主诉 ································· 71
　　(二) 问现病史 ································· 72
　三、问现在症状 ································· 73
　　(一) 问寒热 ································· 73
　　(二) 问汗 ································· 80
　　(三) 问疼痛 ································· 84
　　(四) 问睡眠 ································· 90
　　(五) 问饮食口味 ································· 92
　　(六) 问二便 ································· 97
　　(七) 问头面症状 ································· 102
　　(八) 问胸腹症状 ································· 106
　　(九) 问腰背四肢症状 ································· 108
　　(十) 问男科症状 ································· 109
　　(十一) 问妇科症状 ································· 111
　　(十二) 问儿科症状 ································· 114
　四、问既往史 ································· 116
　　(一) 问既往体质状况 ································· 117
　　(二) 问既往患病情况 ································· 117
　五、问家族史 ································· 117
第四节　切诊 ································· 118
　一、脉诊 ································· 118
　　(一) 诊脉的部位与方法 ································· 119
　　(二) 常脉 ································· 123
　　(三) 病脉 ································· 125
　二、按诊 ································· 131
　　(一) 按诊的方法 ································· 132
　　(二) 按胸腹 ································· 133
　　(三) 按四肢 ································· 136
　　(四) 按腧穴 ································· 137

# 2 Differentiation of syndrome ..... 138

## 2.1 Syndrome differentiation with eight principles ..... 138

### 2.1.1 External and internal differentiation of syndromes ..... 139
2.1.1.1 External syndrome ..... 140
2.1.1.2 Internal syndrome ..... 141
Appendix: Half external and half internal syndrome ..... 142

### 2.1.2 Syndrome differentiation of cold and heat ..... 142
2.1.2.1 Cold syndrome ..... 143
2.1.2.2 Heat syndrome ..... 144

### 2.1.3 Syndrome differentiation of asthenia and sthenia ..... 145
2.1.3.1 Asthenia syndrome ..... 145
2.1.3.2 Sthenia syndrome ..... 147

### 2.1.4 Syndrome differentiation of yin and yang ..... 148
2.1.4.1 Yin syndrome and yang syndrome ..... 148
2.1.4.2 Yin asthenia syndrome and yang asthenia syndrome ..... 150
2.1.4.3 Yin depletion syndrome and yang depletion syndrome ..... 152

### 2.1.5 Relationship among the eight principal syndromes ..... 154
2.1.5.1 Relationship between two principles in a pair ..... 154
2.1.5.2 Relationship between different pairs of principles ..... 167

## 2.2 Syndrome differentiation of qi, blood and body fluid ..... 172

### 2.2.1 Syndrome differentiation of qi disorders ..... 172
2.2.1.1 Qi asthenia syndrome ..... 173
2.2.1.2 Qi sinking syndrome ..... 173
2.2.1.3 Qi stagnation syndrome ..... 174
2.2.1.4 Qi reversion syndrome ..... 175

### 2.2.2 Syndrome differentiation of blood disease ..... 176
2.2.2.1 Blood asthenia syndrome ..... 176
2.2.2.2 Blood stasis syndrome ..... 177
2.2.2.3 Blood cold syndrome ..... 179
2.2.2.4 Blood heat syndrome ..... 180

### 2.2.3 Syndrome differentiation of simultaneous disorder of qi and blood ..... 181
2.2.3.1 Asthenia of both qi and blood ..... 181
2.2.3.2 Qi asthenia and hemorrhagia syndrome ..... 182
2.2.3.3 Depletion of qi with bleeding syndrome ..... 183
2.2.3.4 Qi asthenia and blood stasis syndrome ..... 183

## 第二章 辨证 ......................................................... 138
### 第一节 八纲辨证 ..................................................... 138
#### 一、表里辨证 ....................................................... 139
##### （一）表证 ....................................................... 140
##### （二）里证 ....................................................... 141
##### 附：半表半里证 ................................................... 142
#### 二、寒热辨证 ....................................................... 142
##### （一）寒证 ....................................................... 143
##### （二）热证 ....................................................... 144
#### 三、虚实辨证 ....................................................... 145
##### （一）虚证 ....................................................... 145
##### （二）实证 ....................................................... 147
#### 四、阴阳辨证 ....................................................... 148
##### （一）阴证和阳证 ................................................. 148
##### （二）阴虚证和阳虚证 ............................................. 150
##### （三）亡阴证和亡阳证 ............................................. 152
#### 五、八纲证候间的关系 ............................................... 154
##### （一）同一对纲领间的关系 ......................................... 154
##### （二）不同对纲领间的关系 ......................................... 167
### 第二节 气血津液辨证 ................................................. 172
#### 一、气病辨证 ....................................................... 172
##### （一）气虚证 ..................................................... 173
##### （二）气陷证 ..................................................... 173
##### （三）气滞证 ..................................................... 174
##### （四）气逆证 ..................................................... 175
#### 二、血病辨证 ....................................................... 176
##### （一）血虚证 ..................................................... 176
##### （二）血瘀证 ..................................................... 177
##### （三）血寒证 ..................................................... 179
##### （四）血热证 ..................................................... 180
#### 三、气血同病辨证 ................................................... 181
##### （一）气血两虚证 ................................................. 181
##### （二）气虚失血证 ................................................. 182
##### （三）气随血脱证 ................................................. 183
##### （四）气虚血瘀证 ................................................. 183

## Contents

- 2.2.3.5 Qi stagnation and blood stasis syndrome ········· 184
- 2.2.4 Syndrome differentiation of fluid disorder ········· 185
  - 2.2.4.1 Insufficiency of body fluid ········· 185
  - 2.2.4.2 Phlegm syndrome ········· 186
  - 2.2.4.3 Fluid-retention syndrome ········· 188
  - 2.2.4.4 Edema ········· 189
- **2.3 Syndrome differentiation of viscera** ········· 191
  - 2.3.1 Syndrome differentiation of heart disease ········· 192
    - 2.3.1.1 Asthenia of heart qi ········· 192
    - 2.3.1.2 Heart yang asthenia syndrome ········· 193
    - 2.3.1.3 Sudden loss of heart yang syndrome ········· 195
    - 2.3.1.4 Heart blood asthenia syndrome ········· 196
    - 2.3.1.5 Heart yin asthenia syndrome ········· 196
    - 2.3.1.6 Heart vessels obstruction syndrome ········· 197
    - 2.3.1.7 Exuberance of heart fire syndrome ········· 199
    - 2.3.1.8 Mind confusion by phlegm ········· 200
    - 2.3.1.9 Disturbance of the heart by phlegmatic fire ········· 201
  - 2.3.2 Syndrome differentiation of lung disease ········· 202
    - 2.3.2.1 Pulmonary qi asthenia syndrome ········· 203
    - 2.3.2.2 Lung yin asthenia syndrome ········· 204
    - 2.3.2.3 Syndrome of wind cold encumbering lung ········· 205
    - 2.3.2.4 Wind heat invading lung syndrome ········· 206
    - 2.3.2.5 Syndrome of dryness attacking lung ········· 207
    - 2.3.2.6 Syndrome of accumulation of pathogenic heat in lung ········· 208
    - 2.3.2.7 Syndrome of phlegmatic dampness retention in lung ········· 209
    - 2.3.2.8 Syndrome of confliction of wind and fluid in lung ········· 210
  - 2.3.3 Syndrome differentiation of spleen disease ········· 212
    - 2.3.3.1 Syndrome of asthenia of splenic qi ········· 212
    - 2.3.3.2 Syndrome of asthenia of splenic yang ········· 213
    - 2.3.3.3 Syndrome of sinking of splenic qi ········· 215
    - 2.3.3.4 Syndrome of failure of the spleen to govern blood ········· 216
    - 2.3.3.5 Syndrome of cold and dampness encumbering the spleen ········· 217
    - 2.3.3.6 Syndrome of damp heat encumbering the spleen ········· 218
  - 2.3.4 Syndrome Differentiation of liver disease ········· 219
    - 2.3.4.1 Asthenia syndrome of liver blood ········· 220

（五）气滞血瘀证 …………………………………… 184
　四、津液病辨证 ………………………………………… 185
　　（一）津液不足证 …………………………………… 185
　　（二）痰证 …………………………………………… 186
　　（三）饮证 …………………………………………… 188
　　（四）水肿 …………………………………………… 189
　第三节　脏腑辨证 ……………………………………… 191
　一、心病辨证 …………………………………………… 192
　　（一）心气虚证 ……………………………………… 192
　　（二）心阳虚证 ……………………………………… 193
　　（三）心阳暴脱证 …………………………………… 195
　　（四）心血虚证 ……………………………………… 196
　　（五）心阴虚证 ……………………………………… 196
　　（六）心脉痹阻证 …………………………………… 197
　　（七）心火亢盛证 …………………………………… 199
　　（八）痰迷心窍证 …………………………………… 200
　　（九）痰火扰心证 …………………………………… 201
　二、肺病辨证 …………………………………………… 202
　　（一）肺气虚证 ……………………………………… 203
　　（二）肺阴虚证 ……………………………………… 204
　　（三）风寒束肺证 …………………………………… 205
　　（四）风热犯肺证 …………………………………… 206
　　（五）燥邪犯肺证 …………………………………… 207
　　（六）热邪蕴肺证 …………………………………… 208
　　（七）痰湿阻肺证 …………………………………… 209
　　（八）风水搏肺证 …………………………………… 210
　三、脾病辨证 …………………………………………… 212
　　（一）脾气虚证 ……………………………………… 212
　　（二）脾阳虚证 ……………………………………… 213
　　（三）脾气下陷证 …………………………………… 215
　　（四）脾不统血证 …………………………………… 216
　　（五）寒湿困脾证 …………………………………… 217
　　（六）湿热蕴脾证 …………………………………… 218
　四、肝病辨证 …………………………………………… 219
　　（一）肝血虚证 ……………………………………… 220

2.3.4.2 Syndrome of liver yin asthenia ............................................................ 221
2.3.4.3 Syndrome of liver qi stagnation ............................................................ 222
2.3.4.4 Syndrome of liver fire hyperactivity ..................................................... 223
2.3.4.5 Syndrome of liver yang hyperactivity ................................................... 225
2.3.4.6 Syndrome of endogenous liver wind ..................................................... 226
2.3.4.7 Syndrome of cold stagnation in the liver meridian ............................... 230
2.3.5 Syndrome differentiation of kidney disease ............................................ 231
2.3.5.1 Syndrome of kidney yang asthenia ....................................................... 232
2.3.5.2 Syndrome of edema due to kidney asthenia ......................................... 233
2.3.5.3 Syndrome of kidney yin asthenia .......................................................... 234
2.3.5.4 Syndrome of kidney essence insufficiency ........................................... 235
2.3.5.5 Syndrome of kidney qi weakness .......................................................... 236
2.3.5.6 Syndrome of kidney failing to receive qi ............................................... 238
2.3.6 Syndrome differentiation of stomach disease ......................................... 239
2.3.6.1 Syndrome of stomach cold .................................................................... 239
2.3.6.2 Syndrome of stomach heat .................................................................... 241
2.3.6.3 Syndrome of food retention in the stomach ......................................... 242
2.3.6.4 Syndrome of asthenic stomach yin ........................................................ 243
2.3.7 Syndrome differentiation of gallbladder disease .................................... 244
Syndrome of gallbladder stagnation and phlegm disturbance ......................... 245
2.3.8 Syndrome differentiation of small intestinal disease ............................. 246
Sthenic heat syndrome of small intestine ......................................................... 246
2.3.9 Syndrome differentiation of large intestinal disease .............................. 247
2.3.9.1 Syndrome of large intestinal fluid consumption ................................... 248
2.3.9.2 Syndrome of large intestinal damp-heat ............................................... 249
2.3.10 Syndrome differentiation of bladder disease ........................................ 250
Syndrome of damp heat in the bladder ............................................................. 250
2.3.11 Syndrome differentiation of accompanying diseases of viscera .......... 251
2.3.11.1 Asthenia syndrome of heart and lung qi ............................................. 252
2.3.11.2 Asthenia syndrome of heart and spleen .............................................. 253
2.3.11.3 Asthenia syndrome of heart and kidney yang .................................... 254
2.3.11.4 Syndrome of disharmony between the heart and kidney ................... 255
2.3.11.5 Syndrome of lung and spleen qi asthenia ........................................... 256
2.3.11.6 Syndrome of spleen and kidney yang asthenia ................................... 257
2.3.11.7 Syndrome of kidney and liver yin asthenia ........................................ 258

（二）肝阴虚证 …………………………………………………… 221
（三）肝气郁结证 ………………………………………………… 222
（四）肝火上炎证 ………………………………………………… 223
（五）肝阳上亢证 ………………………………………………… 225
（六）肝风内动证 ………………………………………………… 226
（七）寒凝肝脉证 ………………………………………………… 230
五、肾病辨证 …………………………………………………………… 231
（一）肾阳虚证 …………………………………………………… 232
（二）肾虚水泛证 ………………………………………………… 233
（三）肾阴虚证 …………………………………………………… 234
（四）肾精不足证 ………………………………………………… 235
（五）肾气不固证 ………………………………………………… 236
（六）肾不纳气证 ………………………………………………… 238
六、胃病辨证 …………………………………………………………… 239
（一）胃寒证 ……………………………………………………… 239
（二）胃热证 ……………………………………………………… 241
（三）食滞胃脘证 ………………………………………………… 242
（四）胃阴虚证 …………………………………………………… 243
七、胆病辨证 …………………………………………………………… 244
胆郁痰扰证 ………………………………………………………… 245
八、小肠病辨证 ………………………………………………………… 246
小肠实热证 ………………………………………………………… 246
九、大肠病辨证 ………………………………………………………… 247
（一）大肠液亏证 ………………………………………………… 248
（二）大肠湿热证 ………………………………………………… 249
十、膀胱病辨证 ………………………………………………………… 250
膀胱湿热证 ………………………………………………………… 250
十一、脏腑兼病辨证 …………………………………………………… 251
（一）心肺气虚证 ………………………………………………… 252
（二）心脾两虚证 ………………………………………………… 253
（三）心肾阳虚证 ………………………………………………… 254
（四）心肾不交证 ………………………………………………… 255
（五）肺脾气虚证 ………………………………………………… 256
（六）脾肾阳虚证 ………………………………………………… 257
（七）肝肾阴虚证 ………………………………………………… 258

2.3.11.8 Syndrome of liver fire invading lung ............................... 260
2.3.11.9 Syndrome of imbalance between liver and spleen ............... 261
2.3.11.10 Syndrome of incoordination between liver and stomach ............ 262
2.3.11.11 Syndrome of damp-heat in liver and gallbladder ............... 263
**2.4 Other syndrome differentiation methods** ............................... 265
  2.4.1 Introduction to six-meridians syndrome differentiation ............ 265
    2.4.1.1 Taiyang syndrome ............................................ 266
    2.4.1.2 Yangming syndrome .......................................... 268
    2.4.1.3 Shaoyang syndrome .......................................... 270
    2.4.1.4 Taiyin syndrome ............................................. 271
    2.4.1.5 Shaoyin syndrome ........................................... 271
    2.4.1.6 Jueyin syndrome ............................................. 273
  2.4.2 Introduction to syndrome differentiation of defensive qi, qi, nutrient qi and blood ............................................... 274
    2.4.2.1 Defensive phase syndrome .................................... 275
    2.4.2.2 Qi phase syndrome ........................................... 275
    2.4.2.3 Nutrient phase syndrome ..................................... 276
    2.4.2.4 Blood phase syndrome ........................................ 277

**Postscript** ............................................................... 279

（八）肝火犯肺证 …………………………………………… 260
（九）肝脾不调证 …………………………………………… 261
（十）肝胃不和证 …………………………………………… 262
（十一）肝胆湿热证 ………………………………………… 263
第四节 其他辨证方法简介 ……………………………………… 265
一、六经辨证概要 ………………………………………………… 265
（一）太阳病证 ……………………………………………… 266
（二）阳明病证 ……………………………………………… 268
（三）少阳病证 ……………………………………………… 270
（四）太阴病证 ……………………………………………… 271
（五）少阴病证 ……………………………………………… 271
（六）厥阴病证 ……………………………………………… 273
二、卫气营血辨证概要 …………………………………………… 274
（一）卫分证 ………………………………………………… 275
（二）气分证 ………………………………………………… 275
（三）营分证 ………………………………………………… 276
（四）血分证 ………………………………………………… 277
后记 ……………………………………………………………………… 279

# Introduction 绪 论

Diagnostics of TCM is a subject concentrating on diagnosis of diseases and differentiation of syndromes through examination based on the theory and methodology of TCM. Correct diagnosis and prognosis require thorough understanding of the nature of the disease in question. Therefore, correct diagnosis is prerequisite to the treatment, prognosis and prevention of disease. So diagnostics of TCM serves as a bridge to connect the basic theory of TCM with clinical specialties and is the essential course for all clinical subjects, playing a very important role in TCM.

The diagnostics of TCM has been developed under the guidance of the basic theory of TCM and based on the clinical practice done by numerous doctors in the past thousands of years. It is mainly composed of diagnostic methods and syndrome differentiation. Diagnostic methods are the methods used to examine patients and collect pathological data, mainly including inspection, listening and olfaction, inquiry and pulse-taking, known as the four diagnostic methods. Syndrome differentiation means to synthesize and analyze the pathological data so as to decide the nature of the syndrome. The theory and methods for syndrome differentiation include syndrome differentiation with eight principles, syndrome differentiation of causes, syndrome differentiation of qi, blood and body fluid, syndrome differentiation of viscera, syndrome differentiation of meridians, syndrome differentiation of six meridians, syndrome differentiation of defensive qi, qi, nutrient

中医诊断学是研究运用中医学理论和方法诊察病情、判断疾病、辨识证候的一门学科。要正确治疗疾病和推测预后，必须对疾病的本质有足够的认识，也就是必须先有正确的诊断。因此，正确的诊断是治疗、预后和预防疾病的前提。所以，中医诊断学是沟通中医基础理论与临床各科的桥梁，是中医临床各科的基础，在中医学中占有重要地位。

中医诊断学是在中医基础理论指导下，经过几千年无数医学家临床经验的积累逐步形成和发展起来的。其基本内容包括诊法和辨证两个部分。诊法，即诊察病情，搜集病情资料的方法，主要有望诊、闻诊、问诊和切诊，又称四诊。辨证是对通过四诊获得的病情资料进行综合、分析，判断为某种性质的证候。辨证的理论和方法包括八纲辨证、病因辨证、气血津液辨证、脏腑辨证、经络辨证、六经辨证、卫气营血辨证与三焦辨证等。各种辨证是分析判断病情、认识疾病本质的理论和方

qi and blood as well as syndrome differentiation of triple energizer. Various ways to differentiate syndrome are the theory and methods for analyzing and understanding the nature of disease. They, though with their own characteristics and specific range, supplement each other and together form the syndrome differentiation system in TCM.

Concept of organic wholeness is the main characteristics of the theoretic system of TCM which is thoroughly demonstrated by the diagnostics of TCM. In diagnosing pathological conditions, deciding the category of disease and differentiating syndrome, TCM emphasizes the entirety.

## 1. Examination of entirety

The human body is an organic whole and constantly communicates with the external environment. TCM lays much stress on the characteristics of the human body, such as the integrity, unity and association with the outer world. This idea is summed up as "concept of organic wholeness" which is reflected as examination of entirety in the diagnostics of TCM.

Firstly, the human body is composed of various organs, viscera, meridians, constituents and orifices as well as essence, qi, blood and body fluid. Though possessing different functions, they are not isolated. Such an integral association of the human body is accomplished through the domination of the five zang-organs, supplementation of the six fu organs, association of the five constituents and five sensory organs and nine orifices, the extensive distribution of the meridians and the transportation of essence, qi, blood and body fluid by the net of meridians. Therefore disorder of the viscera, essence, qi, blood and body fluid can be manifested on the superficial tissues and organs. The local pathological changes can affect the whole

法，它们既有各自的特点和应用范围，又相辅相成，密切联系，共同构成中医辨证体系。

整体观念是中医学理论体系的主要特点。中医诊断学充分体现了这个特点，在诊察病情、判断疾病、辨识证候的过程中，强调从整体出发，形成了本学科的特点。

## 1．整体审察

人是一个有机的整体，而且人与外在环境息息相关。中医学非常重视这种人体本身的统一性、完整性及其与外界环境的相互关系。这就是"整体观念"。这种观点在中医诊断学中表现为整体审察的特点。

首先，人体是由许多组织器官所组成，脏腑、经络、形体、官窍和精气血津液等，虽各有不同的功能，但它们之间不是孤立的，而是相互联系的。人体这种整体联系，是以五脏为中心，配合六腑，联系五体、五官九窍等，通过经络纵横广泛地分布，以贯通内外上下，运行精气血津液而实现的。体内脏腑、精气血津液发生病变，可反映于体表组织器官；局部的病变能够影响全

body and vice versa. So by observing the changes of the five sensory organs, shape of the body, complexion and pulse states, we can get to know the pathological changes of the viscera, essence, qi, blood and body fluid. From local changes one can get to know the pathological changes of the whole body. In this way correct diagnosis can be made.

Secondly, there is a close relationship between man and nature. Weather changes and geographical changes may affect the human body. On the other hand, the human body is subjectively adaptable to the natural environment. However, the dysfunction of the regulating ability of the human body or sudden violent changes of the natural environment may lead to diseases. Besides, social environment frequently brings about stimulation to the mind and spirit of human beings, which may affect the visceral functions and lead to diseases. Therefore, natural and social factors must be taken into consideration in the diagnosis of diseases.

Thus, clinical diagnosis of disease must be done under the guidance of concept of organic wholeness and with full attention given to the unity and integration of the human body as well as its close relationship with the environmental factors. Only comprehensive inspection and extensive collection of data with thorough analysis ensures correct diagnosis.

## 2. Combination of disease differentiation and syndrome differentiation

This means to decide the name of the disease and to differentiate the manifestations of the disease.

Disease means a pathological development course

with certain rules caused by destruction of the healthy state due to certain pathogenic factors. This pathological development course manifests several special symptoms and syndromes corresponding to certain stages. Each disease has its own occurrence, development and variation principles. The disease name is the label of the disease in question, such as dysentery, measles and asthma, etc.

Symptom refers to various abnormal manifestations of a disease, including the subjective sensation, such as headache, dizziness and thirst, etc., and the signs observed by other people, such as reddish tongue, yellowish fur and rapid pulse, etc.

Syndrome is a summarization of the development of a disease at a certain stage, including cause, location, nature, pathogenesis and the relevant symptoms and signs. Take "external syndrome due to exogenous wind and cold" for example. It suggests that the cause is the invasion of wind and cold; the location is in the superficies; the nature is cold; the pathogenesis is wind and cold encumbering the superficies and the pulmonary qi failing to disperse. The main symptoms brought about are mild fever, anhidrosis, pain of head and body, stuffy nose with clear nasal discharge, or cough, thin whitish fur as well as floating and tense pulse, etc. This problem can be relieved by expelling wind and dispersing cold or dispersing the lung and relieving superficial pathogenic factors. Otherwise, cold pathogenic factors may enter into the body and transform into heat, therefore worsening the problem.

Symptoms are the evidences for the differentiation of disease and syndrome. Both disease and syndrome

素作用下，健康状态受到破坏，出现具有一定发展规律的演变过程，具体表现出若干特定的症状和各阶段相应证候。各种疾病都有自己发生、发展及演变的规律。病名，即疾病的名称。例如痢疾、麻疹、哮喘等。

症，即症状，是疾病表现的各种异常现象。包括患者自己主观感觉到的异常感觉，如头痛、眩晕、口渴等，和能被他人觉察到的机体疾病变化的客观表现，如舌红、苔黄、脉数等。

证，通常是指证候。即对疾病发展过程中某一阶段的病因、病位、病性、病机、相应的症状、体征及病变趋势等所作的病理概括。例如"外感风寒表证"，提示其病因是感受风寒之邪；病位在表；病性属寒证；病机是风寒束表，肺卫失宣；主要可出现恶寒重发热轻、无汗、头身疼痛、鼻塞流清涕、或咳嗽、苔薄白、脉浮紧等症；如采用疏风散寒、宣肺解表的方法治疗，病可痊愈，否则，寒邪可能化热入里，病势加重。

症状是辨病、辨证的依据。病与证，都是对疾病本质

reflect the understanding of the nature of disease, however, they emphasize on different aspects. Disease reflects the general principles and characteristics of a disease, which is the primary contradiction of a disease. While syndrome reflects the contradiction of a disease at the present stage. At different stages, a disease may manifest several different syndromes known as "the same disease with different syndromes". While different diseases at a certain stage may manifest the same syndrome, known as "different diseases with the same syndrome". Therefore, the differentiation of disease and the differentiation of syndrome refer to the understanding of the nature of a disease from different angles. The differentiation of disease is beneficial to the understanding of the nature of a disease and the grasping of the developing tendency and prognosis from the whole developing course and characteristics. The differentiation of syndrome emphasizes on the changes of a disease at a certain stage and the understanding of the nature of a disease according to the present clinical manifestations to provide evidence for present treatment.

Clinically, combined use of the di-fferentiation of disease and the differentiation of syndrome is made of so as to make them supplement each other for the benefit of revealing the nature of the disease in question and making the diagnosis more accurate, correct and specific.

What should be made clear here is that the differentiation of disease is the main work of all clinical specialties, which is not discussed in detail in this book.

### 3. Synthetic use of all diagnostic methods

This means that, in diagnosing a disease, one must

的认识,但它们的侧重面有所不同。病,反映该疾病发生发展的一般规律和特点,是疾病的根本性矛盾。证,反映疾病当前所处阶段的主要矛盾。一种疾病在其不同的发展阶段,可以出现若干不同的证候,即"同病异证";而不同疾病的一定发展阶段,有可能出现相同的证候,即"异病同证"。因此,辨病与辨证是从不同角度认识疾病的本质。辨病有利于从疾病的全过程和特征上认识疾病的本质,掌握疾病的发展趋势和预后;辨证则重在掌握疾病阶段性变化的具体情况,从疾病当前的临床表现中判断疾病的本质,为当前的治疗提供依据。临床将辨病与辨证相结合,则可相互补充,相得益彰,深化对疾病本质的揭示,使诊断更为全面、准确,则治疗更具针对性。

需要说明的是,辨病是临床各科的主要内容,本书不作阐述。

### 3. 诊法合参

诊法合参,是指在诊察疾

try to collect as detailed as possible the data for comprehensive analysis of the disease. The manifestations of a disease are multiple and complicated. The data collected with the four diagnostic methods are the evidences for the differentiation of both disease and syndrome. Whether the data collected with the four diagnostic methods is accurate or not directly affect the accuracy of the differentiation of both disease and syndrome. The four diagnostic methods are used to examine disease and collect data from different angles. They are significant in diagnosis, however, they still have some limitations and cannot replace each other. So it is improper to stress on one of them and neglect the others. In order to fully understand the pathological conditions of a disease and collect reliable and detailed data, these four methods should be used together and the data collected should be analyzed synthetically.

病时,诸诊并用,全面搜集、综合分析病情资料。疾病的表现是复杂而多样的,四诊搜集的症状是辨病与辨证的依据,四诊所得到的病情资料是否全面可靠,直接影响辨病与辨证的准确性。望、闻、问、切四诊是从各个不同角度诊察疾病,搜集病情资料的,各有其独特的作用和局限性,不能互相取代,也不可以片面强调某一诊法的重要性而忽视其他诊法。因此,为了全面地了解病情,搜集翔实可靠的病情资料,必须诸诊并用,综合分析,才能作出正确的诊断。

# 1  Diagnostic methods

Diagnostic methods are the methods used to collect data related to pathological conditions, including inspection, listening and smelling, inquiry and pulse-taking. Inspection means to examine the external manifestations and excreta; listening and smelling means to examine the speech, breath and odor of the patient; inquiry means to get to know the occurrence, development and treatment of the disease as well as the present symptoms and other information relevant to the disease by asking the patient or the people accompanying the patient; pulse-taking means to examine the pulse and the related regions of the patient.

The human body is a organic whole. Under morbid conditions, local pathological changes may affect the whole body; internal pathological changes can be manifested through the five sensory organs, the four limbs and the superficies. With the examination of the symptoms and signs of a disease by means of the four diagnostic methods, one can understand the cause of the disease and analyze the pathogenesis of the disease so as to provide evidence for deciding treatment based on syndrome differentiation.

The four diagnostic methods are used to examine disease from different angles and they cannot replace each other in diagnosis. So in clinical practice, they are usually used in combination for systematic understanding of a disease in order to ensure comprehensive analysis and correct

# 第一章  诊法

诊法，即诊察疾病，搜集病情资料的方法。包括望诊、闻诊、问诊和切诊，故合称"四诊"。望诊，主要是对患者神、色、形、态的变化及其排出物进行诊察；闻诊，主要是对患者的语言、呼吸等声音变化和散发出的气味进行诊察；问诊，主要是通过对患者或陪诊者的询问，了解疾病的发生发展和治疗经过、当前的症状及其他与疾病有关的情况；切诊，主要是对患者的脉象和有关部位进行诊察。

人体是一个有机整体，发生疾病时，局部的病变可以影响全身；内部的病变，可以从五官、四肢、体表等反映出来。所以通过望、闻、问、切四诊，诊察疾病显现于外的症状和体征，可以了解疾病发生的原因，分析其病变的机理，为辨证论治提供依据。

望、闻、问、切四诊是从不同的侧面诊察病情的四种方法，各有其特定的内容、适用范围和作用，不能相互取代。因此，临床上必须四诊结合运

diagnosis.

## 1.1 Inspection

Inspection means that the doctor use his or her eyes to examine the vitality, colour, shape and posture of the patient's whole body or local region as well as inspect the colour, quantity and texture of the excreta for the purpose of understanding pathological conditions.

Inspection is a convenient and important method for diagnosing disease. It not only enables the doctor to get necessary data, but also provides trace for further diagnosis. Therefore, doctors must have keen powers of observation in clinical practice.

Inspection should be done in the place with full light, especially natural light. If done in the light of lamp, cares should be taken to avoid the influence of the light itself.

The range for inspection is extensive, including all aspects visible to the naked eyes. In general, the aspects for inspection include the whole body, local region and tongue.

### 1.1.1 Inspection of the whole body

Inspection of the whole body, also known as general inspection, refers to purposeful examination of the spirit, colour, shape and posture of the whole body so as to have a general understanding of the disease.

用，并将四诊搜集的病情资料，进行综合分析，才能全面系统地了解病情，并作出正确的诊断。

## 第一节 望诊

望诊，是医生运用视觉，对患者全身和局部的神、色、形、态及其排出物的色、量、质等异常变化进行全面的诊察，以了解病情的一种诊察方法。

望诊是比较方便而又非常重要的诊病方法。通过望诊，不仅能获得有关病情资料，而且能为进一步诊察病情提供线索。因此，临床进行望诊，要求医生具有敏锐的观察力。

望诊须在充足的光线下进行，尤以自然光线为最好。若在灯光下进行，则须注意排除有色灯光的影响。

望诊的范围很广，凡目能所及，皆可进行望诊。概括起来，主要包括望全身情况、望局部情况和望舌等内容。

### 一、望全身情况

望全身情况，即一般望诊，又称"整体望诊"，是对患者全身的神、色、形、态进行诊察，以便对疾病有一个大概的了解。

### 1.1.1.1 Inspection of spirit

Spirit refers to the general manifestations of life activities, including mental states and mental activities.

The material base of spirit is essence. The congenital essence depends on the cereal nutrients to nourish and promote as well as the normal visceral functions to protect. That is why the spirit is said to be the external manifestations of the conditions of visceral essence. Inspection of spirit can enable one to understand whether the essence is exuberant or deficient and whether the visceral functions are strong or weak. Such an understanding is important to the analysis as whether the pathological conditions are light or serious and whether the prognosis is benign or malignant.

Inspection of spirit mainly focuses on the examination of the mental states and emotional conditions, including facial expressions, complexion, eye expressions, speech, breath, physical conditions and response to the external stimulation, etc. Since the visceral essence infuses upward into the eyes and the ocular system is connected with the brain, and also because the eye is the orifice related to the liver, governed by the heart and housing the spirit the inspection of eye expressions is very important. Inspection of spirit means, by examining of the aspects mentioned above, to differentiate whether the spirit is in existence, deficient, lost, false or in disorder for the purpose of deciding whether the healthy qi is abundant or deficient, the visceral functions are strong or weak, the pathological conditions are light or serious and the prognosis is benign or malignant.

#### 1.1.1.1.1 Existence of spirit

The manifestations are mental consciousness, normal vitality, natural facial expressions, ruddy complexion,

（一）望神

神，是指人体生命活动总的外在表现，也包含神志、精神意识活动。

神的物质基础是精气，来源于先天之精气，有赖于后天水谷精气的不断充养，还有赖于脏腑的正常生理功能。因此，神是脏腑精气盛衰的外露征象。通过望神，可以了解精气的盛衰、脏腑功能的强弱，并对于分析病情的轻重、推测预后的良恶有重要意义。

望神主要诊察患者的神志和精神意识状态、表情、面色、眼神、语言、呼吸、形体动态及对外界反应等。由于五脏六腑之精气皆上注于目，目系通于脑，为肝之窍，心之使，神之舍，所以，诊察眼神十分重要。望神，就是通过诊察上述各方面的情况，辨别得神、少神、失神、假神和神乱，以判断正气的盛衰，脏腑功能的强弱，病情的轻重和预后的良恶。

1. 得神

又称"有神"。表现为神志意识清楚，精神尚可，表情

flexible eyes with brightness and vitality, accurate verbal expression and reply, normal voice and breath, normal and natural movement of the limbs. These manifestations suggest non-impairment of healthy qi, normal visceral functions, mild pathological conditions, or favourable prognosis even for serious diseases.

#### 1.1.1.1.2 Lack of spirit, also known as insufficiency of spirit

The manifestations are mental consciousness, dispiritedness, pale complexion, dull expressions of eyes, short of breath, no desire to speak and low voice. These manifestations suggest mild consumption of healthy qi, weak visceral functions, more serious disease and better prognosis. These manifestations are usually seen in patients at the rehabilitating stage or with weak constitution.

#### 1.1.1.1.3 Loss of spirit, also known as depletion of spirit

The manifestations are dispiritedness, pale complexion, dull eye expressions, weak breath or dyspnea, emaciation, difficulty in movement, retard response or even unconsciousness; or coma with delirium and floccitation. The former suggests great impairment of the primordial qi and decline of the visceral functions, usually seen in chronic disease and serious disease with unfavourable prognosis. The latter suggests exuberance of pathogenic factors and serious disturbance of the viscera, often seen in critical pathological conditions with unfavourable prognosis.

#### 1.1.1.1.4 False spirit

False spirit is usually seen in prolonged disease, serious disease and extreme exhaustion of essence with the false manifestations in disagreement with the nature of the disease. For example, dull or pale complexion suddenly

自然，面色荣润，两眼转动灵活、明亮有神，言语对答准确，语声、呼吸如常，肢体活动自如。提示正气未伤，脏腑功能未衰，病情较轻，预后良好。

2. 少神

又称"神气不足"。表现为神志意识清楚，精神不振，面色少华，两眼乏神，少气懒言，语声低弱。提示正气轻度亏损，脏腑功能虚弱，病情比得神者稍重，预后尚好。常见于轻病，或恢复期患者，亦可见于体质虚弱者。

3. 失神

又称"无神"。表现为精神委靡，面色无华，目光晦滞，呼吸气微或喘促，形体羸瘦，动作艰难，反应迟钝，甚则神识不清；或表现为神昏谵语，循衣摸床，撮空理线等。前者提示正气大伤，脏腑功能严重衰减，多见于慢性久病患者，病重，预后不良；后者提示邪气亢盛，脏腑功能严重障碍，病情危重，预后不良。

4. 假神

假神多出现于久病、重病、精气极度衰弱的患者，表现出与病情本质不相符合的假象。如原来面色晦暗，或苍

changes into reddish cheeks; or extreme dispiritedness, mental derangement and retard response suddenly change into excitation but with restlessness; or no desire to speak, low and weak voice and incoherent speech suddenly change into incessant, but simply repeated talking. These phenomena indicate declination of essence and floating of yang due to failure of yin to control yang. This condition is clinically known as "the last radiance of the setting sun" and "sudden spurt of vitality before death", the premonitory signs of death.

Clinically cautions must be taken to differentiate false spirit and improvement of pathological conditions. The manifestation of false spirit is sudden "improvement" in certain aspect which is not in agreement with the whole pathological conditions and immediately turns worse. The improvement of spirit depletion takes place in the course of the improvement of the whole pathological conditions.

#### 1.1.1.1.5 Mental derangement

This condition is usually seen in the case of mania. The usual manifestations are indifferent expression, taciturn and depression, followed by being in a trance, now laughing and then crying due to stagnation of phlegm which confuses the mind; the manifestations like dysphoria, running wildly, shouting, fighting against people or even family members are usually due to disturbance of the heart by phlegmatic fire; the manifestations like sudden coma, drooling, staring upwards, convulsion of limbs and groaning like pig and goat usually indicate epilepsy due to endogenous liver wind and phlegm confusing the mind which can heal automatically.

白，突然两颧泛红如妆；或原来精神极度委靡，意识模糊，反应迟钝，突然神情兴奋，躁烦不安；或原来默默不欲言语，语声低微，时断时续，突然言语不休，且多简单重复等，都属于假神的表现。这是精气衰竭，阴不敛阳，阳失依附而致虚阳外浮，阴阳欲将离绝的表现。临床上通常称为"回光返照"或"残灯复明"，是垂危病人死亡前的先兆。

临床辨证应注意假神与失神患者病情好转的鉴别。假神的表现，是突然在某些方面出现短暂的"好转"假象，与整个病情极不相符，随后则病情迅速恶化。失神患者病情好转，是随着整个病情逐渐全面的好转，而且愈来愈好。

#### 5. 神乱

即精神意识错乱，常见于癫、狂、痫的病人。如表现为表情淡漠，寡言少语，闷闷不乐，继则精神发呆，哭笑无常，多为痰气凝结，阻蔽心神的癫病；若烦躁不宁，登高而歌，弃衣而走，呼号怒骂，打人毁物，不避亲疏，多属痰火扰心的狂病；若突然昏仆，口吐涎沫，两目上视，四肢抽动，口中如作猪羊叫声，一般常能自行恢复，多属痰迷心窍，肝风内动的痫病。

It should be pointed out that the symptoms of mania and mental derangement correspond to the cause and occurrence of these diseases. The clinical syndrome differentiation of these manifestations is different from serious dysfunction of viscera at the advanced stage of serious disease and spirit depletion due to exhaustion of essence.

### 1.1.1.2 Inspection of complexion

Inspection of complexion includes the changes of the colour and luster of the facial skin. The visceral essence flows to the face. So the facial colour and luster are the signs of visceral essence. The facial skin is soft and thin, the luster is visible and easy to observe. Therefore the inspection of complexion is an important part of inspection examination.

The colours of the facial skin are red, white, blue, yellow and black. The changes of these colours can reveal pathological changes of viscera of different nature. The lustre of skin refers to the bright, moist or dull and dry manifestations which can reveal the states of the visceral essence. So inspection of the changes of facial luster can enable one to understand the states of visceral essence, the nature of diseases, the conditions and development of diseases.

#### 1.1.1.2.1 Normal complexion

The normal and healthy complexion is ruddy and lustrous, indicating exuberance of visceral essence and normal functions of the viscera. Due to difference in constitution and the influence of climatic and environmental factors, the normal complexion is further divided into

应当指出，癫、狂、痫患者所出现的精神意识错乱的症状，是由这些疾病的病因、病机和发病规律所决定，其临床辨证意义与重危疾病后期因脏腑功能严重障碍和精气衰竭所引起的失神有本质的不同，应注意区别。

（二）望面色

望面色，包括观察面部皮肤的颜色和光泽的变化。脏腑精气通过经络上荣于面，因此，面部色泽是脏腑精气的外荣征象。面部皮肤薄嫩，色泽变化易显露于外，便于诊察，所以，望面色诊病是望诊的重要内容。

面部皮肤的颜色主要分赤、白、青、黄、黑五种，称为五色，其变化可以反映不同脏腑的病变和疾病的不同性质。皮肤的光泽，即指肤色的鲜明荣润或晦暗枯槁，可反映脏腑精气的盛衰。所以，通过诊察面部色泽的变化，可以了解脏腑精气的盛衰，辨别疾病的性质，分析病情的轻重和判断病情的进退。

1. 常色

人体正常健康状态时面部显示的色泽，称为常色。常色的特征是鲜明润泽，含蓄不露，表示脏腑精气充盛，脏腑功能正常。由于体质禀赋的

dominant complexion and varied complexion.

Dominant complexion refers to the colour of the skin and face that never changes due to racial and constitutional factors.

Varied complexion refers to the changes of the facial and skin color in correspondence to the variations of the seasons and climates. For example, the complexion is slightly bluish in the spring, reddish in the summer, yellowish in the late summer, whitish in the autumn and blackish in the winter. Varied complexion is temporary and unclear.

Besides, drinking liquor, excitement and sports activity may also lead to the changes of complexion. But these changes are not morbid.

#### 1.1.1.2.2 Morbid complexion

Facial colour during the course of disease is called morbid complexion marked by dry and dull colour, or obvious bright colour, or a single colour alone.

The key point in inspecting morbid complexion is to differentiate favourable and unfavourable manifestations of the five kinds of colour and the diseases manifested by these five kinds of colour.

**Favourable and unfavourable manifestations of the five kinds of colour**: Bright and moist colour, no matter what colour it is, indicates mild illness, normal condition of the visceral essence, easiness to cure and better prognosis. While dull and dry colour is malignant colour and indicates serious illness, impairment of the

不同和受气候、环境等影响，常色又有主色、客色之分。

（1）主色：人体终生不变的面色、肤色，称为主色，也称正色。主要与种族和禀赋有关。

（2）客色：随外界季节、气候等变化而发生相应变化的面色、肤色，称为客色。如春季面色稍青，夏季面色稍红，长夏面色稍黄，秋季面色稍白，冬季面色稍黑。客色的变化往往是暂时的，并且不十分明显。

此外，饮酒、七情刺激、运动等因素的影响，面色也会发生暂时的变化，但不属于病色，临证时应予以注意。

2. 病色

疾病过程中，面部所显示的异常色泽，称为病色。病色的特征是色泽枯槁而晦暗，或色泽鲜明暴露，或独呈一色，而无血色相间。

诊察病色的重点，在于辨别五色善恶及五色主病。

（1）五色善恶：不论何色，凡鲜明荣润者为善色，说明病变轻浅，脏腑精气未衰，其病易治，预后较好；凡晦暗枯槁者为恶色，说明病变深重，脏腑精气已伤，病重难治，

visceral essence, difficulty to cure and unfavourable prognosis.

**Diseases indicated by the five kinds of colour**: According to the theory of TCM and clinical experience, the five kinds of colour correspond to disorders of the five zang organs, i.e. blue colour corresponding to the liver, red colour to the heart, white colour to the lung, yellow colour to the spleen, and black colour to the kidney. The disorders of the five zang organs are manifested in correspondence to the kinds of complexion related to them. While the five kinds of colour also demonstrate different nature of diseases. The following is the detailed description:

Red colour: Red colour indicates heat syndrome, also seen in real cold and false heat syndrome.

Red colour results from sufficient blood circulating in the meridians and skins. With heat, blood flows fast. Since heat tends to rise and disperse, the meridians and vessels are dilated and become full. That is why the complexion appears red.

Flushed face is a sign of sthenic heat syndrome due to hyperactivity of visceral yang heat resulting from exogenous fever. Flushed and delicate cheeks indicates asthenia heat syndrome due to endogenous heat resulting from yin asthenia. Pale complexion with occasional migratory reddish luster like makeup in the patient with prolonged illness and serious disease indicates real cold and false heat syndrome due to upward floating of yang caused by predominant yin rejecting yang.

White colour: Indicating asthenia syndrome and cold syndrome.

White colour indicates decline of qi and blood. Pale complexion is caused by insufficiency of qi and blood in the face due to failure of insufficient yangqi to transport blood

预后不良。

（2）五色主病：根据中医学五行理论和临床实践总结，五色分属五脏，青属肝、赤属心、白属肺、黄属脾、黑属肾。五脏的病变可以反映其各主的面色，五色又可反映疾病的不同性质。现将五色主病分述如下：

① 赤色：主热证，亦可见于真寒假热证。

赤色乃血液充盈皮肤脉络所致。血得热则行，且热性升散，致脉络舒张而充盈，因此，面呈赤色。

满面通红，多为外感发热及脏腑阳热亢盛所致的实热证；两颧潮红娇嫩，多为阴虚内热的虚热证。久病、重病患者，面色苍白，时而泛红如妆，游移不定，为阴盛格阳，虚阳上浮所致的戴阳证，即真寒假热证。

② 白色：主虚证、寒证。

白为气血不荣之候。阳气虚衰，无力运血上荣于面；或气血亏虚，不能充盈血脉；

to nourish the face, or due to failure of the asthenia of qi and blood to fill the vessels, or due to coagulation of cold in the meridians and vessels which prevent qi and blood to circulate freely.

Floating whitish complexion and facial dropsy are usually due to insufficiency of yangqi. Light whitish complexion and emaciation are often caused by consumption of qi and blood. Pale complexion is often seen in sthenic cold syndrome, such as interior cold syndrome with sharp abdominal pain. Sudden pale complexion with profuse cold sweating, cold limbs and indistinct pulse is a sign of sudden loss of yangqi.

Yellow colour: Indicating asthenia syndrome and dampness syndrome.

Yellow colour indicates asthenia of the spleen and accumulation of dampness. Yellow complexion may be caused either by malnutrition of muscles due to insufficiency of qi and blood resulting from failure of the spleen to transport, or due to internal accumulation of dampness.

Light yellow, dry and lusterless complexion is called sallow complexion due to gastrosplenic qi asthenia and insufficiency of qi and blood, also seen in chronic hemorrhage, ascariasis and malnutrition, etc. Yellowish complexion with facial dropsy is called yellowish obesity, usually caused by asthenia of splenic qi and internal accumulation of dampness. The state of yellow complexion, eyes and skins is called jaundice due to failure of bile to flow in its normal duct and extravasates in the skins. If the colour is as yellow as tangerine peel, it is called yang jaundice due to steaming of accumulated damp heat and dysfunction of the liver and gallbladder. Sudden onset of disease with deep yellow face, eyes and body, high fever and coma, or even with vomiting, nosebleed and macules, is called acute jaundice or pestilent jaundice, usually caused by in-

或寒凝经脉，气血运行不畅，皆可致面部气血不充而呈白色。

面色㿠白而虚浮，多属阳气不足。淡白而消瘦，多属气血亏虚。面色苍白，多见于实寒证，如里寒证剧烈腹痛；若突然面色苍白，冷汗淋漓，肢冷脉微，则为阳气暴脱之候。

③黄色：主虚证、湿证。

黄色为脾虚、湿蕴的征象。脾虚失运，气血不充，肌肤失养，或湿邪内蕴，皆可致面呈黄色。

面色淡黄，枯槁无华，称为萎黄，多属脾胃气虚，气血不充所致，亦可见于长期慢性失血、虫证、疳积等患者。面色黄而虚浮，称为黄胖，多属脾气虚衰，湿邪内蕴所致。面、目、肌肤俱黄，称为黄疸，由胆汁不循常道外溢肌肤而形成。其中，黄而鲜明如橘皮者，称为阳黄，多因湿热蕴蒸，肝胆疏泄失职所致；若发病急骤，面、目、身深黄，高热神昏，甚则吐衄、发斑者，称为急黄，亦称瘟黄，多因湿热疫毒侵袭，内陷营血，熏蒸肝胆所致；

vasion of damp heat and pestilence deep into blood which steams the liver and gallbladder. Yellowish complexion like being fumigated is called yin jaundice, usually caused by stagnation of cold and dampness or prolonged stagnation of the liver and gallbladder.

　　Bluish complexion: Indicating cold syndrome, pain syndrome, blood stasis syndrome and convulsive syndrome.

　　Bluish colour is a sign of inhibited flow of qi and blood and stagnation of vessels and meridians. The invasion of cold factors causes contraction and stagnation, leading to spasm of meridians and vessels and stagnation of qi and blood. It may be caused either by deficiency of yangqi which fails to warm and transport qi and blood, or by qi stagnation and blood stasis which block meridians and vessels, or by exuberance of pathogenic heat which stagnates blood vessels. Besides, the stagnation of qi and blood in the meridians and vessels will inevitably result in pain. Therefore clinically stagnation of qi and blood is often accompanied by pain syndrome.

　　Pale and bluish complexion, or accompanied by chest pain and abdominal pain, is often due to invasion of cold or yang asthenia and cold exuberance. Bluish and greyish complexion with purplish black lips and chest pain is usually caused by inaction of heart yang and stagnation of heart blood. Cyanotic complexion and lips with asthmatic breath is usually due to stagnation of pulmonary qi, or asthenia of cardiopulmonary qi, or asthenia of pulmonary and kidney qi. Yellowish complexion mingled with bluish colour is called dull jaundice, usually seen in subjugation of the spleen by the liver, tympanites and infantile malnutrition. Cyanotic colour over the part between infantile brows, nose bridge and lips accompanied by high fever is the premonitory signs of convulsion, usually due to exuberance of

黄而晦暗如烟薰者，称为阴黄，多因寒湿郁阻，或肝胆久瘀不化所致。

④ 青色：主寒证、痛证、血瘀证和惊风。

青色是气血运行不畅、经脉瘀阻的征象。寒邪侵袭，寒性收引凝滞，致经脉拘急，气血凝滞；或阳气亏虚，无力温运血脉，血行缓滞；或气滞血瘀，脉络阻滞；或邪热炽盛，血脉壅滞，均可致面色发青。同时，由于气血瘀滞，经脉不利，不通则痛，所以，临床大多伴有痛证。

面色苍白而青，或伴胸腹疼痛，多属寒邪外袭或阳虚寒盛所致。面色青灰，口唇紫暗，心胸部疼痛，多属心阳不振，心血瘀阻所致。面色口唇青紫，气喘息粗，多见于肺气郁闭，或心肺气虚，或肺肾气虚。面色黄中带青，称为苍黄，多见于肝郁乘脾、鼓胀及小儿疳积。小儿眉间、鼻柱、口唇周围青紫，伴高热，为惊风先兆，多因邪热炽盛所致。

pathogenic heat.

Blackish complexion: Indicating kidney asthenia syndrome, cold syndrome, blood stasis syndrome and fluid retention syndrome.

Blackish complexion is the sign of kidney asthenia, yin predomination and exuberance of water or stagnation of qi and blood. The kidney is the organ associating closely with water and fire and is the source of yangqi. Asthenia of kidney yang and retention of fluid will lead to internal exuberance of water cold, loss of warmth in blood, spasm of vessels and meridians and inhibited flow of qi and blood. Blackish complexion may also be caused by consumption of yin by asthenic fire and failure of essence to nourish the face, or by prolonged stagnation of blood in the body.

Light blackish complexion is often caused by asthenia of kidney yang. Dry blackish complexion is usually due to prolonged consumption of kidney essence and asthenic fire consuming yin. Blackish complexion with squamous and dry skin often results from internal retention of blood stasis. Blackish colour of the area around the eye socket indicates retention of fluid due to kidney asthenia and fluid extravasation or leukorrhagia due to downward migration of cold dampness.

### 1.1.1.3 Inspection of body

Inspection of body means to diagnose the patient by examining the physical conditions of the patient.

The body depends on visceral essence to nourish, while the functions of the viscera and the conditions of visceral essence may be reflected by the body. Therefore, inspection of the body may help doctors to understand the functional states of the viscera, the current conditions of qi, blood, yin and yang as well as the conflict between healthy qi and pathogenic factors which may suggest the possibility of contracting certain disease.

#### 1.1.1.3.1 Physical strength and weakness

Inspection of physical strength and weakness may enable one to know the functions of the viscera and the conditions of qi and blood. Generally speaking, the conditions of the body correspond to the conditions of visceral functions and the states of qi and blood. That means internal exuberance ensures external strength and internal decline leads to external weakness.

**Strength**: Strength refers to the strong physique, the manifestations of which are lustrous skin, strong muscles, wide chest and thick bones which indicate sufficiency of qi, powerful functions of the viscera, exuberance of qi and blood and healthy body. Strong body means strong resistance against pathogenic invasion, no liability to contract disease, quick recovery from illness and favourable prognosis.

**Weakness**: Weakness refers to decline of body strength, the manifestations of which are dry skin, lean muscles, thin chest and bones which indicate insufficiency of qi, weak functions of the viscera, deficiency of qi and blood and weak physique. Weakness of the body indicates weak resistance against pathogenic invasion, easiness to catch disease, difficulty in healing and unfavourable prognosis.

#### 1.1.1.3.2 Physical obesity and emaciation

Inspection of physical obesity and emaciation may suggest the possibility to contract certain diseases.

**Obesity**: Obesity is characterized by round head, short and thick neck, wide and flat shoulders, wide-short-round chest, big belly, smaller body, flabby muscles, dispiritedness and lassitude which are the signs of predo-

盛衰、邪正的消长，并能提示易患某些疾病的可能性。

**1. 形体强弱**

通过诊察形体强弱，可以概括得知脏腑功能的强弱和气血的盈亏。一般地说，机体形体的强弱，与脏腑功能的强弱和气血的盛衰是一致的，内盛则外强，内衰则外弱。

（1）强：指身体强壮。如表现为皮肤润泽，肌肉结实，胸廓宽厚，骨骼粗大等，为形气有余。表示内脏坚实，气血充盛，身体强壮。其抗病力强，不易患病，病则易愈，预后较好。

（2）弱：指身体衰弱。如表现为皮肤干燥，肌肉瘦削，胸廓狭窄，骨骼细小等，为形气不足。表示内脏脆弱，气血亏少，身体衰弱。其抗病力弱，容易患病，病则难治，预后较差。

**2. 形体胖瘦**

通过诊察形体胖瘦，可提示易患某些疾病的可能性。

（1）胖：指形体肥胖。如表现为头圆形，颈短粗，肩宽平，胸廓宽短呈圆形，大腹便便，身体偏矮，肌肉松软，肤白

mination of the body and asthenia of qi, suggesting insufficiency of yangqi and internal exuberance of phlegmatic dampness as well as susceptibility to vertigo, apoplexy and obstructive syndrome of the chest. That is why it is said that "obese people are predominant in dampness" and "obese people are susceptible to wind stroke".

**Emaciation**: Emaciation is characterized by long head, thin and long neck, narrow shoulders, narrow and flat chest, small belly, higher body, thin muscles and dryness of skin which suggest asthenia of blood and internal exuberance of asthenic fire usually seen in patients with pulmonary tuberculosis and internal impairment by asthenic overstrain. That is why it is said that "thin people are predominant in fire" and "thin people are susceptible to cough due to pulmonary tuberculosis".

If the whole body is extremely emaciated and the patient lies in bed and cannot rise up again, it is usually caused by chronic disease, severe disease and declination of visceral essence as well as unfavourable prognosis.

#### 1.1.1.3.3 Deformity

Deformity includes chicken chest and tortoise back The former refers to the evident protrusion of the lower part of sternum marked by longer posterior and anterior diameter and shorter left and right diameter of the thoracic cavity, usually seen in children. The latter refers to protrusion of the spinal column. Both cases are caused by congenital defects or postnatal malnutrition which lead to insufficiency of kidney essence and maldevelopment of the bones.

### 1.1.1.4 Inspection of postures

Inspection of postures means to examine the patient's postures in tranquility and action as well as abnormal activities.

The postures of the patient in tranquility and action is

closely related to the conditions of yin and yang of the body as well as natures of the illness as being cold or heat or asthenia or sthenia. The movement of the limbs is under the control of the heart spirit and in close relation with the functions of the bones, muscles, tendons and vessels. Therefore, the postures of the patient in tranquility and action as well as the abnormal activities are all the external manifestations of disease. Different diseases may be reflected by different postures and activities. Inspection of postures is helpful for deciding the natures of diseases and diagnosis of certain diseases.

### 1.1.1.4.1 Inspection of postures in tranquility and action

Yang governs action and yin tranquility. The sitting, lying and walking postures of the patient may be summarized like this: movement, supination and extension indicate that the disease of yang nature, usually manifesting as external syndrome, heat syndrome and sthenia syndrome; quietness, pronation and bending indicate the disease of yin nature, usually manifesting as internal syndrome, cold syndrome and asthenia syndrome.

**Sitting:** Sitting with the head bending down, shortness of breath and no desire to speak usually indicates asthenia of pulmonary qi or failure of the kidney to receive qi; sitting with the head rising up and asthmatic breath signifies adverse flow of qi due to pulmonary sthenia; asthma with inability to lie down indicates pulmonary distension and retention of fluid in the chest and abdomen.

**Lying:** Lying on bed facing the outward with the ability to turn the body freely usually indicates yang syndrome, heat syndrome and sthenia syndrome; lying on bed facing the inward with inability to turn the body freely indicates yin syndrome, cold syndrome and asthenia sydrome; lying on a supine position with the extension of

的阴阳盛衰和病性的寒热虚实密切相关。肢体的活动受心神的支配,并与骨骼、肌肉、筋脉等组织器官的功能密切相关。因此,患者的动静姿态、肢体的异常动作都是疾病的外在反映。不同的疾病,可表现出不同的体位和动态。通过望姿态,有助于判断病性的寒热虚实和某些疾病的诊断。

1. 望动静姿态

阳主动,阴主静。患者坐、卧、行走的姿态,可概括为动者、仰者、伸者,病属阳,多为表证、热证、实证;静者、俯者、屈者,病属阴,多为里证、寒证、虚证。

(1)坐姿:患者坐而俯首,气短懒言,多为肺气虚或肾不纳气;坐而仰首,气喘息促,多属肺实气逆;喘而但坐不得卧,卧则气逆喘甚,多为肺胀、饮停胸腹的病证。

(2)卧姿:患者卧时面常向外(朝亮处),身体能自转侧,多为阳证、热证、实证;面常向里(背光),身体不能自转侧,多为阴证、寒证、虚证。卧时仰面伸肢,常欲揭去衣被,

the limbs and refusal to cover quilt and put on clothes indicates the syndrome of predominant yang and sthenic heat; huddling up when lying on bed with preference to put on more clothes indicates yin sthenia and yang asthenia or abdominal pain; inability to lie down due to cough usually occurs in autumn and winter, often caused by internal retention of fluid; lying on bed with inability to sit up (sitting up causes dizziness) indicates asthenia of both qi and blood.

**Walking**: Unstable walking with tremor of the limbs usually occurs together with dizziness, usually caused by internal disturbance of liver wind or impairment of tendons and bones.

Besides, deformity of the lower limbs, trauma and injury of joints all can lead to abnormal walking postures. In this case, diagnosis should be made with the aid of other ways of examination.

#### 1.1.1.4.2 Inspection of abnormal movements

Abnormal movements of the patient's limbs usually indicate the signs of certain diseases. For example, spasm of the limbs, stiff necks and opisthotonus indicate internal disturbance of liver wind due to extreme heat generating wind, usually seen in exogenous febrile disease at the stage of exuberant heat; tremor or peristalsis of fingers and toes indicates internal disturbance of asthenic wind, seen at the advanced stage of exogenous febrile disease due to deficiency of body fluid and malnutrition of tendons and vessels. Such a problem seen in chronic disease due to internal impairment is often caused by insufficiency of qi and blood and malnutrition of the tendons and vessels. Pain of the limbs and joints, inflexibility of the joints or spasm of the hands and feet as well as swelling, stiffness and deformity of the joints usually suggest obstructive syndrome. Flabbiness of the limbs and difficulty in moving

多为阳盛实热证；卧时蜷缩成团，喜加衣被，多为阳虚阴盛或腹有疼痛的病证。咳逆倚息不得卧，好发于秋冬，多为内有伏饮。但卧不能坐，坐则眩晕，多为气血两虚的病证。

（3）步态：步态不稳，肢体颤动不宁，常与眩晕并见，多属肝风内动，或筋骨受损。

此外，下肢畸形、外伤及关节损害等皆可引起步态异常，需配合有关检查作出诊断。

**2. 望异常动作**

患者肢体的异常动作，往往反映了某些疾病的特征。如四肢抽搐、颈项强直、角弓反张，为肝风内动，多因热极生风而致，常见于外感温热病热盛期。指、趾颤动或蠕动，为虚风内动，见于外感温热病后期，因阴液亏虚，筋脉失养而致；见于内伤久病，则多因气血不足，筋脉失养而成。肢体骨节疼痛，屈伸不利，或手足拘挛，关节肿胀、强直、变形，多属痹证。肢体软弱，行动不便，或肌肉萎缩，属痿证。单侧肢体行动不便，或麻木不仁，则属中风偏瘫。

or atrophy of muscles are usually of flaccidity syndrome. Difficulty in moving or numbness of unilateral limbs indicates hemiplegia due to wind stroke.

### 1.1.2 Inspection of local regions

Inspection of local regions is used to closely examine some regional areas to obtain necessary clinical data on the basis of general inspection according to the pathological conditions in question.

The pathological changes of the tissues and organs in the human body are mainly reflected by external manifestations (such as luster, color and postures), functions and sensation. These external manifestations indicate either the disorders of the tissues and organs or the regional reflection of the pathological changes of visceral qi and blood. Therefore, inspection of local regions is not only helpful for diagnosing the pathological changes of the local tissues and organs, but also helpful for understanding the pathological conditions of the viscera.

Inspection of local regions include various aspects, among which the inspection of tongue is discussed in another section. The other aspects are discussed in the following.

#### 1.1.2.1 Inspection of head and hair

The head is the region where all yang meridians converge. Besides, the conception vessel, thoroughfare vessel and many branches or collaterals of the yin meridians extend to the head. Therefore, essence of all viscera come up to nourish the head. Inside the head stores the brains (cerebral marrow) and marrow, which is governed by the kidney. The kidney also governs bones. The devel-

## 二、望局部情况

望局部情况，又称为"分部望诊"，是在整体望诊的基础上，根据病情及诊断的需要，对患者的某些局部进行重点、细致的诊察，以进一步获取与疾病诊断相关的临床资料。

人体各部组织器官的病变，主要反映在外形（色泽、形态）、功能和感觉三方面的变化。其中有的是局部组织器官本身的病变，有的是全身脏腑气血病变在局部的表现。因此，通过望局部情况，不仅有助于对各局部组织器官病变的诊断，而且可以了解所应脏腑的病变情况。

望局部情况的内容很多，其中望舌另作专述，这里主要阐述以下内容。

### （一）望头与发

头为诸阳之会，任脉、冲脉以及许多阴经的分支或络脉也上行于头部，故脏腑精气皆上荣于头。头中内藏脑髓，髓为肾所主。肾又主骨。颅骨和脑髓的生长发育，全赖肾精充养。发为血之余，肾之外

opment of the skull and brains all depend on kidney essence to nourish. The hair is the extending part of blood and the external manifestation of the kidney. The spleen and the stomach are the sources of qi and blood. Therefore, inspection of head and hair is helpful for understanding the conditions of the kidney, spleen and stomach as well as qi and blood.

#### 1.1.2.1.1 Inspection of head

Inspection of head means to examine the external shape and movement of the head.

**Shape of head**: Bigger head with smaller face, downward looking of the eyes and low intelligence in children is usually caused by insufficiency of kidney essence and retention of fluid, often seen in children with fluid retention in the brain. Smaller head with round top, earlier closure of fontanel and low intelligence in children is frequently caused by insufficiency of kidney essence and maldevelopment of the brain. Protrusion of forehead and temporal regions with flat top of head in children often results from congenital insufficiency of kidney essence, or postnatal improper regulation of the spleen and stomach and maldevelopment of the skull, usually seen in rickets.

**Fontanel**: Inspection of fontanel must be done in examining the infants under the age of 1 year and a half. Sunken fontanel indicates asthenia syndrome, usually caused by excessive vomiting which impairs body fluid, or by weakness of the spleen and stomach and prolapse of the gastrosplenic qi, or by congenital insufficiency and malnutrition of the brains. Protrusion of fontanel indicates sthenia syndrome, usually caused by virulent heat in exogenous febrile disease attacking the upper part of the body, or by fluid retention and blood stasis in the skull. Retard closure of fontanel and non-closure of the bone fissure is

华。脾胃为气血生化之源。所以,通过望头与发,可以了解肾、脾胃和气血的盛衰情况。

1. 望头

主要诊察头的外形和动态。

(1) 头形:小儿头形过大,颜面较小,两目下视,伴智力低下,多因肾精不足,水液停聚所致,常见于水饮停于脑的患儿。小儿头形过小,头顶部尖圆,颅缝闭合过早,伴智力低下,多因肾精不足,颅脑发育不良所致。小儿头颅前额、两颞部突出,头顶平坦呈方形,称为方颅,多因先天肾精不足,或后天脾胃失调,颅骨发育不良所致,常见于佝偻病患儿。

(2) 囟门:1岁半以内的婴幼儿,尤须诊察囟门。囟门凹陷,称为囟陷,为虚证,多因吐泻伤津,或脾胃虚弱,中气下陷,或先天不足,脑髓失养所致。囟门高突,称为囟填,为实证,多因外感温热病火毒上攻,或颅内水停血瘀所致。囟门迟闭,骨缝不合,称为解颅,多因先天肾精不足,或出生后久病失养所致。

frequently caused by congenital insufficiency of kidney essence, or by chronic disease and malnutrition after birth.

**Shaking**: Involuntary shaking or tremor in both children and adults means internal disturbance of liver wind.

#### 1.1.2.1.2  Inspection of hair

The inspection of head and hair mainly examines the luster, shape, growth and loss of hair.

**Luster and shape**: In the yellow race, black, dense and lustrous hair is the sign of sufficient kidney essence and exuberance of qi and blood. Yellowish, dry, thin, soft and brittle hair is the sign of insufficiency of kidney essence and asthenia of qi and blood which fail to nourish hair. White hair in young people without pathological changes is usually related to congenital constitution and is not a morbid condition. If white hair is accompanied by aching and weak loins and knees, tinnitus and amnesia, it is caused by asthenia of liver and kidney yin and lack of essence. If white hair is accompanied by insomnia and poor appetite, it is caused by overstrain of the heart and spleen as well as deficiency of qi and blood. Appearance of infantile hair like tassels with yellowish lusterless dryness is usually seen in malnutrition due to impairment of the spleen and stomach by improper feeding.

**Loss of hair**: Sparse, yellow and dry hair is caused by insufficient kidney essence, asthenia of qi and blood which fail to nourish hair, usually seen in patients after serious illness and chronic disease. Sparse hair in young people often results from blood heat or consumption of kidney essence. Greasy hair with obvious loss of hair at the top of the head accompanied by pruritus and desquamation is usually caused by internal accumulation of damp heat. Sudden patch loss of hair with round or elliptic exposed head scalp is known as alopecia areata due to blood

（3）动态：无论大人或小儿，头摇不能自主者，皆为肝风内动。

**2. 望头发**

主要诊察头发的色泽、形态和生长脱落情况。

（1）色泽形态：黄色人种头发色黑，浓密润泽，是肾精充足，气血旺盛的表现。头发色黄干枯，细软，脆而易断，是肾精不足，气血亏虚，发失荣养所致。青年白发而无病象，常与先天禀赋有关，不属病态。若伴腰膝酸软、耳鸣、健忘，多是肝肾阴虚精少所致；若伴心悸失眠、纳少，是属劳伤心脾，气血亏少所致。小儿发结如穗，枯黄无泽，多见于疳积，多因喂养不当，脾胃虚损所致。

（2）脱发：头发稀疏易落，色黄而枯，多属肾精不足，气血亏虚，发失荣养所致，常见于大病后和慢性虚损病患者。青壮年头发稀疏易落，多由于血热，或肾精亏损所致。头发油腻，头顶部脱发明显，伴头皮瘙痒、脱屑，多因湿热内蕴所致。突然片状脱发，显露圆形或椭圆形光亮头皮，称

asthenia and wind attack, or caused by anxiety and nervousness which lead to qi stagnation and fire depression as well as blood heat generating wind.

### 1.1.2.2 Inspection of the five sense organs

The five sense organs refer to the eyes, ears, nose, mouth and tongue which are closely related to the viscera. Each organ itself is directly or indirectly related to several viscera and its functions are also associated with the heart spirit. Therefore, the inspection of the five sensory organs is not only helpful for the selection of treatment of the sensory organs themselves based on syndrome differentiation, but also helpful for understanding the pathological changes of the viscera. The inspection of tongue is discussed in another section. The following is the discussion of the inspection of the eyes, ears, nose, mouth, lips, gums and throat.

#### 1.1.2.2.1 Inspection of the eyes

The eyes are the orifices related to the liver. However, all the visceral essence flows upward into the eyes. In the ancient time, people divided the eye into five parts in the "theory of five wheels", corresponding to the five zang organs, i. e. the eyelids pertaining to the spleen known as muscle wheel, the canthi pertaining to the heart known as blood wheel, the white part pertaining to the lung known as qi wheel, the black part pertaining to the liver known as wind wheel and the pupil pertaining to the kidney known as water wheel. According to the theory of five wheels, inspection of the abnormal changes of different parts of the eyes can reveal the disorders of the related viscera.

**Colour of the eyes:** Redness of the eyes indicates heat. To be specific, red canthus indicates heart fire,

为斑秃,多因血虚受风所致,也可因忧虑、紧张等精神因素导致气滞火郁,血热生风而形成。

（二）望五官

五官,指目、耳、鼻、口、舌等五种器官。五官与内脏有着密切而复杂的关系,每一器官都与多个脏腑存在着直接或间接的关系,其功能又与心神有关。因此,诊察五官的异常变化,不仅有助于对其本身病变的辨证施治,而且可以了解脏腑的病变。这里主要阐述目、耳、鼻、口、唇、龈和咽喉的望诊,望舌另作专述。

1. 望目

目为肝之窍,但五脏六腑精气皆上注于目,前人有"五轮学说"把目的各个部分与五脏相联属,分为五轮,即上下眼睑为肉轮,属脾;目两眦血络为血轮,属心;白睛为气轮,属肺;黑睛为风轮,属肝;瞳仁为水轮,属肾。根据五轮学说,诊察目之不同部位的异常变化,可以了解相应脏腑的病变。

望目,除诊察眼神外,还应注意目色、目形及动态的异常。

（1）目色:目赤为热,其中眦赤为心火,白睛赤为肺

redness of the white part indicates pulmonary fire, redness of the white part with reddish veins signifies exuberant fire due to yin asthenia, redness of the whole eyes shows wind heat in the liver meridian, and red, swelling and ulcerated eyelids indicates splenic fire or damp heat. For example, yellowish change of the white part is a sign of jaundice and pale canthus and eyelids shows insufficiency of blood.

**Shape of the eyes**: Sunken orbit is often due to loss of body fluid resulting from excessive vomiting and diarrhea, or due to decline of visceral essence resulting from chronic diseases. Dropsy of the eyelids and cheeks usually indicates edema; prolapse of the lower eyelid in the middle-aged is not morbid. Exophthalmus accompanied by swelling neck is goiter.

**Movements of the eyes**: Staring straight upward and obliquely during the course of a disease mostly indicates internal disturbance of liver wind. Immobile straight staring is a severe condition of the declination of visceral essence. Slight fixation of the vision is usually due to internal retention of phlegmatic heat. Open eyes during sleep is often caused by weak functions of the spleen and stomach. Platycoria and no reaction to light are critical signs of kidney essence exhaustion, also seen in poisoning. Miosis results from exuberant fire in the liver and gallbladder or asthenic impairment of the liver and kidney and up-flaming of asthenic fire, or poisoning. Anisocoria suggests blood stasis or phlegm and fluid retention in the brain.

#### 1.1.2.2.2 Inspection of the ears

The ears are the orifices related to the ears and the places where all meridians converge. Besides, the shaoyang meridians of both the hand and the foot flows anterior

火,白睛显红络为阴虚火旺,全目红肿为肝经风热,眼胞红肿湿烂为脾火或湿热。如白睛变黄是黄疸之征,目眦和睑内淡白是血亏之兆。

(2) 目形:目窠内陷,多因剧烈吐泻,伤津脱液,或久病脏腑精气虚衰所致。眼睑浮肿如卧蚕状,伴面部浮肿,多为水肿病;中老年人眼下睑微肿下垂,一般不属病态。两目突出,伴颈部肿大,多是瘿瘤。

(3) 目态:疾病过程中,两目上视、斜视,多见于肝风内动。两目直视,不能转动,目睛正圆,多属脏腑精气衰竭的重证。目睛微定,多为痰热内闭。睡眠露睛,多属脾胃虚弱。瞳仁散大,对光反应消失,多属肾精耗竭,为濒死危象,也可见于中毒患者。瞳仁缩小,则多属肝胆火炽,或肝肾虚损,虚火上炎,或为中毒。两侧瞳仁不等大,提示颅内有瘀血或痰饮。

**2. 望耳**

耳为肾之窍,又为宗脉之所聚,手足少阳经行耳之前后,手足太阳和阳明经之脉也

to the ears and the taiyang and yangming meridians distribute over the ears. So the ears are closely connected with the whole body through meridians and collaterals. Therefore, many visceral disorders can be reflected over the ears. Generally speaking, inspection of the ears is chiefly helpful for understanding the conditions of the kidney essence and the pathological changes of the gallbladder.

Inspection of the ears should concentrate on the colour, shape and inner part of the ears.

**Colour and shape of the ears**: Ears of healthy people are characterized by rich flesh, slight yellow, reddish and moist luster, which are the signs of sufficiency of kidney essence. Whitish colour of the whole ears indicate cold syndrome; bluish and blackish colour of the ears is usually seen in pain syndrome. Thin and dry ears are a sign of insufficiency of kidney essence; scorching dry and black colour of the ears signifies extreme loss of kidney essence.

**Pathological changes inside the ears**: Pathological changes in the ears are mainly otorrhea of pus. Otorrhea of yellowish pus and white pus is all due to prolonged stagnation of damp heat in the liver and gallbladder.

#### 1.1.2.2.3 Inspection of the nose

The nose is the orifice related to the lung, corresponding to the spleen meridian and connecting with the stomach meridian. So inspection of the changes of the nose is helpful for understanding changes of the lung, spleen and stomach.

Inspection of the nose mainly concentrates on examining the excreta as well as the colour and shape of the nose.

**Colour and shape of the nose**: Reddish swelling with sore of the nose is usually caused by exuberant heat in the stomach or blood heat. Enlargement of the nose tip with thickened skin, bulging surface like acne or wart is called rosacea caused mostly by accumulation of heat in the lung and stomach. Ulceration and sinking of the nose bridge is usually seen in syphilis; sinking of nose bridge with the loss of brows is usually a critical condition in leprosy.

Asthma with flapping nose wings is usually caused by retention of pathogenic heat or phlegm in the lung in new disease and is a critical condition of the exhaustion of pulmonary and renal essence in chronic disease.

**Nasal excreta**: See the section of inspecting excreta.

#### 1.1.2.2.4　Inspection of mouth and lips

The spleen opens to the mouth, flourishes on the lips and is internally and externally related with the stomach. The spleen and the stomach are the production source of qi and blood. So, inspection of mouth and lips is helpful for understanding the functions of the spleen and stomach as well as the pathological changes of qi and blood in the whole body.

Inspection of mouth and lips mainly focuses on inspecting the luster, colour, dryness, moisture and shape.

**Colour, luster, dryness and moisture**: The normal colour of lips is reddish, fresh and moist. Deep red and dry lips indicates consumption of fluid by exuberant heat; purplish and brownish dry lips indicates extreme exuberance of stagnant heat; bright red lips indicates yin asthenia and exuberant fire; lips as red as cherry usually indicates poisoning by coal gas; pale lips is caused by asthenia of both qi and blood; purplish lips indicates qi stagnation and blood stasis; blackish colour around the mouth indicates kidney qi on verge to exhaust; dry and fissured lips indicate impairment of fluid; swelling and painful lips or lips with ulceration and sores are often caused by fumiga-

厚，表面隆起，高低不平，状如赘疣，或生粉刺，称为酒齄鼻，多由肺胃蕴热所致。鼻柱溃陷，多见于梅毒；鼻柱塌陷，伴眉毛脱落，常为麻风恶候。

喘而鼻翼煽动，新病多属热邪或痰饮壅阻肺气所致；久病多为肺肾精气虚竭的危重证。

（2）鼻内分泌物：见望排出物。

**4. 望口、唇**

脾开窍于口，其华在唇，与胃互为表里。脾胃为气血生化之源。所以，诊察口与唇，可以了解脾胃的功能和全身气血的病变。

望口与唇，主要诊察口唇的色泽、润燥和形态。

（1）色泽、润燥：唇色以红而鲜润为正常。唇色深红而干，为热盛伤津；唇色绛紫而干焦，为瘀热盛极；唇色鲜红为阴虚火旺；唇色如樱桃红，常见于一氧化碳中毒；唇色淡白多属气血两虚；唇色青紫多为气滞血瘀；环口黑色者是肾气将绝。唇干燥皲裂是津液已伤。唇红肿疼痛，或有糜烂、唇边生疮，多因脾胃蕴热上蒸所致。

tion of heat accumulating in the spleen and stomach.

**Shape**: During the course of a disease, constant opening of mouth indicates that pulmonary and splenic qi is on verge to exhaust and that the syndrome is asthenic; difficulty in opening mouth is lockjaw seen in convulsion in sthenia sydnrome.

#### 1.1.2.2.5　Inspection of gums

Gums are connected with the collaterals of yangming meridian. So inspection of gums is helpful for understanding the pathological changes of the stomach. Inspection of gums mainly concentrates on examining the colour of gums. Nomrally, gums are light red and moist. Pale gums indicates blood asthenia; reddish swelling and painful gums indicate exuberance of gastric fire; slight swelling gums without pain indicate up-flaming of asthenic fire; bleeding and reddish swelling gums indicate impairment of the collaterals by gastric fire; bleeding gums without reddish swelling suggest impairment of the collaterals by asthenic fire.

#### 1.1.2.2.6　Inspection of throat

The throat is the door to the lung and stomach, the pathway for breathing and eating and the region over which the kidney meridian circulates. So inspection of throat is helpful for examining the pathological changes of the lung, the stomach and the kidney.

Inspection of throat mainly concentrates on the colour and shape of the throat. Reddish swelling and pain of throat is due to virulent wind heat attacking the upper or due to stagnant heat in the lung and stomach to fumigate the upper; reddish swelling and ulceration of the throat indicates extreme exuberance of heat virulence; bright red and tender throat with slight swelling and pain is due to up-flaming of asthenic fire resulting from deficiency of kidney yin; unilateral or bilateral reddish and painful

（2）形态：疾病过程中，口开而不闭者，为口张，是肺脾之气将绝，属虚证；口闭而难张者，为口噤，多见于痉病或惊风，属实证。

#### 5. 望齿龈

齿龈为阳明脉络所系，所以，诊察齿龈的异常变化，可以了解胃的一些病变。望齿龈，主要诊察色泽的变化。色淡红而润泽是为正常。龈色淡白，是血虚不荣；齿龈红肿疼痛，是胃火炽盛；齿龈微肿而痛不红，是虚火上炎。齿龈出血且红肿，是胃火伤络；出血而不红肿，是虚火伤络。

#### 6. 望咽喉

咽喉为肺胃之门户，呼吸、饮食之通路，又系肾经循行之处。故望咽喉主要可以了解肺、胃、肾的病变。

望咽喉主要诊察咽喉色泽、形态的变化。咽喉红肿疼痛，多为风热邪毒上攻，或肺胃郁热上蒸；红肿溃烂，为热毒盛极；鲜红娇嫩，肿痛不甚，多为肾阴亏虚，虚火上炎。咽喉一侧或两侧突突起肿块，状如乳突，色红且痛，称为乳蛾，是肺胃积热，或风热上攻而成；

lumps like mastoid process is due to accumulation of heat in the lung and stomach or due to wind heat attacking the upper; reddish swelling and ulceration with erasable yellowish white pus-like substance or suppurative points is called tonsillitis due to exuberant virulent heat as well as heat fumigation and muscle decaying; false whitish membrane on the throat that is not erasable, bleeding when rubbed heavily and reappearing is diphtheria due to accumulation of pestilent factors in the lung and stomach that fumigates the throat and must be treated in isolation.

#### 1.1.2.3　Inspection of neck

Neck is the part connecting the head with the trunk of the body; the anterior part is called neck and the posterior part is called nape. Normal neck should be erect and symmetrical with the trachea located on the middle. Laryngeal protuberance is prominent in the male and invisible in the female. The neck can be rotated, bent and raised freely in standing and sitting position. So inspection of neck concentrates on the shape and movement of the neck.

##### 1.1.2.3.1　Changes of the shape

The commonly seen changes are:

**Goiter**: Goiter refers to unilateral or bilateral lumps like tumor below the laryngeal protuberance which is either small or large and movable with swallowing, usually caused by stagnation of liver qi and retention of phlegm, sometimes due to local climate and environment.

**Scrofula**: Scrofula refers to cervical clustered nodules, usually caused by asthenic fire scorching phlegm into nodules due to asthenia of lung and kidney yin, or by accumulation of qi and blood in the neck due to attack by wind fire and seasonal pestilence.

##### 1.1.2.3.2　Changes of movement

Abnormal changes of the movement of the neck

若红肿溃烂出现黄白色脓样物或脓点，拭之易去，属烂乳蛾，是热毒炽盛、热灼肉腐而致。如咽部出现灰白色假膜，擦之不去，重擦出血，随即复生，则是白喉，为疫病之毒，蕴积肺胃，上蒸咽喉所致，急需隔离治疗。

#### （三）望颈项

颈项是联接头颅和躯干的部分，其前部称颈，后部为项。正常人的颈项端直，两侧对称，气管居中，男性喉结较突出，女子喉结不显露，站立或正坐位时，摇转俯仰自如。颈项部的望诊应注意外形和动态变化。

1. 外形变化

其外形异常变化常见的有：

（1）瘿瘤：颈前颔下喉结的一侧或两侧有肿块如瘤，或大或小，可随吞咽移动，称为瘿瘤。多由肝郁气结痰凝所致，或与地方水土有关。

（2）瘰疬：颈侧颔下肿块如垒，按之累累如串珠，称为瘰疬。多由肺肾阴虚，虚火灼津结成痰核，或感受风火时毒，致气血壅滞，结于颈项。

2. 动态变化

其动态的异常变化主

include the following aspects:

**Flaccidity of the neck**: Weakness of the neck unable to support the head is called flaccidity of the neck. Flaccidity of the neck in the babies over 4 months old is due to congenital deficiency, insufficiency of essence and marrow, or due to postnatal improper feeding which leads to asthenia of qi and blood and malnutrition of the skeleton. Flaccidity of the neck with dispiritedness in chronic and severe diseases is due to exhaustion of essence.

**Stiff neck**: Stiff neck refers to spasm of the muscles and sinews over the neck, making it difficult for the neck to bend, raise and rotate. Stiffness of the neck after sleep is due to improper posture in sleep or due to wind cold attacking the neck. Stiffness of neck with high fever, headache and vomiting is usually due to heat virulence in febrile disease attacking the upper; stiffness of neck and back with posterior bending of the head, stretching of the trunk, bending of the spine and spasm of the limbs is called opisthotonus, usually seen in tetanus and exogenous febrile disease with wind generated by extreme heat.

### 1.1.2.4 Inspection of skin

Skin is distributed over the surface of the body, connected with the lung with weiqi circulating inside. Skin is the defending barrier of the body and nourished by qi, blood and body fluid through meridians. So the disorders of the skin itself and the disorders of viscera can be reflected by the skin. Inspection of the skin is not only helpful for diagnosing skin disorders, but also helpful for understanding the nature of the disease, the conditions of the viscera and the states of qi and blood.

要有：

（1）项软：颈项软弱，无力支撑头颅，称为项软。婴儿出生4个月后项软，不能抬头，系先天禀赋不足，精亏髓少，或后天失养，气血亏虚，骨骼失充所致。久病、重病后项软，神疲乏力，多为精气衰竭的表现。

（2）项强：项部筋脉肌肉拘急强硬，不能前俯后仰、左右转动者，称为项强。睡眠后，颈项强痛，不能转侧，或一侧颈项拘急疼痛，称为落枕，多因睡姿不当，或颈部感受风寒所致。项强，兼壮热、头痛、呕吐，多属温病热邪上攻。项背强直拘急，头向后仰，躯干前挺，背脊反折如弓，兼四肢挛急，称为角弓反张，多见于破伤风、外感热病热极生风等，须结合其他检查作出诊断。

### （四）望皮肤

皮肤居一身之表，内合于肺，卫气循行其间，是机体的屏障，气血津液通过经络外荣皮肤。因此，不仅皮肤本身的多种病变，而且脏腑病变亦反映于皮肤，引起皮肤发生异常变化。通过望皮肤，不仅有助于皮肤病证的诊断，还可以了解疾病的性质，脏腑的虚实，气血的盛衰。

The normal skin colour of the yellow race is similar to complexion and appears reddish and yellowish, moist and lustrous, elastic and smooth, which are signs of sufficiency of body fluid and essence.

Inspection of skin mainly concentrates on the colour, shape and pathological changes of the skin, such as macules, eruption, miliaria alba, abscess, carbuncle, boil and furuncle.

#### 1.1.2.4.1 Inspection of colour

The diagnostic significance of inspection of skin is similar to that of inspection of complexion.

#### 1.1.2.4.2 Inspection of shape

Dropsy of skin is due to spreading of dampness; dry skin is due to consumption of body fluid or depletion of essence and blood; dry and rough skin like scales is called squamous skin due to mixture of blood asthenia with blood stagnation and malnutrition of the muscles and skin.

#### 1.1.2.4.3 Inspection of skin disorders

Many skin diseases and general diseases may bring about the changes of the colour and shape of the skin. The following are some of the commonly encountered ones.

**Inspection of macules**: Macules refer to reddish or purplish uneven patches on the skin and can be divided into yang macules and yin macules.

Reddish or purplish and silk texture or cloud like macules with fever, dysphoria and fast pulse is called yang macules, usually seen at the exuberant heat stage in

黄色人种正常人的皮肤与面色相似，肤色红黄隐隐，荣润而有光泽，富有弹性，柔韧光滑。是津液充沛，精气旺盛的征象。

望皮肤，主要诊察患者皮肤的色泽、形态和表现于皮肤的病证，如斑、疹、白痦、痈、疽、疔、疖等。

**1. 望色泽**

皮肤色泽变化的诊断意义，与望面色类同，可参见望面色，不再赘述。

**2. 望形态**

皮肤虚浮肿胀，多属水湿泛溢为病；皮肤干瘪枯燥，多为津液耗伤，或精血亏损；皮肤干燥粗糙，形如鳞甲，称为肌肤甲错，多由血虚挟瘀，肌肤失养所致。

**3. 望皮肤病症**

许多皮肤病和全身性疾病皆可引起皮肤色泽、形态发生变化，而表现为特殊的皮肤病证，临床常见的有以下几种：

（1）斑：皮肤出现色红或紫，点大成片，大小不一，平铺于皮下，抚之不碍手，压之不退色者，称为斑。有阳斑、阴斑之分。

色红或紫，形似锦纹、云片，兼身热、烦躁、脉数等症，为阳斑，常见于外感温热病热

exogenous febrile disease due to exuberant heat scorching blood and driving blood to extravasate. Bright red macules appearing on the chest and abdomen first and gradually extending to the four limbs with freshment of the spirit after abatement of fever is the sign of outgoing of pathogenic factors, suggesting favourable prognosis. Thick, deep red or purplish macules, or appearing first on the four limbs and gradually extending to the chest and abdomen with continuous high fever and even coma, is a sign of extreme exuberance of virulent heat and internal sinking of pathogenic factors, suggesting unfavourable prognosis.

Light colored or purplish thin macules with varied size, unfixed location, occasional appearance and disappearance, pale tongue and weak pulse are yin macules, usually seen in miscellaneous diseases of internal impairment resulting from failure of qi to control blood and extravasation of blood.

**Inspection of eruptions**: Eruptions refer to reddish points like millet or petals that can be felt by hands and fade when pressed. Eruptions may appear in various diseases, such as measles, rubella and urticaria.

Measles is an acute epidemic eruptive disease in pediatrics, usually due to attack by exogenous morbillous toxin. Measles is characterized by pink pockmarks which appear first over the hairline and face, gradually extending to the trunk and four limbs and disappearing after full eruption. Pink-colored and evenly-distributed measles with orderly eruption, orderly disappearance, abatement of fever and desquamation after eruption is favourable, suggesting that healthy qi dominates over pathogenic factors and that the prognosis is favourable. Deep red or purplish and thick or evenly mixed or unevenly erupting or sudden vanishing measles accompanied by high fever and asthmatic

盛期,因热炽营血,迫血妄行所致。若斑少而色泽红活,先出现于胸腹,后延及四肢,同时热退神清,是邪气外透的征象,为顺证,提示病情较轻,预后较好。斑多稠密,色深红或紫暗,或先见于四肢,后延及胸腹,同时高热不退,甚至神志昏迷,是热毒盛极,邪气内陷之征,提示病情深重,预后不良。

色浅淡或紫暗,大小不一,隐而稀少,发无定处,时隐时现,兼面白、舌淡、脉弱等症,为阴斑,常见于内伤杂病,多因气不摄血,血溢脉外所致。

(2)疹:皮肤出现色红,点小如粟,或如花瓣,高出皮肤,抚之碍手,压之退色者,称为疹。疹可见于多种病证,如麻疹、风疹、瘾疹等。

麻疹是小儿科常见急性发疹性传染病。多因外感时邪麻毒所致。其出疹特点是,疹色桃红形似麻粒,先见于发际颜面,渐延及躯干四肢,全身疹透齐全后逐渐消退,退后脱屑。若疹色红润,分布均匀,疹出顺序而齐全,并依出疹顺序逐渐消退,疹出热退,为顺证,提示正胜邪却,病轻,预后好;若疹点深红或紫暗,稠密,甚或融合成片,或透发

breath is unfavourable, suggesting that pathogenic factors dominate over healthy qi and that the prognosis is unfavourable.

   Rubella is a commonly encountered acute epidemic disease in pediatrics, usually caused by exogenous virulent heat. Rubella is characterized by light red colour, small size, sparse distribution, more distribution on face and neck, less distribution on four limbs, itching skin and no desquamation after disappearance of eruption.

   Urticaria is a cutaneous disease caused by internal accumulation of damp heat complicated by invasion of pathogenic wind which is stagnated in the skin. It may be caused by allergy. Its eruption is marked by various size of macules which are in the size of pockmarks or soybean, protruding on the skin, occasionally emerging and disappearing. It is quite itching and appears in patches after being scratched.

   **Miliaria alba**: Miliaria alba refers to a kind of small whitish blisters on the skin characterized by brightness like millet, protrusion over the skin and unchanged colour over the root. There is serous fluid in miliaria alba which comes out when scatched. The blisters are distributed over the neck, chest and abdomen, occasionally over the four limbs and never on the head. There is desquamation after disappearance of miliaria alba. It is usually caused by retention of exogenous damp heat in the skin and inhibited sweating, often seen among patients with damp and febrile disease. Miliaria alba with bright colour and full serous fluid is called crystal miliaria alba, suggesting sufficiency of fluid, capability of healthy qi to dominate over pathogenic factors, outgoing of damp heat and favourable prognosis. Miliaria alba with white and dry colour and no serous fluid is called dry miliaria alba, suggesting insufficiency of fluid, failure of healthy qi to dominate over path-

不齐，或突然隐没，伴见高热、喘息等症，多属逆证，提示邪盛正虚，病重，预后不良。

风疹亦是小儿科常见急性发疹性传染病。多因外感风热时邪所致。其出疹特点是疹色淡红，细小稀疏，面颈部较多，躯干四肢较少，伴皮肤瘙痒，疹退后无脱屑。

瘾疹是一种皮肤病，多因内蕴湿热，复感风邪，郁于皮腠而发，或由于对某些物质过敏所致。其出疹特点是皮肤出现大小不等的丘疹，小如麻粒，大如豆瓣，高出皮肤，时隐时现，甚痒，搔之成片。

（3）白痦：白痦是皮肤上出现的一种白色小疱疹。其特点是：晶莹如粟，高出肤面，根部肤色不变，内含浆液，擦破流水，多分布于颈项胸腹，偶见于四肢，唯不见于头面部，消退时脱屑。多因外感湿热之邪，郁于肌肤，汗出不彻，蕴酿而成。常见于湿温病患者。若晶莹饱满、颗粒清楚，为晶痦，提示津气充足，正能胜邪，湿热外达，属顺证，预后好；色白而枯、干瘪无浆，为枯痦，提示津气不足，正不胜邪，属逆证，预后不良。

ogenic factors and unfavourable prognosis.

**Carbuncle, phlegmon, boil and furuncle**: Carbuncle, phlegmon, boil and furuncle appear on the surface of the body and are usually treated in surgery.

Carbuncle: Carbuncle refers to local swelling with tense root and accompanied by hot sensation and pain. Carbuncle is of yang syndrome and is characterized by quick onset, susceptibility to ulceration and liability to healing. It is usually caused by internal accumulation of damp heat and virulent heat, stagnation of qi and blood as well as exuberance of heat and decaying of muscles.

Phlegmon: Phlegmon refers to extensive swelling without tip, changes of skin, fever and pain. It is of yin syndrome marked by gradual onset, longer duration, difficulty in dispersing, ulcerating and healing. It is usually caused by asthenia of qi and blood, stagnation of cold and phlegm, or internal accumulation of virulence of wind which migrates in the muscles, deepens into tendons and bones as well as stagnates qi and blood.

Boil: Boil appears like millet at first with hard deep root, numbness or itching, white top and pain, followed by bright redness, pyrexia, aggravation of swelling and sharp pain. It is usually caused by accumulation of heat in the viscera, complicated by virulence attacking the skin, resulting in stagnation of qi and blood.

Furuncle: Furuncle appears superficially on the skin with small and round size, red swelling, pyrexia, mild pain, susceptibility to suppurate and ulcerate and liability to healing after ulceration. It is usually caused by internal accumulation of virulent heat, or by stagnation of summer-heat dampness in the skin which stagnates qi and blood.

### 1.1.2.5 Inspection of infantile index finger veins

Inspection of infantile index finger veins means to

（4）痈疽疔疖：痈、疽、疔、疖都是发于体表、有形可诊的外科疮疡疾患。

痈：局部红肿高起，范围较大，根盘紧束，伴有焮热疼痛者，称为痈，属阳证。具有发病迅速，易溃易敛的特点。多因湿热火毒内蕴，气血瘀滞，热盛肉腐而成。

疽：患处漫肿无头，肤色不变，不热少痛者，称为疽，属阴证。其起病缓慢，病程长，不易消散，难溃难敛。多由气血亏虚，寒痰凝滞，或风毒内积，流注肌肉，内陷筋骨，气血瘀阻而成。

疔：初起如粟，根脚坚硬而深，麻木或痒，顶白而痛，继则焮红发热，肿势渐增，疼痛剧烈者，称为疔。多因脏腑蕴热，复感邪毒阻于皮内，致气血瘀滞而成。

疖：发于皮肤浅表，形小而圆，红肿热痛不甚，易脓易溃，溃后即愈者，称为疖。多由内蕴热毒或外感暑湿郁阻于肌肤，致局部气血壅滞而成。

（五）望小儿食指脉络

望小儿食指脉络，是诊察

examine the length, colour and shape of the veins along the palmar margin to detect pathological changes. This method is applicable for the diagnosis of infants under the age of three. Since artery over cunkou in infants is short and infants tend to cry in clinical examination and affect the accuracy of pulse taking, inspection of index finger veins is usually used to help diagnose because infantile skin is thin and tender and veins are visible.

Infantile index finger vein is divided into wind pass, qi pass and life pass. The first stem of the index finger, the part between metacarpophalangeal transverse lines and the transverse lines on the second stem, is wind pass; the second stem, the part between the transverse line on the second stem and the transverse ine on the third stem, is qi pass; and the third stem, the part between the transverse line on the third stem and the top of the index finger, is life pass (see Fig. 1).

患儿食指掌面前缘脉络的长短、色泽和形态等，以了解病情的一种诊法。望小儿食指脉络诊法适用于3岁以内的幼儿，这是因为幼儿寸口脉部位短小，诊病时又常易哭闹，影响脉象的真实性，且幼儿皮肤薄嫩，脉络显而易见。因此，常以望食指脉络辅助诊断。

小儿食指脉络分为风、气、命三关。食指的第一节，即掌指关节横纹向远端至第二节横纹之间，为风关；第二节，即第二节横纹至第三节横纹之间，为气关；第三节，即第三节横纹至食指末端，为命关。（见图1）

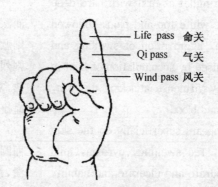

Fig. 1　Three passes of infantile index finger vein
图1　小儿食指脉络三关图

The normal infantile index finger vein is light red and slightly purplish, dimly visible within the wind pass, usually not quite clear or even indistinct. The vein usually

正常小儿食指脉络，色泽淡红略紫，隐现于风关之内，大多不浮露，甚至不明显，多

appears oblique, singular, moderate in thickness, thicker and longer in hot weather, thinner and shorter in cold weather. It is longer in infants under the age of one and becomes shorter with the increase of age.

**Methods for inspecting infantile index finger vein.** The parent carries the infant to the place with full light and the doctor grasps the end of the infantile index finger with the left hand and pushes the infantile index finger from the anterior palmar margin of the index finger to the palm direction for several times with the side of the right thumb. The pushing should be moderate in strength and make the vein clearer for observation.

**Content of the inspection of infantile index finger vein.** The inspection mainly concentrates on the length, colour, floating or sinking, lightness or stagnancy and shape of the vein.

Length: During the course of a disease, appearance of the index finger vein on the wind-pass indicates that the disease is mild; if it extends to the qi-pass, it means that the disease is serious; if it extends to the life-pass, it shows that the disease is very serious; if it stretches directly to the tip of the finger, it indicates critical condition and unfavourable prognosis.

Colour: Light-coloured and whitish vein indicates insufficiency of qi and blood; reddish vein indicates exogenous wind and cold; deep red or purplish vein indicates internal exuberance of heat; bluish vein indicates pain syndrome or convulsion; cyanotic or purplish dark vein indicates stagnation of blood collaterals and critical condition.

Floating and sinking: Visible and floating vein indicates that the pathogenic factors are in the superficial and that the disease has just occurred; deep and indistinct vein means that the pathogenic factors are in the interior as in

为斜形、单枝，粗细适中，天热时稍粗稍长，天寒时变细缩短。1岁以内稍长，随年龄增长而缩短。

**1. 望小儿食指脉络的方法**

令患儿家属将患儿抱向光线明亮处，医生用左手握住患儿食指末端，以右手拇指侧部从患儿食指掌面前缘指端向手掌方向推动数次，用力须适中，使脉络更加明显，便于观察。

**2. 望小儿食指脉络的内容**

望小儿食指脉络应注意长短、色泽、浮沉、淡滞和形态等变化。

长短：在疾病过程中，食指脉络显于风关者，为病情较轻；脉络至气关者，病情较重；脉络达于命关者，病情严重；脉络直达指端者，谓之"透关射甲"，病情凶险，预后不良。

色泽：脉络色淡白者，多为气血不足；色鲜红者，多为外感风寒；色深红或紫红者，多为内热炽盛；色青者，多为痛证或惊风；色青紫或紫黑者，多为血络瘀闭，病情危重。

浮沉：脉络浮现明显者，为病邪在表，多见于外感病初起；脉络沉隐不显者，为病邪在里，多见于外邪入里或内伤

the case of internal invasion of pathogenic factors or internal impairment.

Lightness and stagnancy: Light-coloured vein indicates insufficiency of qi and blood; deep and dull colour of vein indicates excess of pathogenic factors and stagnaton of qi and blood.

Form: Thin vein indicates asthenia and cold syndromes; thick vein indicates sthenia and heat syndromes; single and oblique vein indicates mild disease; multiple and curled vein indicates serious disease; gradual extension of vein indicates progression of disease; gradual shrinkage of vein indicates alleviation of disease.

In a word, inspecting infantile index finger vein includes three aspects: estimation of the state of diseases by inspecting three passes, discrimination of cold and heat by inspecting color reddness and purpleness, and determination of asthenia and sthenia by inspecting lightness and stagnancy.

### 1.1.2.6 Inspection of excreta

Excreta refers to the secretion and excreta from the human body, including tears, spittle, snivel, sweating, saliva, urine, stool, menstruation, leukorrhea, sputum and vomitus, etc. Excreta is produced by the functional activities of the viscera. Normally, the excretion of tears, spittle, snivel, sweating, saliva, urine, stool, menstruation, leukorrhea and sputum follow certain rules. However, under morbid conditions, there may be some changes in its colour, quality, volume and form. The production of sputum and vomitus is due to the dysfunction of the viscera. So inspection of excreta is helpful for understanding the location and nature of disease as well as the functional states of the viscera.

Inspection of excreta mainly includes examination of

病证。

淡滞：脉络色浅淡者，多为气血不足；色深暗滞者，多为邪气有余，气血郁闭。

形态：脉络较细者，多为虚证、寒证；增粗者，多为实证、热证。单枝、斜形，多为病轻；多枝、弯曲，多为病重。脉络日渐增长者，为病进；日渐缩短者，为病退。

总之，望小儿食指脉络，以三关测轻重，红紫辨寒热，浮沉分表里，淡滞定虚实为其概要。

### （六）望排出物

排出物是人体分泌物和排泄物的总称，主要包括泪、唾、涎、涕、汗、二便、月经、带下及痰、呕吐物等。排出物是脏腑功能活动的产物。正常情况下，泪、唾、涎、涕、汗、二便、月经、带下等都有一定的排出规律，当脏腑发生病变时，可引起其在色、质、量、形等方面发生异常变化；痰和呕吐物则是脏腑功能失调的产物。因此，通过望排出物，可以了解病变部位及相关脏腑功能的盛衰和疾病的性质。

望排出物，主要诊察其

its colour, quality, volume and form. Generally speaking, whitish or light-coloured and thin excreta indicates cold syndrome and asthenia syndrome due to retention of dampness resulting from stagnation of pathogenic cold or insufficiency of yangqi and weakness in transportation and transformation; yellowish or deep-coloured and thick excreta indicates heat and sthenia syndrome due to fumigation by pathogenic heat which condenses body fluid.

Inspection of excreta is rich in content, the following mainly describes the inspection of sputum, snivel, spittle, saliva and vomitus. Sweating, urine, stool, menstruation and leukorrhea will be discussed in the chapter of inquiry.

#### 1.1.2.6.1 Inspection of sputum

Sputum is a kind of sticky fluid, substance produced by disturbance of fluid metabolism, excreted from the lung and trachea due to dysfunction of the lung and the spleen. That is why it is said that "the spleen is the source of sputum, while the lung is the container of sputum". The production of sputum may bring about various diseases. So it is said that "sputum is produced by diseases, but sputum further worsens diseases".

Yellowish and sticky, or hard and coagulated sputum is heat-sputum produced by exogenous wind-heat, or by accumulation of endogenous heat which fumigates the lung. Whitish, thin or blackish sputum is cold-sputum due to consumption of yangqi by cold, failure of qi to transform fluid and accumulation of dampness. Thin and frothy sputum is wind-sputum due to pathogenic wind attacking the lung. Whitish, slippery and easily expectorated sputum is damp-sputum due to asthenia of the spleen and exuberance of dampness. Scanty, sticky sputum difficult to expectorate, or with unproductive cough, is dry sputum due to pathogenic dryness attacking lung and consuming fluid in exogenous disease; in diseases due to internal

色、质、量、形等情况。一般地说,排出物色白或淡、清稀,多属寒证、虚证,这是因为寒邪凝滞,或阳气不足,运化无力,使水湿不化之故;色黄或深、稠浊,多属热证、实证,是由热邪薰灼,煎熬津液所致。

望排出物的内容较多,其中,汗、二便、月经、带下等将在问诊中介绍,这里重点阐述痰、涕、唾、涎及呕吐物的望诊。

#### 1. 望痰

痰是由肺和气道排出的粘液,属机体水液代谢障碍的产物,其形成主要由肺、脾的功能失常所致,故前人有"脾为生痰之源,肺为贮痰之器"之说。痰形成后,又可导致多种疾病,故又有"痰因病生,病以痰著"之说。

痰黄粘稠,或坚而成块,为热痰,多因外感风热,或内热壅盛,肺受薰灼所致。痰白质稀或有灰黑点,为寒痰,多因寒伤阳气,气不化津,聚湿成痰。痰清稀而多泡沫,为风痰,多因风邪袭肺所致。痰白滑量多而易咯,为湿痰,多因脾虚湿盛所致。痰少而粘,难以咯出,甚则干咳无痰,为燥痰,在外感病中,多因燥邪犯肺伤津;内伤病中,则因肺阴虚损,虚火灼肺所致。若痰少

impairment, sputum results from consumption of pulmonary yin and asthenia-fire scorching the lung. If sputum is mingled with fresh blood, it means that the pulmonary collaterals are impaired due to invasion of dry-heat into the lung as well as asthenia of yin and exuberance of fire. If sputum appears like purulent blood or chyle with foul smell, it is usually seen in pulmonary abscess due to accumulation of heat toxin in the lung and suppuration of the decayed resulting from blood stasis.

#### 1.1.2.6.2 Inspection of spittle and saliva

Spittle refers to thick secretion in the mouth, while saliva refers to the thin part of secretion in the mouth. Spittle is related to the kidney and also to the spleen and stomach; while saliva is related to the spleen.

Reduced spittle and dry mouth and throat are usually caused by exhaustion of body fluid or failure of body fluid to flow upwards, often seen in consumption of body fluid in exogenous disease, or internal impairment and prolonged disease marked by asthenia of spleen qi, failure of qi to transform fluid or insufficiency of kidney yin. Frequent salivation from the corners of the mouth in infant is usually due to failure of the asthenic spleen to control fluid or due to attack of wind-heat. Distorted mouth with inability to close the mouth and spontaneous drooling in adult is usually seen in wind stroke. Frequent regurgitation of clear and thin fluid in the mouth is often caused by asthenic cold in the middle energizer; or insufficiency of kidney yang and disorder of qi transformation; or by internal exuberance of cold dampness and upward flow of pathogenic dampness.

#### 1.1.2.6.3 Inspection of snivel

Snivel refers to sticky fluid discharged from the nose. Snivel is related to the lung. Inspection of snivel is helpful for understanding the conditions of pulmonary qi

而粘，甚则痰中带血，血色鲜红，是肺中血络受损，多因燥热犯肺，或阴虚火旺所致。痰如脓血，或脓痰如糜粥而腥臭，多见于肺痈，因热毒壅肺，热壅血瘀，化腐成脓所致。

### 2. 望唾、涎

唾为口腔内分泌的唾液中之稠厚者，涎为口腔内分泌的唾液中之清稀者。唾为肾之液，然亦关乎脾胃；涎为脾之液。

唾液减少，口舌干燥，多因津液枯乏，或津液不能上承所致，常见于外感病伤津，或内伤久病，脾气亏虚，气不化津，或肾阴不足。小儿经常口角流涎，称为滞颐，多因脾虚不能摄津，或受风热所致。成人口角歪斜不能闭合，涎自流出，多见于中风病。经常口泛清水，多因中焦虚寒，或肾阳不足，气化失司；或寒湿内盛，水湿之邪上泛所致。

### 3. 望涕

涕是鼻中分泌的粘液，为肺之液。望涕可以了解肺气的虚实，以及所受邪气的

and the nature of the pathogenic factors.

Stuffy nose with clear snivel indicates exogenous wind-cold. Turbid and yellowish snivel indicates exogenous wind-heat or wind-cold transforming into heat. Persistent discharge of turbid yellowish pus-like snivel with foul smell indicates nasosinusitis due to accumulation and retention of damp-heat. Snivel mingled with blood is usually caused by dry-heat impairing collaterals; frequent discharge of snivel with bloody streaks probably indicates malignant syndrome of nasal cavity and further examination is necessary.

### 1.1.2.6.4 Inspection of vomitus

Vomiting is caused by upward adverse flow of gastric qi. Inspection of vomitus is helpful for understanding the cause of upward adverse flow of gastric qi and the nature of disease.

Thin vomitus without foul smell indicates cold syndrome due to consumption of gastrosplenic yang or invasion of pathogenic cold in the stomach. Turbid and sour vomitus indicates heat syndrome due to exuberant heat in the stomach or liver fire attacking the stomach. Sour and fetid vomitus with indigested food accompanied by unpressable abdominal distension and pain is caused by retention of food due to intemperance of food and indigestion. Vomiting of indigested food without sour and fetid smell is caused by asthenic cold in the spleen and stomach. Vomiting of clear fluid, sputum and saliva is usually due to dysfunction of the spleen due to retention of fluid in the stomach. Vomiting of yellowish and greenish bitter fluid is due to accumulation of damp heat in the liver and gallbladder or due to adverse flow of liver and gallbladder qi which invades the stomach. Vomiting of fresh blood or purplish blood with clot or with food dregs is often due to impairment of the collaterals by stomach heat and liver fire or

性质。

鼻塞流清涕,是外感风寒。鼻流浊涕色黄,是外感风热,或风寒化热。久流浊涕,涕黄如脓,腥臭难闻,为鼻渊,是湿热蕴阻所致。涕中夹血,多为燥热伤络;经常涕中带血丝,当慎防鼻腔恶候,须作进一步检查。

### 4. 望呕吐物

呕吐是由胃气上逆而致。通过望呕吐物,可以帮助了解胃气上逆的原因和病性的寒热虚实。

呕吐物清稀无臭,为寒证,多因脾胃阳气亏虚,或寒邪犯胃所致。呕吐物秽浊酸臭,为热证,多因胃热炽盛,或肝火犯胃所致。呕吐物酸腐夹杂不消化食物,兼见脘腹胀痛、拒按,属食积,多因暴饮暴食,宿食不化所致。若呕吐不消化食物而无酸腐气,多属脾胃虚寒。呕吐清水痰涎,多因脾失健运,胃有停饮所致。呕吐黄绿苦水,多为肝胆湿热蕴结,或肝胆之气横逆犯胃所致。吐血鲜红或紫暗有块,或夹食物残渣,多因胃热肝火伤络,或血瘀胃脘所致。呕吐物脓血混杂,为胃痈,多因胃中热毒蕴蓄,气血瘀滞化腐

blood stasis in the epigastrium. Vomitus with pus and blood indicates stomach abscess due to accumulation of heat toxin in the stomach and putrefaction of blood stasis.

### 1.1.3 Inspection of tongue

Inspection of tongue, an important part of inspection diagnosis in TCM, is a diagnostic method by means of observing the changes of the body and fur of the tongue.

The tongue is closely related to the viscera and meridians. The tongue is the external part of the heart and is connected with the heart meridian. The tongue also manifests the conditions of the spleen because it is connected with the spleen meridian. The kidney stores essence and the kidney meridian reaches both sides of the tongue. The liver stores blood and governs tendons, the liver meridian also extends to the tongue. The lung reaches the throat and is connected with the tongue. The tongue fur is produced by gastric qi fumigating cereal nutrients.

The tongue depends on qi and blood to nourish and body fluid to moisten. So the form, texture and color of the tongue are closely related to the state and circulation of qi and blood. The moisture and dryness of the tongue coating and body are related to the quantity and distribution of body fluid. That is why the tongue can reveal the states of the viscera, qi, blood, yin, yang, pathogenic factors and healthy qi as well as the progress of diseases. So examination of the tongue can enable one to understand internal pathological changes.

#### 1.1.3.1 Methods for inspection of tongue

The patient is asked to sit down or lie in supination, exposed to the light source. The tongue is protruded naturally and the tip of the tongue is kept slightly downwards.

而成。

## 三、望舌

望舌，又称舌诊，是观察舌体与舌苔的变化，以测知病情变化的一种诊察方法。是望诊的重要组成部分，是中医诊法的特色之一。

舌与脏腑经络关系密切。舌为心之苗，手少阴心经之别系舌本；舌为脾之外候，足太阴脾经连舌本、散舌下；肾藏精，足少阴肾经挟舌本；肝藏血，主筋，其经脉络于舌本；肺系上达咽喉，与舌根相连。舌苔是由胃气蒸化谷气上承于舌而成。

舌体有赖于气血的濡养和津液的滋润。舌体的形质和舌色与气血的盈亏和运行状态有关；舌苔和舌体的润燥与津液的多少及其输布状况有关。因此，人体脏腑的虚实、气血阴阳的盈亏、邪正的消长、病情的顺逆等，都可从舌象变化上反映出来。所以诊察舌象可测知体内的病变。

### （一）望舌的方法

望舌时应让患者取坐位或仰卧位，面向光源，自然伸舌于口外，舌体平展，舌尖略

The mouth is opened wide to make the tongue exposed fully.

The sequence of inspection of the tongue begins from the tip of the tongue, then the middle and margin of the tongue, and finally the root of the tongue. The inspection begins with the tongue body first and then moves to the tongue fur. The inspection should be complete and quick.

In the inspection of tongue, trials should be made to exclude various false manifestations, such as "dyed tongue fur" due to light, diet and drugs.

Inspection of the tongue mainly includes the examination of the tongue proper and the tongue fur.

The body of the tongue is composed of muscles and vessels. In the ancient times some people believed that the surface of the tongue corresponded to the viscera. That is to say the tip of the tongue reflects the pathological changes of the heart and lung, the center of the tongue reflects the pathological changes of the spleen and stomach, the root of the tongue reflects the pathological changes of the kidney and the margins of the tongue reflect the pathological changes of the liver and gallbladder (see Fig. 2). Such an idea about the correspondence of the tongue to the viscera is clinically practical. However, the analysis should be comprehensive and based on the changes of the tongue body and tongue fur.

向下,尽量张口使舌体充分暴露,时间不宜过长。

望舌的顺序,一般是先看舌尖,再看舌中、舌侧,最后看舌根部;先看舌体,后看舌苔。应力求全面而迅速。

望舌时须注意排除各种因素所造成的假象。如光线的影响、饮食或药品形成的"染苔"等。

望舌主要诊察舌体与舌苔两方面的变化。

舌体是全舌的肌肉脉络组织。前人有舌面分部内应脏腑之说。即舌尖多反映上焦心、肺的病变,舌中部多反映中焦脾、胃的病变,舌根部多反映下焦肾的病变,舌两侧多反映肝、胆的病变(见图2)。这种舌面分候脏腑理论具有一定的临床参考价值,但必须结合舌体、舌苔变化综合判断,不可过于拘泥。

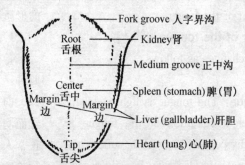

Fig. 2　Correspondence of the tongue to the viscera
图2　舌诊脏腑部位分属图

Inspection of the body of the tongue includes the colour, shape, texture and movement of the tongue, which reflect the conditions of the viscera, qi and blood.

The tongue fur or coating refers to the lichen-like material formed on the surface of the tongue. Inspection of the colour of the tongue and fur can reveal the conditions and nature of pathogenic factors as well as the interaction between healthy qi and pathogenic factors.

### 1.1.3.2 Normal states of the tongue

The conditions of the tongue among healthy people are the normal states of the tongue marked by suitable size, softness, flexibility, light-red colour, luster and moisture; even and whitish thin fur which is neither dry nor greasy and slippery, closely attached to the surface of the tongue, distributed more on the center and root and less on the margins and tip. The normal conditions of the tongue is usually described as "light-reddish tongue with thin and whitish fur" (see colour Fig. 1), suggesting normal functions of the viscera, sufficiency of qi, blood and body fluid as well as superabundance of gastric qi.

### 1.1.3.3 Inspection of the tongue body

The body of the tongue is in close relation with the visceral qi and blood through meridians. By means of inspection, one can understand the conditions of the viscera, qi and blood.

Inspection of the body of the tongue includes the colour, shape and movement of the tongue.

#### 1.1.3.3.1 Colour of the tongue

It includes the four changes as follows:

**Light-reddish tongue**: The tongue is light-reddish, moist and lustrous. Such a condition of the tongue is usually seen among healthy people, suggesting sufficiency of qi and blood. Sometime it is also seen in mild cases,

望舌体包括诊察舌的颜色、形质和动态，主要反映脏腑的虚实、气血的盛衰。

舌苔是舌面上附着的苔状物。望舌苔包括诊察苔质和苔色，主要反映病邪的浅深、性质，以及邪正的消长。

### （二）正常舌象

人体在健康状况下表现的舌象，为正常舌象。正常舌象的特征是舌形不大不小，舌体柔软，活动自如，舌色淡红而荣润；舌苔薄白均匀，不干不燥，不滑不腻，紧贴舌面，中、根部较多，边、尖部较少。常描写为"淡红舌，薄白苔"（见彩图1）。提示脏腑功能正常，气血津液充盈，胃气旺盛。

### （三）望舌体

舌体通过经络与脏腑气血密切联系。因此，通过诊察舌体，可以了解脏腑的虚实、气血的盛衰。

望舌体主要诊察舌色、舌的形质和动态。

**1. 舌色**

舌体颜色的变化有以下四种：

（1）淡红舌：舌体颜色淡红而润泽，称为淡红舌。见于正常人，为气血充盈而调和的征象；亦见于轻病，如外感病

such as primary stage of exogenous disease, mild pathological conditions, or mild internal impairment, indicating that qi, blood, yin, yang and viscera are not involved.

**Light-whitish tongue:** The colour of the tongue is lighter than that in normal condition, more white and less red, or even showing no signs of blood (see colour Fig. 2). Such a condition suggests deficiency of qi and blood or asthenia of yangqi.

Malnutrition of the tongue due to asthenia of qi and blood: The tongue is light-white due to asthenia of qi and blood or asthenia of yangqi which fails to transport blood to nourish the tongue. For example, light-white and thin tongue is due to deficiency of qi and blood; light-white and bulgy tongue is due to asthenia of yangqi.

**Red and deep-red tongue:** The tongue is redder than that in the usual condition (see colour Fig. 3). The deep or dull red tongue is called deep-red tongue (see colour Fig. 4). Red and deep-red tongue both indicates heat syndrome. The redder the tongue, the severer the heat.

Red or deep-red tongue is caused by superabundance of blood in the vessels of the tongue due to hyperactivity of the tongue. Slightly red tongue or reddish margins and tip of the tongue indicates exogenous superficial heat syndrome; reddish tongue tip indicates up-flaming of heart fire; deep-red tongue with fur indicates sthenia-heat syndrome frequently seen at the superabundant heat stage of exogenous disease, or in relative predominant visceral heat in miscellaneous diseases due to internal impairment; deep-red tongue with scanty fur or without fur indicates asthenia-heat syndrome seen at the advanced stage of exogenous febrile disease with consumption of yin fluid or in patients with yin asthenia and superabundance of fire due to internal impairment and chronic disease.

初起,病情轻浅,或内伤轻病,尚未伤及气血阴阳和脏腑。

(2) 淡白舌：舌色较正常舌浅淡,白多红少,甚至全无血色,称为淡白舌(见彩图2)。主气血亏虚或阳气虚弱。

气血亏虚,舌失荣养；或阳气虚弱,无力温运血液上荣于舌,则致舌淡白。如舌淡白而瘦小者,属气血亏虚；舌淡白而胖嫩者,多属阳气虚弱。

(3) 红、绛舌：较正常舌色红,舌呈鲜红色,称为红舌(见彩图3)。较红舌色深或略带暗红色,称为绛舌(见彩图4)。红、绛舌均主热证,舌色愈红提示热势愈甚。

邪热亢盛,致气血沸涌,上壅于舌,脉络充盈则舌红或绛；阴虚水涸,虚火上炎于舌络,亦可致舌红或绛。如舌稍红或仅边尖红,多为外感表热证；舌尖红赤,多为心火上炎。舌红绛而有苔者属实热证,多见于外感病热盛期,或内伤杂病脏腑阳热偏盛的患者；舌红绛少苔或无苔者属虚热证,多见于外感温热病后期,阴液受损,或内伤久病,阴虚火旺的患者。

**Cyanotic and purplish tongue**: The tongue is completely cyanotic or purplish, or cyanotic and purplish or purplish macules on the surface of the tongue (see colour Fig. 5), indicating inhibited circulation of qi and blood.

Cyanotic and purplish tongue is caused either by internal exuberance of yin cold and obstruction of vessels; or by superabundance of pathogenic heat and obstruction of vessels; or by decline of yangqi, weak transportation of blood and inhibited flow of blood; or by failure of the liver to disperse and convey as well as qi stagnation and blood stasis. Light-purplish or dull purplish tongue with moisture is caused by inhibited flow of qi and blood due to yang asthenia and yin exuberance; purplish red or deep-purplish and dry tongue is caused by superabundant heat consuming fluid and stagnation of qi and blood; dull purplish tongue or tongue with purplish macules is caused by internal retention of blood stasis. Besides, cyanotic and purplish tongue is also seen in cases of congenital heart disease or intoxication by drugs or food.

#### 1.1.3.3.2  Shape of tongue

Shape of tongue mainly includes several changes as follows:

**Rough tongue and tender tongue**: Rough tongue is marked by rough or curved texture, dry surface and dull colour; while tender tongue is characterized by fine texture, moistened and lustrous surface, light colour and bulgy appearance.

Inspecting to see whether the tongue is rough or tender is helpful for understanding whether the disease is of asthenia or sthenia. Rough tongue usually indicates sthenia syndrome and heat syndrome due to hyperactivity of yang-heat and consumption of body fluid. Tender tongue

（4）青紫舌：舌见青、紫色，称为青紫舌。可表现为全舌青或紫，或青紫相间，或舌上见紫色斑点（见彩图5），均主气血运行不畅。

青紫舌或因于阴寒内盛，血脉瘀滞；或因于热邪炽盛，血脉壅滞；或因于阳气虚弱，运血无力，血行缓滞；或因于肝失疏泄，气滞血瘀而形成。如舌淡紫或紫暗而湿润者，属阳虚阴盛，气血运行不畅；舌紫红或绛紫而干者，属热盛伤津，气血壅滞；舌色紫暗或舌上有紫色斑点，则为瘀血内阻之征。此外，青紫舌还可见于某些先天性心脏病或药物、食物中毒等。

**2. 舌形**

舌体形质的变化主要有以下几种：

（1）苍老舌与娇嫩舌：舌体纹理粗糙或皱缩，舌面干燥，舌色较暗，形质坚敛苍老，称为苍老舌；舌体纹理细腻，舌面湿润，舌色浅淡，形质浮胖娇嫩，称为娇嫩舌。

诊察舌质的苍老与娇嫩，可以概括得知病证的虚实。苍老舌多主实证、热证。多因阳热亢盛，伤津耗液，致舌体失润而苍老所形成。娇嫩舌

usually signifies asthenia syndrome and cold syndrome due to failure of asthenia yang to transport dampness, or due to qi asthenia and deficiency of yin-essence, which fail to nourish the tongue.

**Bulgy tongue**: The tongue is bigger than usual (see colour Fig. 6), usually indicating internal retention of dampness and phlegm.

Bulgy tongue is caused either by qi asthenia or yang asthenia which fail to warm and transform fluid, leading to stagnation of fluid or accumulation of dampness into phlegm in the tongue collaterals. Light-white and bulgy tongue with moist and slippery fur is due to asthenia of spleen and kidney yang which fails to transform body fluid and leads to internal retention of dampness and phlegm. Light-red or red and bulgy tongue with yellowish greasy fur is usually due to damp-heat in the spleen and stomach.

**Swollen tongue**: Swollen tongue means that the tongue is swollen, usually suggesting sthenia syndrome.

Swollen tongue is either caused by superabundant heat in the heart and spleen, or by mixture of febrile pathogenic factors with alcoholic toxin attacking on the upper, or by intoxication which leads to stagnation of qi and blood in the tongue collaterals. Deep-red and swollen tongue is due to superabundant heat in the heart and spleen. Purplish, dull and swollen tongue is due to alcoholism or intoxication.

**Thin and emaciated tongue**: The tongue is thinner than usual (see colour Fig. 7), indicating asthenia of qi and blood or consumption of yin fluid.

Thin tongue is usually due to asthenia of qi and blood, or consumption of yin fluid and insufficient moisture and nutrition of the tongue. Light-coloured and thin

多主虚证、寒证。多因阳虚不运,水湿内停,舌体被水湿侵淫所形成,或因气虚、阴精亏损,舌失滋养而形成。

(2) 胖大舌:舌体较正常舌胖大,称为胖大舌(见彩图6)。多主水湿、痰饮内停。

胖大舌多因气虚或阳虚,无以温化水液,水湿停滞,或湿聚成痰饮,阻滞舌络而形成。如舌色淡白而胖嫩,舌苔水滑,多属脾肾阳虚,津液不化,水湿、痰饮内停;舌淡红或红而胖大,舌苔黄腻,多属脾胃湿热。

(3) 肿胀舌:舌体肿胀,甚则盈口满嘴,称为肿胀舌。主实证。

肿胀舌或因心脾热盛,或因温热病邪挟酒毒上攻,或因中毒,致气血壅滞于舌络而形成。如舌深红而肿胀,多为心脾热盛;舌紫暗而肿胀,多见于酒毒上攻或中毒。

(4) 瘦薄舌:舌体较正常舌瘦小而薄,称为瘦薄舌(见彩图7)。主气血亏虚,或阴液亏损。

气血亏虚,或阴液亏损,舌失濡润充养,致舌体瘦薄。如舌色浅淡而瘦薄,多为气血

tongue is caused by deficiency of qi and blood; deep-red and thin tongue is caused by exuberant heat consuming yin or by superabundance of fire due to yin asthenia.

**Fissured tongue**: There are various fissures on the tongue (see colour Fig. 8), indicating deficiency of fluid or essence and blood.

Fissured tongue is usually due to consumption of body fluid or asthenia of essence and blood. Deep-red and fissured tongue is due to exuberant heat consuming fluid; light-coloured and fissured tongue is due to asthenia of essence and blood.

However, fissured tongue may be seen in some healthy people, known as congenital fissured tongue. Such a tongue is marked by fine fissures and covered with tongue fur.

**Prickly tongue**: The tongue is covered with reddish prickles (see colour Fig. 9), suggesting superabundance of pathogenic heat.

Prickly tongue is due to superabundance of heat in the viscera, invasion of heat into blood and accumulation of heat in the tongue collaterals. The location of prickles may indicate the location of pathogenic heat. Prickles on the tongue tip indicate hyperactivity of heart fire; prickles on the tongue center indicate superabundance of heat in the stomach and intestines; prickles on the margins indicate exuberance of liver and gallbladder fire. The more the prickles and the deeper the colour, the severer the pathogenic heat.

**Tooth-marked tongue**: The margins of the tongue are printed with tooth marks (see colour Fig. 10), indicating qi asthenia or yang asthenia and internal retention of

亏虚；舌色红绛而瘦薄，则为热盛伤阴或阴虚火旺。

（5）裂纹舌：舌面上出现各种形状的裂纹，称为裂纹舌（见彩图8）。裂纹可深浅不一，多少不等。主阴津或精血亏虚。

阴津耗损，或精血亏虚，致舌体失养，则舌有裂纹。如舌色红绛而裂，多为热盛伤津；舌色淡白而裂，则为精血亏虚。

此外，少数正常人可出现先天性裂纹舌，其裂纹较细，且有舌苔覆盖，此无辨证意义。

（6）芒刺舌：舌体上有红色凸起如刺，抚之棘手，称为芒刺舌（见彩图9）。主邪热亢盛。

脏腑热盛，热入营血，充斥舌络，则致舌生芒刺。根据芒刺所生部位，可分辨邪热所在部位。如舌尖有芒刺，多属心火亢盛；舌中有芒刺，多属胃肠热盛；舌边有芒刺，则为肝胆火盛。芒刺愈多，颜色愈深，提示邪热愈盛。

（7）齿痕舌：舌体边缘有牙齿压迫的痕迹，称为齿痕舌（见彩图10）。主气虚或阳虚，

dampness.

The spleen governs transportation and transformation. The decline of the spleen qi or spleen yang will lead to dysfunction in transportation and transformation as well as internal retention of dampness in the tongue, resulting in bulgy tongue which is squeezed by teeth. That is why tooth-marked tongue and bulgy tongue appear simultaneously.

However, tooth-marked tongue is also seen among some healthy people, characterized by constant existence of slight tooth-marks and no bulging manifestation.

#### 1.1.3.3.3 Movement of the tongue

This mainly includes the examination of the changes of movement of the tongue. Normally the tongue is soft and flexible, indicating sufficiency of qi and blood, normal circulation of vessels and meridians as well as normal functions of the viscera. There are four kinds of different movement of the tongue.

**Stiff tongue**: The tongue is not soft; it is inflexible or stiff and immobile. Such a change of the tongue is usually seen in exogenous diseases due to exuberant heat consuming body fluid, or due to invasion of heat into the pericardium, or due to phlegm and turbid substance confusing the heart. It is also seen in miscellaneous diseases due to internal impairment caused by wind phlegm obstructing the collaterals.

Stiff tongue seen in exogenous diseases is caused either by hyperactivity of pathogenic heat which consumes body fluid and leads to malnutrition of the tongue and inflexibility of the tongue; or by invasion of heat into the pericardium involving the spirit; or by phlegm and turbid substance confusing the heart and affecting the tongue. Stiff tongue seen in miscellaneous diseases due to internal

水湿内停。

脾主运化,脾气或脾阳虚衰,运化失职,水湿内停,阻滞于舌,致舌体胖大,受齿缘挤压而形成齿痕舌。故齿痕舌常与胖嫩舌同见。

此外,少数健康人可出现先天性齿痕舌,其舌体不胖大,有轻微齿痕,且长期存在,不易消失,这无辨证意义。

3. 舌态

主要诊察舌体活动的变化。正常舌态表现为舌体柔软,活动灵便,伸缩自如,提示气血充盛,经脉通调,脏腑功能健旺。常见的舌态变化有以下几种:

(1) 强硬舌:舌体失其柔和,卷伸不利,甚或僵硬强直,不能活动,称为强硬舌。见于外感病,多属热盛伤津,或热入心包,或痰浊蒙闭心窍;见于内伤杂病,则属风痰阻络。

强硬舌见于外感病,或因邪热亢盛,灼伤阴津,致舌脉失养,舌体失其柔和;或因热入心包,扰及神明;或因痰浊蒙闭心窍,致舌失其主而成。见于内伤杂病,多因肝风挟痰,上阻舌络而致。如舌色红

impairment is caused by obstruction of the tongue collaterals due to liver wind complicated by phlegm. Deep-red stiff tongue with scanty fluid is due to exuberant heat consuming body fluid or invasion of heat into the pericardium, frequently seen at the severe heat stage of exogenous diseases. Stiff tongue with greasy and thick fur seen in miscellaneous diseases due to internal impairment is caused by wind-phlegm obstructing collaterals. If the tongue suddenly becomes stiff, accompanied by aphasia, numbness of the limbs and dizziness, it is the premonitory sign of wind stroke.

**Shivering tongue**: The tongue is involuntarily tremoring, indicating endogenous liver wind.

Shivering tongue is caused either by consumption of blood or body fluid which fails to nourish the tendons and vessels; or by extreme heat generating wind due to exuberant heat scorching the liver meridian; or by liver yang transforming into wind. Light-whitish and shivering tongue is due to asthenia of qi and blood and endogenous asthenia-wind, usually seen in internal impairment, chronic diseases and severe diseases; reddish shivering tongue with scanty dry fur is due to consumption of yin fluid, malnutrition of the tendons and vessels and endogenous wind, usually seen at the advanced stage of exogenous febrile diseases; deep-red and shivering tongue is due to extreme heat generating wind, frequently seen at the severe heat stage of exogenous diseases; reddish and shivering tongue is due to liver yang transforming into wind, often seen in miscellaneous diseases due to internal impairment accompanied by headache and dizziness.

**Deviated tongue**: The tongue is deviated to one side (see colour Fig.11), suggesting wind stroke or premonitory sign of wind stroke due to liver wind complicated

绛少津而强硬,属热盛伤津,或热入心包,多见于外感病热盛期。内伤杂病见舌强硬苔厚腻,属风痰阻络,若突然舌强硬,语言謇涩,伴肢体麻木、眩晕欲仆者,多为中风先兆。

(2) 颤动舌:舌体不自主地颤动,称为颤动舌。是肝风内动的表现之一。

血虚或阴液亏损,筋脉失养,或邪热亢盛,热极生风,或肝阳化风,均可致舌体颤动不宁。如舌色淡白而颤动,属气血虚衰,虚风内动,多见于内伤久病、重病患者;舌红少苔而干,舌体颤动,属阴液亏损,筋脉失养,虚风内动,多见于外感温热病后期阶段;舌红绛而颤动,见于外感病热盛期,为热极动风的表现;舌红颤动,见于内伤杂病,伴头痛、眩晕,多为肝阳化风。

(3) 歪斜舌:舌体不正,伸舌时舌体歪向一侧,称为歪斜舌(见彩图11)。是中风或

by phlegm or liver wind complicated by stagnation in the collaterals of the tongue.

**Flaccid tongue**: The tongue is too weak to protrude and withdraw, suggesting extreme consumption of fluid or decline of qi and blood.

Flaccid tongue is caused by extreme consumption of yin fluid, or by decline of qi and blood as well as malnutrition of musculature and vessels of the tongue. Deep-red and flaccid tongue with scanty fur in chronic disease due to internal impairment is due to extreme predominance of fire resulting from yin asthenia; light-whitish and flaccid tongue is due to decline of qi and blood. Reddish dry and flaccid tongue at the advanced stage in exogenous febrile diseases is due to consumption of yin by heat.

**Shrunk tongue**: The tongue is contracted and cannot protrude, or cannot even reach the teeth, usually indicating critical condition. Such a syndrome is either of cold or of heat nature.

Shrunk tongue is caused either by invasion of pathogenic cold; or by stagnation of endogenous cold in the musculature and vessels of the tongue; or by extreme heat consuming fluid and causing spasm of the musculature and vessels; or by stagnation of liver wind with phlegm in the vessels of the tongue. Light-whitish or cyanotic, purplish, moist and shrunk tongue is due to stagnation of cold in the musculature and vessels of the tongue; deep-red, dry and shrunk tongue is due to extreme heat consuming fluid; bulgy and shrunk tongue with greasy fur is due to liver wind complicated by phlegm.

However, congenital short sublingual frenum also prevents the tongue from protruding.

**Protruding and wagging tongue**: The tongue that

中风先兆。由肝风挟痰或挟瘀阻滞舌体经络而致。

（4）痿软舌：舌体软弱，伸缩无力，称为痿软舌。主阴液虚极，或气血虚衰。

阴液虚极，或气血虚衰，舌体筋脉失养，则致舌体痿软。如内伤久病出现舌红绛少苔而痿软，为阴虚火旺已极；舌淡白而痿软，则为气血虚衰。若外感温热病后期，出现舌干红而痿软，为热灼阴伤。

（5）短缩舌：舌体卷缩、紧缩，不能伸出口外，严重者伸舌不能抵齿，称为短缩舌。多为病情危重的征象，其证候性质有寒热之分。

短缩舌，可因寒邪侵袭，或阳虚生寒，凝滞筋脉，致舌脉挛缩；或因热盛伤津，致筋脉拘急；或因肝风挟痰，阻滞舌脉而形成。如舌淡白或青紫、湿润而短缩，属寒凝筋脉；舌红绛、干燥而短缩，属热盛津伤；舌胖大而短缩，苔腻者，则属肝风挟痰所致。

此外，先天性舌下系带过短亦可影响舌体伸出口外，此无辨证意义。

（6）吐弄舌：舌伸出口

protrudes out but is unable to retreat is called protruding tongue; the tongue that frequently protrudes out but immediately draws back or licks the lips or corners of the mouth is called wagging tongue. Both conditions suggest heat in the heart and spleen. In severe cases, protruding tongue indicates invasion of pestilence into the heart or healthy qi on the verge to exhaust. Wagging tongue is the premonitory sign of endogenous wind, also seen in children with maldevelopment of intelligence.

#### 1.1.3.4　Inspection of tongue fur

Normally the tongue fur is caused by fumigation of the gastric qi and moistening of gastric fluid. Morbid tongue fur is caused by upward flow of gastric qi with pathogenic factors. Inspection of the tongue fur is helpful for understanding the location and nature of disease as well as the relation between healthy qi and pathogenic factors. Inspection of the tongue fur includes examination of the nature and colour of the tongue fur.

##### 1.1.3.4.1　Nature of the tongue fur

This includes examination of the thickness, moistness, greasiness, putridity, dryness, exfoliation and root of the tongue fur.

**Thickness**: The standard for examining the thickness of the tongue is whether it is "bottom visible" or "bottom invisible". That means the tongue fur with dimly visible body of the tongue is thin fur, while the tongue fur with invisible body of the tongue is thick fur.

The thickness of the tongue fur reflects the degree and severity of the pathogenic factors as well as the development of disease. Generally speaking, thin tongue fur is seen at the primary stage of exogenous disease, suggesting that the pathogenic factors are superficial and the disease is mild; it is also seen in diseases due to internal

外,不能缩回者,称为吐舌;舌时时稍微伸出口外,立即缩回,或舐唇上下、口角左右,反复转弄者,称为弄舌。两者均属心脾有热。但在病情危重时,吐舌提示疫毒攻心或正气将绝。弄舌多为动风之兆,亦可见于小儿智能发育不良。

#### (四) 望舌苔

正常舌苔由胃气上薰,胃津上潮而生;病苔是胃气挟邪气上泛而成。通过诊察舌苔,可以了解病位的浅深、病邪的性质及邪正的消长。望舌苔主要诊察苔质和苔色。

**1. 苔质**

即舌苔的形质。望苔质主要诊察舌苔的薄厚、润燥、腻腐、剥落及有根与无根等变化。

(1) 薄厚:苔质的薄厚以"见底"和"不见底"为标准,即透过舌苔能隐隐见到舌体的为薄苔,不能见到舌体的为厚苔。

苔的厚薄,反映病邪的深浅、多少及病情的进退。一般地说,薄苔多见于外感病初起,提示病邪在表,病情轻浅;亦见于内伤病正气亏虚,尤其是脾胃虚弱的患者。厚苔则

impairment with deficiency of healthy qi, especially with hypofunction of the spleen and stomach. Thick tongue fur is the sign of exuberance of pathogenic factors, frequently due to internal invasion of exogenous pathogenic factors, or due to internal stagnation of phlegm, dampness and food retention as well as fumigation of gastric qi with turbid substance and pathogenic factors.

During the course of a disease, the change of the tongue fur from thinness to thickness indicates gradual exuberance of pathogenic factors, development of pathogenic factors from the exterior to the interior and progress of pathological conditions from mildness to severity; the change of the tongue fur from thickness to thinness suggests predomination of healthy qi over pathogenic factors, elimination of pathogenic factors internally and externally as well as development of the pathological conditions from severity to mildness.

**Moistening and dryness of tongue fur**: The tongue fur that is moist with moderate dampness is called moist tongue fur. The tongue fur with excessive dampness and slipperiness is called slippery tongue fur. The tongue fur that is dry, without fluid or even fissured is called dry tongue fur. The tongue fur that is dry, rough and sandy is called rough tongue fur.

The moistening and dryness of the tongue fur reflect the conditions and distribution of body fluid. Moist tongue fur indicates sufficiency and upward distribution of body fluid. Slippery tongue fur indicates cold-dampness, or retention of fluid and internal invasion of cold-dampness, or asthenia of yangqi and failure of qi to transform fluid. Dry and rough tongue fur indicates consumption of fluid by exuberant heat or consumption of yin fluid. The drier and rougher the tongue fur, the severer the consumption of

为邪盛于里的征象,多因外感病病邪入里,或因痰湿、食积内阻,胃气挟食浊邪气上蒸所致。

疾病过程中,舌苔由薄渐厚,表示病邪渐盛,由表入里,病情由轻转重,为病进;舌苔由厚渐薄,则表示正气胜邪,邪气得以内消外达,病情由重转轻,为病退。

(2)润燥:根据苔的润燥,可分为以下几种:舌苔润泽,干湿适度,称为润苔。舌面水分过多,扪之湿滑,伸舌欲滴,称为滑苔。舌苔干燥,扪之无津,甚则舌苔干裂,称为燥苔。苔质干燥、粗糙如砂石,扪之糙手,称为糙苔。

苔的润燥,反映津液的盈亏和输布情况。润苔表示津液充盈而上承。滑苔为寒湿,或水饮内停,寒湿内侵,或阳气虚衰,气不化津而致。燥苔、糙苔均为热盛伤津,或阴液亏耗。干燥、粗糙的程度愈甚,提示津伤液耗的程度愈重。多见于外感温热病的中、

body fluid. Such a condition is usually seen at the medium and advanced stages of exogenous febrile diseases. Besides, internal stagnation of pathogenic dampness, obstruction of yangqi or asthenia of yangqi and failure of qi to transform fluid may also lead to dry tongue fur, the manifestation of which is light-whitish tongue accompanied by chest oppression and dry mouth without desire to drink.

During the course of a disease, the change of the tongue fur from moisture to dryness indicates consumption of body fluid and severity of heat; while the change of tongue fur from dryness to moisture suggests abatement of pathogenic heat and gradual restoration of body fluid.

**Greasy and putrid tongue fur:** Tongue fur compact and difficult to exfoliate which is thick on the center and thin on the margins is called greasy tongue fur (see colour Fig. 12). While the tongue fur loose, sparse and easy to exfoliate with thickness on both the center and margins is called putrid tongue fur.

The greasiness and putridity of the tongue fur reflect the decline and development of yangqi and turbid dampness. Greasy tongue fur is usually caused by internal exuberance of dampness and obstruction of yangqi, often seen in syndromes due to dampness, phlegm, retention of food and damp-febrile factors. Putrid tongue fur is usually caused by fumigation of excess of yang-heat, often seen in syndromes due to retention of food in the stomach and intestines or accumulation of phlegm and turbid substance.

**Exfoliating tongue fur:** Exfoliating tongue fur means that the fur on the tongue has exfoliated partially or completely during the course of a disease. Partial exfoliation of tongue fur is divided into anterior exfoliated tongue fur, medium exfoliated tongue fur and patched exfoliated tongue fur (see colour Fig. 13). If the tongue fur is completely exfoliated, it is called mirror-like tongue.

后期阶段。此外，若湿邪内郁，阻遏阳气，或阳气亏虚，气不化津上承，亦可致舌苔较为干燥，其多表现为舌质淡白，并伴胸闷、口干不欲饮等症。

疾病过程中，舌苔由润转燥，表示津液已伤，热势加重；舌苔由燥转润，则表示热邪渐退，津液渐复。

（3）腻腐：苔质颗粒细腻而致密，边薄中厚，紧贴舌面，刮之不易脱落，称为腻苔（见彩图12）；苔质颗粒较大而疏松，边中皆厚，刮之易脱，称为腐苔。

苔的腻腐，反映阳气与湿浊的消长。腻苔多因湿浊内盛，阳气被遏所致，多见于湿浊、痰饮、食积内停及湿温等病证。腐苔多因阳热有余，蒸腾腐浊之气上泛而成，故多见于食积胃肠，或痰浊内蕴的病证。

（4）剥落：舌面本有苔，病程中舌苔部分或全部剥落，称为剥落苔。部分舌苔剥落者，根据舌苔剥落部位的不同，可分为前剥苔、中剥苔和花剥苔（见彩图13）。若舌苔全部剥落，舌面光洁如镜，称

Exfoliation of the tongue fur is usually due to failure of deficient gastric qi to fumigate the tongue or due to failure of the exhausted gastric yin to moisten the tongue. Therefore the exfoliation of the tongue fur can tell whether the gastric qi and yin still exist or not and how the prognosis of a disease will be. Exfoliated tongue fur and deep-red tongue indicate consumption of yin by exuberant heat; exfoliated tongue fur and light-coloured tongue indicate consumption of both qi and yin; mirror-like tongue suggests severe consumption of gastric qi and is a sign of the exhaustion of gastric yin. If the tongue fur is patched and greasy, it suggests that phlegm is not resolved, healthy qi is consumed and the pathological conditions are complicated. During the course of a disease, if the tongue fur is completely exfoliated, it means insufficiency of gastric qi and yin, gradual decline of healthy qi and gradual worsening of the pathological conditions; if the tongue fur reappears thin and white after exfoliation, it indicates gradual restoration of gastric qi and favourable recovery from the disease.

The tongue fur with or without root: The tongue fur with root means that the fur is closely attached to the surface of the tongue and is not easy to exfoliate. It is also called real tongue fur. The tongue fur without root means that the tongue fur appears floating or painted on the tongue and is easy to exfoliate. It is also called false tongue fur.

**The tongue fur with root is formed by accumulation of gastric qi with turbid pathogenic factors on the tongue**; the tongue fur without root is due to failure of gastric qi too exhausted to produce new fur and inability of the original fur to continue on the tongue. Inspecting whether the tongue fur is with or without fur is helpful for

为镜面舌。

剥落苔均因胃气匮乏,不能上薰于舌,或胃阴枯涸,不能上潮于舌而成。因此,苔的剥落,反映胃气、胃阴的存亡,并可据此推测疾病的预后。如舌苔剥落,舌红绛而干,为热盛伤阴;舌苔剥落而舌淡者,为气阴两伤;镜面舌则为胃气大伤,胃阴枯涸之重证的征象。若苔花剥而兼有腻苔,则提示痰浊未化,正气已伤,病情较为复杂。

疾病过程中,舌苔从全至剥,表示胃气、胃阴不足,正气渐衰,病情渐重;若舌苔剥落后,复生薄白苔,表示胃气渐复,疾病向愈。

(5) 有根苔与无根苔:舌苔坚敛着实,紧贴舌面,刮之不易脱去,即为有根苔,又称真苔。舌苔不着实,似浮涂于舌上,刮之易去,即为无根苔,又称假苔。

understanding whether gastric qi still exists or not and whether the pathogenic factors are exuberating or declining. Such an understanding enables one to know whether the disease is serious or not and whether the prognosis is favourable or unfavourable. The tongue fur with root at the primary and medium stages of a disease indicates that pathogenic factors are in predomination but the healthy qi is still vigorous enough to resist pathogenic factors and that the prognosis is favourable. The appearance of tongue fur with root at the advanced stage or in chronic disease suggests that gastric qi is still in predomination or gradually restores, signifying favourable prognosis. If the tongue fur without root appears in such a case, it indicates deficiency of gastric qi, decline of healthy qi, severity of pathological conditions and unfavourable prognosis.

#### 1.1.3.4.2 The colours of tongue fur

The colours of tongue fur commonly seen are white, yellow and grayish black which may appear singularly or simultaneously. The examination of the colours of tongue fur should be done together with the analysis of the texture, colour and shape of the tongue proper.

**White tongue fur**: Apart from normal tongue fur, white tongue fur is usually seen in external syndrome and cold syndrome. But white tongue fur is not only confined to external syndrome and cold syndromes.

Thin and white tongue fur is often seen at the primary stage of exogenous disease and diseases due to internal impairment without fever. At the primary stage of exogenous diseases, pathogenic factors attack the superficies but have not invaded the interior, the tongue fur does not have obvious changes. That is why thin and white tongue fur indicates external syndrome. Light-red tongue with thin, white and moist tongue fur indicates wind-cold external syndrome; tongue with reddish margins and tip as well as thin, white and moistless fur indicates wind-heat external syndrome. Light-white tongue with thin and white fur is usually seen in internal asthenia-cold syndrome.

Whitish greasy tongue fur is usually due to internal retention of damp turbid substance, phlegm and fluid or due to food retention without transforming into heat (see colour Fig. 14). Powder-like thick and white tongue fur that does not feel dry is called powder tongue fur, frequently caused by mixture of exogenous fetid pathogenic factors and heat toxin, usually seen in pestilence and internal abscess.

**Yellow tongue fur:** Yellow tongue fur usually indicates internal syndrome and heat syndrome.

During the course of a disease, the change of tongue fur from white to yellow suggests that the pathogenic factors have transformed into heat and transmitted to the interior. The yellower the tongue fur, the severer the pathogenic factors. Light-yellow tongue fur indicates mild heat, deep-yellow tongue fur signifies severe heat and sallow tongue fur suggests extreme heat. That is why yellow tongue fur usually appears simultaneously with red and deep-red tongue (see colour Fig. 15).

Thin and yellow tongue fur indicates mild pathogenic heat, usually seen in wind-heat external syndrome, or inward invasion of heat transformed from wind-cold, or mild heat progress in internal heat syndrome. Yellow and white tongue fur suggests that the pathogenic factors are transmitted from the exterior to the interior and cold transforms into heat in exogenous disease. Yellow and greasy tongue fur is usually due to accumulation of damp-heat, or due to phlegm and fluid retention transforming into heat, or due to food retention and heat putrefaction. Yellow and

寒证。

苔白腻，多属湿浊、痰饮内停，或食积尚未化热（见彩图14）。苔白厚如积粉，扪之不燥，称为积粉苔，多因外感秽浊湿邪与热毒相结而致，多见于瘟疫或内痈。

（2）黄苔：苔见黄色，称为黄苔。多主里证、热证。

疾病过程中，白苔转黄，提示邪已化热入里，一般说，苔色愈黄，提示邪热愈甚。淡黄为热轻，深黄为热重，焦黄为热极。故黄苔常与红、绛舌同见（见彩图15）。

薄黄苔，为邪热未甚，多见于风热表证，或风寒化热初入里，或里热证热势尚轻。黄白相兼苔，提示外感病正处于病邪由表入里、由寒化热的过程中。黄腻苔，多为湿热蕴结，或痰饮化热，或食积热腐。黄糙苔，多为邪热伤津，或肠腑热结之证。但若苔黄滑润，舌质淡白胖嫩者，则为阳气虚

rough tongue fur is often caused by pathogenic heat consuming body fluid or by retention of heat in the intestines. But if the tongue fur is yellow, slippery and moist and the tongue is light-white and bulgy, it is due to decline of yangqi and failure of dampness and water to transform.

**Grayish black tongue fur:** Grayish black tongue fur suggests severity of internal heat syndrome or internal cold syndrome. The moisture and dryness of the tongue texture are the evidences to differentiate the nature of cold and heat (see colour Fig. 16 and 17).

Grayish tongue fur is light-black tongue fur. So grayish tongue fur and blackish tongue fur are the same. The colour of the tongue fur corresponds to the degree of the pathological conditions. The deeper the tongue fur colour, the severer the pathological conditions. Grayish black tongue fur in cold syndrome usually develops from white tongue fur. For example, grayish black and moist tongue fur with light-white tongue signifies yang asthenia and cold exuberance, or cold dampness and internal retention of phlegm and fluid. Grayish black tongue fur in heat syndrome evolves from sallow tongue fur. For instance, grayish black and dry fur with deep-red tongue or even prickly tongue is due to extreme heat consuming fluid.

### 1.1.3.5 Comprehensive analysis of the body of the tongue and tongue fur

Disease is a complicated course. The changes of the tongue and the tongue fur are the reflections of the complicated pathological conditions of the body. These changes reflect different aspects of the disease in question. As mentioned before, the body of the tongue mainly reflects the conditions of the viscera, qi and blood; the tongue fur mainly indicates the degree and nature of the disease and the relation between the pathogenic factors and healthy qi. So after fully understanding the common changes of

衰,水湿不化而致。

（3）灰黑苔：苔见灰黑,称为灰黑苔。主里热或里寒证的重证。其苔质润燥是辨别寒热性质的依据（见彩图16、17）。

灰苔为浅黑苔,故灰黑苔为同类。苔色浅深与疾病程度相应,即苔色愈深,提示病情愈重。寒证的灰黑苔常由白苔发展转化而成,如苔灰黑而湿润,舌淡白,为阳虚寒盛,或寒湿、痰饮内停。热证的灰黑苔常由焦黄苔发展转化而成,如苔灰黑而干燥,舌红绛,甚则生芒刺,为热极津伤。

### （五）舌体与舌苔的综合分析

疾病是一个复杂的过程,舌体与舌苔的变化都是机体复杂病变的反映,但它们是从不同的侧面反映疾病的情况。如前所述,舌体主要反映脏腑的虚实、气血的盛衰;舌苔主要反映病邪的浅深、性质和邪正的消长。因此,在分别掌握舌体、舌苔的常见变化及其主

the body of the tongue and the tongue fur and their indications, we have to further understand the relation between the body of the tongue and the tongue fur and make comprehensive analysis of the changes of the body of the tongue and the tongue fur.

Usually the changes of the body of the tongue and the tongue fur are the same, and so is their pathogenesis and indications. For example, the tongue is red and the tongue fur is yellow and dry in sthenia-heat syndrome; the tongue appears light-white and the tongue fur appears white and moist in asthenia-cold syndrome. But sometimes the changes of the tongue and the tongue fur are different. In such a case, comprehensive analysis should be made of the causes, pathogenesis and the interrelation. For example, if the tongue is light-white and the tongue fur is yellow and greasy, light-white tongue indicates deficiency of qi and blood, while yellow and greasy tongue fur suggests internal accumulation of damp-heat. Comprehensive analysis shows that such changes of the tongue and the tongue fur suggests asthenia-sthenia complex syndrome due to deficiency of qi and blood complicated by exogenous damp-heat attack. For instance, if the tongue is deep-red and the tongue fur is white and greasy, deep-red tongue indicates exuberance of internal heat or yin asthenia and fire superabundance, while white and greasy tongue fur suggests internal exuberance of phlegm-dampness or internal retention of food. In exogenous febrile disease, such an analysis indicates heat in the nutrient phase and dampness in the qi phase; in miscellaneous diseases due to internal impairment, it suggests frequent yin asthenia and fire exuberance accompanied by phlegm-dampness or retention of food. The above analysis shows that difference of changes in the tongue and the tongue fur usually suggests two or more pathological changes in the

病的同时，还应注意舌体与舌苔之间的相互关系，并将舌体与舌苔的变化进行综合分析。

一般情况下，舌体与舌苔的变化是一致的，其病机相同，主病一致。如：实热证出现舌体红，苔黄而干；虚寒证出现舌体淡白，舌苔白润。但是，也有舌体与舌苔变化不一致的情况，则应综合分析其病因、病机及其相互关系。如：舌淡白苔黄腻，舌淡白提示气血亏虚；苔黄腻，为湿热内蕴。综合分析可知，此属气血亏虚而又感受湿热之邪的虚实夹杂证。又如：舌红绛苔白腻，舌红绛为内热炽盛或阴虚火旺；苔白腻为痰湿内盛或食积内阻。因此，在外感温热病，提示营分有热，气分有湿；在内伤杂病，提示素体阴虚火旺，又兼痰湿，或饮食积滞。由此可知，当舌体与舌苔变化不一致时，往往提示病体同时存在两种或两种以上的病理变化，病情较为复杂，其辨证意义为两者的综合。

body. Syndrome differentiation of such a complicated case should be careful analysis of both aspects of pathological changes.

## 1.2 Listening and olfaction

Listening and olfaction means listening to various sounds and noises made by the patient and smelling the odor and excreta from the body of the patient so as to understand the pathological conditions of the patient. Since various sounds and noises as well as odor all come from the activities of the viscera, listening to sounds and smelling odors are helpful for examining the morbid conditions of the viscera.

### 1.2.1 Listening to sounds

Voice is produced by vibration of air in the cavity and tube organs. The voice made in the mouth is in close relation to the lung, throat, epiglottis, tongue, teeth, lips and nose. All kinds of voice (sounds) are made by means of the activities of the lung and the lung governs qi and respiration. That is why the ancient people believed that "the lung is the governor of qi and the kidney is the root of qi", "the lung is the door of voice" and "the kidney is the root of voice". Since the pathological changes of the other viscera may affect the functions of the lung and the kidney in producing sounds and because the other viscera are under the domination of the heart spirit, listening to sounds not only can examine the conditions of the organs directly related to voice, but also further diagnose visceral disease according to the changes of voice (sounds).

## 第二节 闻诊

闻诊是通过听取患者发出的各种声音和嗅察患者身体及其排出物散发出的气味以了解病情的诊察方法。因为各种声音和气味都产生于脏腑活动,所以通过听声音和嗅气味,可以诊察脏腑的病变。

### 一、听声音

声音是由体内的气流通过空腔、管道器官产生振动而发出,从口发出的声音直接与肺及喉、会厌、舌、齿、唇、鼻等器官有关。又因各种声音的发出,主要是气的活动,而肺主气、司呼吸,肾主纳气,故前人有"肺为气之主,肾为气之根","肺为声音之门","肾为声音之根"等说法。此外,由于其他脏腑的病变亦可以影响肺、肾的功能而引起声音的变化,而各脏腑功能均受心神的主宰,因此,通过听声音不仅可以诊察与发音直接有关器官的病变,而且还可根据声音的变化,进一步诊察内脏的病变。

## 1.2.1.1 Speech

In listening to speech, cares should be made to detect whether the speech is strong or weak, whether the words are coherent and whether the expression is clear and fluent. The speech of normal people is natural in pronunciation, smooth in tone, clear in expression and consistent in words. Since the viscera, constitution and physical building are different from person to person, the voice is either high or low, loud or small and clear or full. For example, male voice is low and full, female voice is high and clear, children's voice is sharp and melodious, and voice of the aged is low and deep. Generally speaking, high and sonorous voice in healthy people is a manifestation of sufficiency of primordial qi and pulmonary qi.

There is close relation between speech and emotions. For example, the voice in joy is lively and cheerful, the voice in rage is stern and quick, the voice in sorrow is sad and disjointed. These are the normal changes of voice.

### 1.2.1.1.1 Voice

The abnormal changes of voice are either strong or weak, heavy or deep, hoarseness or aphonia.

**Strong and weak voice:** Generally speaking, sonorous voice with restlessness and polylogia indicates sthenia syndrome and heat syndrome; low, weak and disjointed voice with quietness and oligologia indicates asthenia syndrome and cold syndrome.

**Deep and heavy voice:** Deep and heavy voice is usually caused by failure of pulmonary qi to disperse and obstruction of the nose due to exogenous pathogenic wind, cold and dampness, or by obstruction of the airway due to stagnation of dampness.

**Hoarseness and aphonia:** Hoarseness means harsh-voice, while aphonia means complete loss of voice.

## （一）语言

听语言,应注意语声的强弱、语言内容是否言与意符、语言是否清晰流利。正常人的语言,具有发音自然,音调和畅,言语清楚流利,言与意符等特点。但是,由于各人的脏腑、形质、禀赋有所差异,故正常的声音也有大小、高低、清浊的不同。如男性多声低而浊,女性多声高而清,儿童则声尖清脆,老人则声浑厚低沉。一般认为,正常人声音高亢洪亮,是元气和肺气充沛的表现。

语言与情志的变化也有密切关系。如喜时发声欢悦而和畅,怒时发声忿厉而急疾,悲哀时则声悲而断续,这些一般均属正常范围。

### 1. 语声

语声的异常,主要有强弱、重浊、音哑和失音等变化。

（1）语声强弱:一般来说,患者语声高亢有力,烦躁多言,多属实证、热证;语声低微,声音断续,静而少言,多属虚证、寒证。

（2）语声重浊:语声重浊多由外感风、寒、湿邪,致使肺气不宣,鼻窍不利,或湿浊阻滞,气道不畅所致。

（3）音哑和失音:音哑,是指语声嘶哑;失音,是指完

Hoarseness is similar to aphonia in pathogenesis. If hoarseness is very serious, it will develop into aphonia. Hoarseness or aphonia in new disease pertains to sthenia syndrome due to exogenous pathogenic factors attacking on the lung or due to failure of the pulmonary qi to disperse resulting from stagnation of phlegm. Such a pathological condition is known as "a solid bell cannot ring (dysphonia or hoarseness due to sthenia syndrome of the lung)". Hoarseness or aphonia in a chronic disease pertains to asthenia syndrome due to exhaustion of fluid and impairment of the lung caused by asthenia of lung and kidney yin and asthenia-fire scorching metal (lung). Such a pathological condition is known as "a broken bell cannot ring (hoarseness due to impaired function of the lung)". Hoarseness or aphonia may be caused by prolonged speaking or singing or shouting with rage, which impairs both qi and yin and deprives the throat of moisture. Hoarseness at the advanced stage of pregnancy is due to pressure of the fetus on the uterine collaterals which obstructs the kidney meridian and prevents kidney essence to be transported to the upper. It will heal automatically after delivery.

#### 1.2.1.1.2 Paraphasia

**Delirium**: Delirium means raving with high and sonorous voice in coma. Such a morbid condition pertains to sthenia syndrome due to heat disturbing the mind seen in invasion of pathogenic factors into the pericardium in seasonal febrile disease or sthenia syndrome of yangming fu-organ.

**Fading murmuring**: Fading murmuring is marked by unconsciousness, repeated and incoherent murmuring in a low voice. It is caused by excessive consumption of heart qi and is an asthenia syndrome of mental derangement, usually seen in patients with chronic and prolonged diseases.

**Soliloquy**: Soliloquy is marked by mental depres-

全发不出音。声音嘶哑与失音的病因病机基本相同，失音为声音嘶哑之甚。新病音哑或失音，属实证，多是外邪袭肺，或痰浊壅滞，以致肺气不宣，即所谓"金实不鸣"。久病音哑或失音，多属虚证，常是肺肾阴虚，虚火灼金，以致津枯肺损，声音难出，即所谓"金破不鸣"。长时说唱或暴怒叫喊，致使气阴两伤，咽喉失润，也可导致音哑或失音。妊娠末期出现声音嘶哑，是由于胎体增大，胞脉受压，使肾脉不通，肾之精气不能上承所致，分娩后则可自愈。

### 2. 语言错乱

言为心声，语言错乱多属心神病变。

（1）谵语：神志昏迷，胡言乱语，声高有力，称为谵语。多属热扰心神之实证，可见于温病邪入心包或阳明腑实证。

（2）郑声：神志不清，语言重复，时断时续，声音低弱，称为郑声。属于心气大伤，精神散乱的虚证，多见于久病、重病患者。

（3）独语：情志抑郁，自

sion, talking to oneself, murmuring and incoherent speech, usually caused by coagulation of phlegm confusing the mind or by severe impairment of heart qi. Such a morbid condition is usually seen in epilepsy.

**Raving:** Raving is marked by manic movement, shouting and sonorous voice usually due to phlegm fire attacking the heart.

**Paraphasia:** Paraphasia means that the patient speaks nonsense in consciousness and is aware of it afterwards. Such a morbid state is often due to insufficiency of heart qi and malnutrition of the spirit. Such a morbid condition is often seen among patients with chronic disease or of the aged.

### 1.2.1.1.3 Slurred speech

Slurred speech is marked by unclear and slow expression without fluency, usually seen in wind stroke or sequela of wind stroke. It is due to obstruction of the collaterals by wind-phlegm and malnutrition of the tongue musculature and vessels, which make the tongue inflexible. Slurred speech at the advanced stage of febrile disease is due to heat consuming yin and malnutrition of the tongue.

### 1.2.1.2 Respiration

The lung governs qi and respiration, while the kidney governs the reception of qi. So the disorders of respiration are usually due to the pathological changes of the lung and kidney. The following is a brief description of the abnormal changes in respiration.

### 1.2.1.2.1 Rapid and weak respiration

Generally speaking, the disease with acute onset and rapid breath and high voice pertains to heat syndrome and sthenia syndrome; the disease with long duration, weak breath and shortness of breath in movement pertains to asthenia syndrome and cold syndrome.

言自语,喃喃不休,语无伦次,见人则止,称为独语。多属痰气凝结,蒙蔽心神,或心气大伤所致,多见于癫病。

(4) 狂言:狂躁妄动,骂詈号叫,声高有力,称为狂言。多见于痰火扰心的狂病。

(5) 错语:患者神志清醒而语言错乱,言后自知说错,称为错语。多因心气不足,神失所养而致,多见于久病或老年人。

### 3. 语言謇涩

说话不流利,含糊不清,缓慢涩滞,称为语言謇涩。多见于中风或中风后遗症,是风痰阻络,舌体筋脉失于濡养,致舌失柔软和灵动。若见于热病后期,是热灼阴伤,舌体失养所致。

### (二) 呼吸

肺主气、司呼吸,肾主纳气。故呼吸异常多见于肺、肾的病变。呼吸异常常见以下几种:

### 1. 气粗与气微

一般来说,发病急,呼吸气粗声高,多属热证、实证;病程长,呼吸气微,动则气短,多属虚证、寒证。

#### 1.2.1.2.2 Dyspnea and bronchial wheezing

Dyspnea refers to difficulty in breath, shortness and rapidity in breath, or even opening the mouth, raising the shoulders and flapping the nose wings in breathing as well as inability to lie flat. Dyspnea is either of asthenia or sthenia nature. Sthenia-dyspnea is marked by rapidity, deep breath and quick exhalation, usually due to sthenia pathogenic factors in the lung and inhibited flow of qi; asthenia-dyspnea is marked by slow and weak breath, less inhalation and more exhalation, discontinued breath, dyspnea in movement and preference for deep breath, usually caused by asthenia-impairment of the lung and kidney as well as insufficient reception of qi.

Bronchial wheezing is marked by rapid breath like dyspnea, stridor in the throat, repeated relapse and difficulty in cure, usually caused by internal retention of phlegm complicated by exogenous pathogenic factors' attacks which stirs up the latent retention of fluid; or by excessive intake of sour, salty, uncooked and cold food.

Clinically dyspnea is not necessarily to occur together with wheezing. Simultaneous appearance of dyspnea and wheezing is called asthma.

#### 1.2.1.2.3 Shortness of breath and weak breath

Shortness of breath means that the breath is not continuous like dyspnea and that the patient raises the shoulders when breathing. Usually there is no sputum. Such a morbid condition is usually seen in various diseases of asthenia or sthenia nature. The asthenia syndrome is marked by shortness of breath and low voice, usually accompanied by dispiritedness, lassitude and spontaneous sweating due to weakness and chronic disease which consumes primordial qi and thoracic qi; sthenia syndrome is marked by shortness of

2. 喘与哮

喘,是指呼吸困难,短促急迫,甚者张口抬肩,鼻翼煽动,不能平卧。喘有虚实之分,实喘发作急骤,气粗声高息涌,惟以呼出为快,多属肺有实邪,气机不利;虚喘发病徐缓,喘声低微,吸少呼多,息短不续,动则喘甚,但得引长一息为快,是肺肾虚损,气失摄纳所致。

哮,呼吸急促似喘,喉中有哮鸣音,称为哮。多反复发作,缠绵难愈。多因内有痰饮,复感外邪,引动伏饮而发,亦可因过食酸咸生冷食物而诱发。

临床上喘不一定兼哮,但哮多兼喘,哮、喘同时出现,称为哮喘。

3. 短气与少气

短气,指呼吸短促而不相接续,气短不足以息,似喘而不抬肩,气急而无痰声。可见于多种疾病,证有虚实之分。虚证以气短声低息微为特征,常伴神疲乏力、自汗等症,多因体弱、久病,元气耗损,宗气不足所致;实证以气短声粗为特征,常伴胸闷、咳嗽喘息等症,多因痰饮停滞,气机不利

breath and hoarseness of voice accompanied by chest oppression, cough and dyspnea due to stagnation of phlegm and retention of fluid as well as inhibited flow of qi.

Weak breath is marked by feeble and short breath and low voice. It is not discontinuous like the manifestation in shortness of breath. Weak breath is usually due to insufficiency of visceral qi, especially asthenia of lung and kidney qi.

Besides, This conditions is accompanied by sighs due to chest oppression and depression resulting from emotional upsets and depression of liver qi.

### 1.2.1.3　Cough

Cough is due to failure of the lung to disperse and descend and upward adverse flow of pulmonary qi, usually seen in lung disorders. Cough may be caused by the disorders of other viscera. Cough is usually related to sputum. So in diagnosis, cares should be taken to analyze the characteristics of voice in cough, understand the time and duration of cough and differentiate the syndromes in the light of the colour, nature and quantity of sputum as well as other complications.

Deep cough with whitish thin sputum and nasal obstruction is usually due to wind-cold attacking the lung, or due to retention of pathogenic cold in the lung which prevents the lung from normal dispersing and descending. Low cough with profuse whitish sputum easy to expectorate accompanied by chest oppression and epigastric fullness is often due to stagnation of phlegm and dampness in the lung which stop the lung from normal dispersing and descending. Low cough with yellowish thick sputum easy to expectorate accompanied by dry pain of throat and hot sensation in the nose in breathing is due to invasion of pathogenic heat into the lung which consumes pulmonary fluid and inhibits flow of pulmonary qi. Dry cough without sputum or with scanty and sticky sputum and dry throat is due to invasion of pathogenic dryness into the lung or due to deficiency of pulmonary yin, consumption of pulmonary fluid and failure of the lung to depurate and clear. Weak cough accompanied by shortness of breath or dyspnea is due to lung asthenia or due to consumption of pulmonary qi in chronic diseases.

Besides, cough like barking of a dog accompanied by hoarseness usually indicates diphtheria due to asthenia of lung and kidney yin, pestilent factors attacking the throat and obstruction of the airway. Infantile paroxysmal and continuous cough like the crying of an egret in the end is called "whooping cough" or pertussis, usually caused by mixture of pathogenic wind with latent phlegm which transforms into heat and obstructs the airway.

### 1.2.1.4 Hiccup and belching

Hiccup and belching are all caused by upward adverse flow of gastric qi.

#### 1.2.1.4.1 Hiccup

Hiccup is marked by upward rise of qi and involuntary gurgling noise in the throat. Syndrome differentiation of hiccup is done according to the hiccup sounds, duration and other complications.

Repeated hiccup with sonorous voice is due to retention of pathogenic heat in the stomach. Deep, long and weak hiccup is due to weakness of the spleen and stomach. Sonorous hiccup with normal sounds, short duration and no other complications is due to urgency in eating or due to postcibal attack by wind-cold. This kind of hiccup is regarded as normal. Sudden hiccup with weak voice and long intermittence in chronic diseases or serious diseases indicates decline of gastric qi and worsening of pathological

清肃所致。咳声低微无力，兼气短或喘，多属肺虚，因久病肺气虚损所致。

此外，咳声如犬吠，常兼音哑，多为白喉，因肺肾阴虚，疫毒攻喉，闭塞气道所致。小儿咳嗽阵作，连声不绝，终止时作鹭鸶叫声，称"顿咳"，也称"百日咳"，多因风邪与伏痰搏结，郁而化热，阻遏气道所致。

### （四）呃逆与嗳气

呃逆与嗳气都由于胃气上逆所导致。

#### 1. 呃逆

呃逆，表现为气逆上冲，致咽喉部呃呃有声，不能自制。根据呃声的高低、间歇时间的长短及其兼症的不同进行辨证。

呃声频频，连续不断，声高有力，多是邪热客胃所致。呃声低沉而长，气弱无力，是脾虚胃弱所致。呃声清亮，不高不低，持续时间短暂，无其他兼症，多因咽食匆促，或食后偶感风寒所致，不属病态。久病、重病，突然出现呃逆，其声低弱，良久一声，是胃气衰

conditions.

#### 1.2.1.4.2 Belching

Belching refers to deep, long and slow noise made in the throat due to upward rise of qi from the stomach. Syndrome differentiation of belching should be made according to whether the voice is high or low, whether there is acid and putrid odor and whether there are other complications.

Sonorous belching with acid and putrid odor accompanied by unpressable epigastric and abdominal distending pain as well as thick and greasy tongue fur is due to retention of food in the stomach. Repeated sonorous belching accompanied hypochondriac and epigastric pain and taut pulse to be alleviated after belching is due to emotional upsets caused by invasion of liver qi into the stomach. Belching with deep voice and acid-putrid odor accompanied by no taste for food, light-coloured tongue and weak pulse is due to weakness of the spleen and stomach, usually seen in chronic diseases or the aged. Occasional belching after meal is usually due to overeating and is not morbid.

### 1.2.2 Olfaction

Normally there is no abnormal odor in the healthy people whose visceral functions are normal and circulation of blood and qi is smooth. Under pathological conditions, the visceral functions are affected, qi, blood and body fluid are encumbered and fumigated by pathogenic factors, or the transportation and transformation of food and water become abnormal, giving rise to the production of strange odor. So smelling the patient's body and the excreta is helpful for understanding the pathological changes.

Attention should be paid to different odors so as to understand their nature. Generally speaking, slight stinking odor or odor without foul smell indicates asthenia

败,病情转危之兆。

2. 嗳气

嗳气,是气从胃中上逆,致咽喉部发出沉长而缓的声音。闻诊时应根据嗳气声之高低、有无酸腐气及其兼症之不同进行辨证。

嗳气声响,有酸腐气味,伴脘腹胀痛拒按,苔厚腻,为食滞胃脘而成。嗳气频作,其声响亮,每与情志不舒有关,伴胁胀脘痛,脉弦,嗳气后胁胀脘痛减轻,乃肝气犯胃所致。嗳气声低沉,无酸腐气味,伴纳谷不馨,舌淡脉弱,为脾胃虚弱所致,多见于久病或老人。饮食之后,偶有嗳气,多因饮食过饱所致,不属病态。

### 二、嗅气味

正常人脏腑功能正常,气血流畅,不产生异常气味。患病后,脏腑功能失调,气血津液为病邪困扰、薰蒸,或水谷运化失常,则可产生异常气味。因此,通过嗅察病体及其排出物的气味,可以了解疾病的情况。

嗅气味需注意嗅察气味的不同种类,以辨别病证的不同性质。一般来说,气味微腥

syndrome, cold syndrome or cold-dampness syndrome. Heavy stinking or foul odor indicates sthenia syndrome, heat syndrome or dampness syndrome. Sour and putrid odor usually suggests retention of food. Blood smell suggests bleeding disease. Putrid odor suggests ulceration and sore.

In differentiating odors, attention should be paid to examine the source of odors so as to decide the location of the disease. And syndrome differentiation should be made in the light of the difference in odors.

### 1.2.2.1 Smelling body odor
#### 1.2.2.1.1 Foul breath
Foul breath is seen in oral diseases, such as caries. Foul breath is usually due to stomach heat. Sour odor from the mouth indicates retention of food; putrid odor from the mouth suggests internal abscess.

#### 1.2.2.1.2 Sputum and snivel odor
Stinking and foul sputum with pus and blood is usually seen in exuberance of heat toxin or accumulation of heat toxin into lung abscess. Odorless thin sputum and snivel are usually seen in exogenous disease due to windcold. Frequent discharge of foul and thick snivel suggests nasosinusitis due to lung heat or damp-heat in the gallbladder meridian.

#### 1.2.2.1.3 Body odor
Foul and putrid body odor suggests ulceration and sore. Bromhidrosis is due to fumigation by damp-heat.

#### 1.2.2.1.4 Odor of feces and urine
Clear urine without stinking odor indicates asthenia and cold syndrome, also seen among healthy people. Scanty reddish and stinking urine indicates

或无臭，多属虚证、寒证，或寒湿；气味浊腥或臭秽，多属实证、热证，或湿热；气味酸腐、馊臭，常因宿食停积所致；嗅到血腥气，提示患者患有出血性疾病；嗅到腐臭气，则提示患者患有溃腐疮疡。

嗅气味尚需注意审察气味之来源，以确定病变的部位，并且结合气味种类的不同进行辨证。

### （一）嗅病体之气
**1. 口臭**

口臭，多见于口腔不洁，或有龋齿。口气臭秽多因胃热所致；口出酸馊气，是内有宿食；口出腐臭气，提示多患有内痈。

**2. 痰涕之气**

咳吐腥臭浊痰脓血，多见于热毒炽盛，瘀结成痈之肺痈。痰涕清稀无气味，常见于外感风寒。经常流臭秽浊涕，多为鼻渊，因肺热或胆经湿热所致。

**3. 身臭**

身体发出腐臭气，提示患有溃腐疮疡。身发狐臭气，是因湿热郁蒸所致。

**4. 二便之气**

小便清而无臊气，多属虚、寒证，亦见于正常健康人；小便短赤而臊，多是湿热下

downward migration of damp-heat. Loose and stinking stool suggests asthenia-cold in the spleen and intestines. Sour, putrid and foul odor of stool or foul flatus indicates retention of food and indigestion.

#### 1.2.2.1.5 Menstruation odor

Thin and stinking menorrhea and leukorrhea indicate asthenia-cold or cold-dampness syndrome. Yellowish thick and foul leukorrhea is due to downward migration of damp-heat. In dealing with leukorrhea with stifling foul odor, cares should be taken to exclude the possibility of cancer.

### 1.2.2.2 Odor in the room

Putrid and foul odor or corpse odor in the patient's room suggests deterioration of the viscera and critical pathological conditions; blood smell in the patient's room suggests hemorrhage. Besides, strong smell of urine in the patient's room is usually seen at the advanced stage of edema; bad apple smell is usually seen in severe diabetes, indicating critical pathological conditions.

## 1.3 Inquiry

Inquiry means investigating into the occurrence, development and treatment of the disease as well as the present manifestations and other related problems by means of inquiring the patient or other people accompanying the patient.

The occurrence, development and treatment of the disease as well as the present manifestations are important evidences for diagnosis. Such information can only be obtained by inquiry. So inquiry is the main method used to understand the medical history and subjective symptoms of the patient.

In doing inquiry, the doctor should comprehen-sively and purposefully ask the chief complaint and the related aspects. It is forbidden to suggest and induce the patient in doing inquiry. The doctor should use simple language to talk with the patient, avoiding using medical terms.

Inquiry includes general information, chief complaint, present disease history, present symptoms, past medical history and family history.

## 1.3.1 General information

General information includes name, sex, age, marital status, nationality, profession, one's place of origin, present address and date of first visit.

The information mentioned above is helpful for doctors to get necessary data related to the disease and provides evidences for the diagnosis and treatment. For example, woman tends to have problems related to menstruation, leukorrhagia, pregnancy, delivery and child-feeding; man tends to have problems of seminal emission, spontaneous spermatorrhea, immature ejaculation and impotence; infants are delicate in viscera and tend to contract measles, variella and diphtheria; young people and people in the prime of life are superabundant in qi and blood and tend to develop sthenia syndrome; the aged are deficient in qi and blood and tend to have asthenia syndrome because their viscera are weak; the middle-aged

觉症状的主要方法，它在中医四诊中占有十分重要的地位。

在询问病情时，医者要善于围绕患者的主要病痛，进行有目的、有步骤的询问，既要突出重点，又要全面了解，以避免遗漏病情。此外，不可凭个人主观意愿去暗示和诱导患者，语言应通俗易懂，切忌使用患者听不懂的医学术语，以避免所获病情资料的片面或失真，影响正确的诊断。

问诊的内容包括一般情况、主诉、现病史、现在症状、既往史、家族史等。

## 一、问一般情况

一般情况包括患者的姓名、性别、年龄、婚姻、民族、职业、籍贯、现住址、就诊日期等。

了解上述情况，医者可以获得与疾病有关的一般资料，为诊断治疗提供一定的依据。如女子可患有月经、带下、妊娠、产育、哺乳等方面的病变；男子可有遗精、滑精、早泄、阳痿等病证；小儿脏腑娇嫩，易患麻疹、水痘、白喉等病；青壮年气血充盛，抗病力强，病多实证；老年人气血衰少，脏腑虚损，病多虚证；癌症、胸痹、中风等病，多见于中老年人；长期从事某些工作易患某些

and aged are easy to have cancer, chest oppression and wind stroke; those who are engaged in a certain kind of work for a long time tend to have profession disease; and in some specific areas certain kinds of endema and epidemic diseases are commonly encountered.

Besides, the information mentioned above is also important for writing medical record, recording and surveying the procedure of diagnosis and treatment as well as keeping contact with the patients and their relatives.

## 1.3.2 Inquiry of chief complaint and history of present illness

Chief complaint and history of present illness are the main aspects included in inquiry and are important for diagnosis, treatment and syndrome differentiation.

### 1.3.2.1 Inquiry of chief complaint

Chief complaint refers to the most serious symptoms and signs and their duration felt by the patients when they come to the doctor. Chief complaint is the main reason why the patient comes to the doctor and the chief symptom of the illness.

Accurate chief complaint is key to further understanding of the pathological conditions of the patient. So chief complaint is helpful for primary classification and diagnosis of the disease. And it is also an important evidence for investigation, cognition, analysis and treatment of diseases.

Careful recording must be made of the symptoms included in the chief complaint or the location, nature, degree and time of signs. The recording to the chief complaint must be concise and avoid any ambiguity.

职业病；有的地区由于特定的自然条件，某些地方病、流行病较多。

此外，依据上述情况，也便于书写病历，记录、查阅诊治疾病的经过，以及与患者或其家属联系和随访。

## 二、问主诉与现病史

主诉与现病史是问诊的主要内容，问主诉与现病史对诊断疾病、辨别病证有重要意义。

### （一）问主诉

主诉是指患者就诊时最感痛苦的症状、体征及其所持续的时间。主诉常是患者就诊的主要原因，也是疾病的主要矛盾所在，即主症。

确切的主诉常可为进一步深入诊察病情指明方向。根据主诉，可以初步估计疾病的范畴和类别，病势的轻重缓急。因此，主诉具有重要的诊断价值，是调查、认识、分析、处理疾病的重要线索。

对于主诉所述症状或体征的部位、性质、程度、时间等，要逐一询问清楚。记录主诉时，文字应简明扼要，不能含糊、笼统。

### 1.3.2.2 Inquiry of the history of present illness

The history of present illness refers to the whole course of the onset, development and changes of illness from its occurrence to the time that the patient comes to the doctor. The inquiry of the history of present illness includes three aspects: occurrence, pathological changes and course of diagnosis and treatment.

#### 1.3.2.2.1 Occurrence

Occurrence includes the time of onset, whether the onset is sudden or gradual, cause of onset, initial symptoms and their nature and location as well as primary treatment. The understanding of such aspects is important for differentiating the cause and location and nature of disease.

#### 1.3.2.2.2 Development of disease

Inquiry of the development of disease includes the pathological changes from the onset of disease to the time that the patient comes to the doctor. Specifically speaking, it includes the nature, degree and changes of the main symptoms, the time of alleviation or aggravation, when there are new pathological changes, and whether there is any rules in the pathological changes. Such an inquiry is important for the understanding of the struggle between healthy qi and pathogenic factors as well as the tendency of the development of pathological changes.

#### 1.3.2.2.3 Procedure of diagnosis and treatment

Inquiry of the procedure of diagnosis and treatment includes whether the patient consults the doctor after onset, what test has been made, what the result is, what the diagnosis is made, what treatment has

## （二）问现病史

现病史是指围绕主诉，从起病到此次就诊时疾病的发生、发展和变化的全部过程，以及诊治经过等。现病史应从起病情况、病情演变、诊治经过等三个方面进行询问。

**1. 起病情况**

主要包括起病的时间，突然发病或缓慢起病，发病原因或诱因，最初的症状及其性质、部位，当时曾作何处理等。了解上述情况，对于辨别疾病的原因、病位、病性等有重要的作用。

**2. 病情演变**

按时间顺序，询问自发病后至就诊时病情演变的主要情况，其主要症状的性质、程度有何变化，何时好转或加重，何时有什么新的病情出现，病情的变化有无规律等。通过询问病情演变，对于了解疾病的邪正斗争情况，以及病情发展趋势有重要意义。

**3. 诊治经过**

询问患病后是否曾经就医，做过哪些检查，结果怎样，当时的诊断结论如何，经过哪些治疗，疗效怎样等。这些既往诊治情况，可作为当前诊断

been taken and what the curative effect is, etc. Such data above the diagnosis and treatment made in the past can be taken as a reference for the present diagnosis and treatment.

### 1.3.3 Inquiry of the present symptoms

Inquiry of the present symptoms includes the present sufferings, discomfort and other information related to the disease.

The present symptoms are the reflections of the present pathological changes and are the important evidences for the diagnosis and syndrome differentiation. Inquiry of the present symptoms (including the location, nature, degree, occurrence and duration as well as the conditions for aggravation or alleviation) is helpful for understanding the cause, location and nature of disease as well as the state of healthy qi and pathogenic factors.

Each disease has its specific main symptoms and secondary symptoms. So inquiry of the present symptoms should concentrate on both the systemic content of inquiry and the basis of chief complaint and the main symptoms.

Inquiry of the present symptoms includes inquiry of fever and cold, sweating, pain, sleep, diet and appetite, defecation and urine and symptoms over the head and face as well as back and limbs. It also covers the symptoms in the andriatry, gynecology and pediatrics.

#### 1.3.3.1 Inquiry of fever and cold

Inquiry of fever and cold means asking the patient

与治疗的参考。

## 三、问现在症状

问现在症状，是指对患者目前所感到的痛苦和不适，以及与病情相关的全身情况进行全面、系统的询问。

现在症状是机体当前病变的具体反映，是诊病辨证的主要依据，也是问诊的重要内容。通过询问现在症状的特征，即症状的具体部位、性质、程度、出现和持续的时间、加重或减轻的条件等，可以了解疾病的病因、病位、病性、邪正盛衰等情况，对于疾病的诊断有重要作用。

每一病证都有其特定的主要症状与次要症状。因此，问现在症状时既要注意问诊内容的系统性，又要在重视患者现病主诉的基础上，围绕主症，有目的、有重点地询问。

问现在症状包括问寒热、问汗、问疼痛、问睡眠、问饮食口味、问二便、问头面症状、问胸腹症状、问腰背四肢症状、问男科症状、问妇科症状及问儿科症状等内容。

### （一）问寒热

问寒热是询问患者有无

whether he or she has the sensation of fever and aversion to cold. Fever and cold are the common symptoms seen in the course of a disease and are the evidences for differentiating the nature of pathogenic factors and the states of yin and yang in the body.

Aversion to cold is a subjective sensation, including disliking cold and fearing cold. If the patient feels cold and such sensation cannot be relieved after putting on more clothes and quilt or staying near fire, it is called disliking cold; if the patient feels cold and such sensation can be relieved after putting on more clothes and quilt or staying near fire, it is called fearing cold. Fever means that the body temperature is higher than usual, also including subjective sensation of general or local fever like feverish sensation over the five centers (palms, soles and chest) which does not necessarily mean the increase of body temperature. The occurrence of fever and cold lies in the nature of pathogenic factors as well as decline and predomination of yin and yang in the body, reflecting or signifying the result of the struggle between healthy qi and pathogenic factors as well as the changes of yin and yang. Generally speaking, in the disease due to pathogenic factors, pathogenic cold leads to disliking of cold and pathogenic heat leads to fever; in the cold and fever caused by the predomination and decline of yin and yang in the body, exuberance of yang leads to fever and superabundance of yin leads to cold, asthenia of yin brings about fever and asthenia of yang results in cold. So inquiry of cold and fever is helpful for understanding the nature of pathogenic factors and differentiating the states of yin and yang in the body.

In inquiring fever and cold, the doctor should make sure whether there is cold and fever or not, whether cold and fever appear simultaneously, whether fever and cold is serious or mild, what time it appears and how it lasts as

怕冷与发热的感觉。寒与热是疾病过程中的常见症状,是辨别病邪性质和机体阴阳盛衰的重要依据。

怕冷是患者的主观感觉,有恶寒和畏寒的区别。凡患者自觉怕冷,多加衣被,近火取暖,仍感寒冷不缓解的,称为恶寒;若患者怕冷,加衣覆被,或近火取暖而能缓解的,称为畏寒。发热除指体温高于正常外,还包括患者自觉全身或某一局部发热,如五心烦热,但体温不一定升高。寒与热的产生,主要决定于病邪的性质和机体阴阳的盛衰两个方面,是机体邪正交争、阴阳盛衰变化的反映和结果。一般来说,邪气致病,寒邪多致恶寒,热邪多致发热;机体阴阳盛衰所致的寒热,阳盛则热,阴盛则寒,阴虚则热,阳虚则寒。因此,通过问寒热可以了解病邪的性质和辨别机体阴阳之盛衰。

问寒热,必须问清寒热的有无,寒热是否同时出现,寒热的轻重,出现的时间和持续的时间,以及其他兼症等。

well as other complications.

Clinically the types of cold and fever include aversion to cold and fever, cold sensation without fever, fever without cold sensation, and alternate cold and fever.

#### 1.3.3.1.1 Aversion to cold and fever

Aversion to cold and fever means that the patient dislikes cold and the body temperature increases, usually seen at the primary stage of exogenous disease which pertains to external syndrome due to retention of pathogenic factors in the superficies and struggle between defensive yang and pathogenic factors. Aversion to cold is caused by invasion of pathogenic factors in the skin which affects the function of defensive yang to warm the muscles; fever is caused by pathogenic factors encumbering the superficies and resistance of defensive qi against pathogenic factors. When the pathogenic factors are in the superficies, there is difference in aversion to cold and fever due to the difference of pathogenic factors in nature. Generally there are three types of aversion to cold and fever according to their degree.

**Serious aversion to cold and mild fever**: Serious aversion to cold and mild fever indicate external syndrome due to wind-cold. Cold is a pathogenic factor of yin nature. When pathogenic cold invades the superficies, defensive yang is stagnated and the superficies lacks warmth, leading to serious aversion to cold. Cold tends to coagulate. So when defensive yang is stagnated and when pathogenic factors struggle with healthy qi, fever is caused.

**Serious fever and mild aversion to cold**: Serious fever and mild aversion to cold indicate external syndrome due to wind-heat. Wind-heat is a pathogenic factor of yang nature. When pathogenic factor of yang nature causes

临床常见的寒热类型有恶寒发热、但寒不热、但热不寒、寒热往来等。

**1. 恶寒发热**

恶寒发热是指患者恶寒,同时体温升高而发热,多见于外感病初起阶段,属表证,为外邪客于肌表,卫阳与邪气相争的反映。外邪侵袭肌表,影响卫阳"温分肉"的功能,肌腠失煦则恶寒;邪气外袭,卫气抗邪则发热。由于感受外邪性质的不同,当外邪在表时,其恶寒发热的情况亦各有区别。以恶寒发热的轻重而言,可分为以下三种类型。

(1) 恶寒重发热轻:主风寒表证。寒为阴邪,寒邪袭表,卫阳被遏,肌表失煦则恶寒重;寒性凝滞,卫阳郁闭失宣,邪正相争,故发热。

(2) 发热重恶寒轻:主风热表证。风热为阳邪,阳邪致病则阳盛,所以发热较重;风热袭表,腠理开泄,故轻微

disease, yang is usually superabundant. That is why fever is serious. When wind-heat invades the superficies, the muscular interstices become loose. That is why aversion to cold is mild.

**Mild fever and aversion to wind**: Mild fever and aversion to wind indicate external syndrome due to wind attack. Aversion to wind means sensation of cold in contact with wind and is relieved after avoiding wind, usually caused by exogenous pathogenic wind. Since wind tends to open, muscular interstices become loose when attacked by wind. That is why there are mild fever and aversion to wind.

The degree of aversion to cold and fever in external syndrome is not only related to the nature of pathogenic factors, but also to the relation between pathogenic factors and healthy qi. For example, if both the pathogenic factors and healthy qi are in predomination, aversion to cold and fever are all serious, signifying drastic struggle between healthy qi and pathogenic factors. When both pathogenic factors and healthy qi are deficient, aversion to cold and fever are all mild, indicating slight struggle between healthy qi and pathogenic factors. When pathogenic factors are superabundant and healthy qi is deficient, aversion to cold is serious and fever is mild, suggesting failure of healthy qi to control pathogenic factors.

#### 1.3.3.1.2 Cold without fever

Cold without fever means that the patient only feels cold but there is no fever. It is usually caused by direct invasion of pathogenic cold into the interior which stagnates yangqi and prevents it from moving outwards; or by decline of yangqi and lack of warmth of the body. According to the onset, duration, cause and pathogenesis, cold without fever can be further divided into aversion to cold in new disease and fear of cold in chronic disease.

恶寒。

（3）发热轻而恶风：主伤风表证。恶风是指遇风觉冷,避之可以缓解,多因外感风邪所致。由于风性开泄,腠理疏松,所以发热轻而恶风。

表证恶寒发热的轻重,不仅与病邪的性质有关,而且与邪正盛衰密切相关。如邪正俱盛者,恶寒发热皆较重,是正邪剧争的表现；邪轻正衰者,恶寒发热均较轻,属正邪斗争不甚；邪盛正衰者,恶寒重发热轻,是正不胜邪的征象。

**2. 但寒不热**

但寒不热是指患者只感怕冷而不觉发热。多因寒邪直接侵犯于里,阳气被遏,不能外达；或阳气虚衰,形体失于温煦所致。但寒不热根据发病缓急,病程长短及病因病机,有新病恶寒与久病畏寒的区别。

**Aversion to cold in new disease**: Aversion to cold in new disease is caused by serious invasion of cold directly into the viscera which stagnates yangqi and deprives the body of warmth. Sudden aversion to cold with cold limbs accompanied by cold abdominal pain or dyspnea with sputum rale pertains to cold syndrome of internal sthenia.

**Fear of cold in chronic disease**: Fear of cold in chronic disease is usually caused by decline of yangqi and lack of warmth of the body. The patient frequently fears cold and the limbs are not warm, usually relieved with warmth, with light-coloured and tender tongue as well as deep, slow and weak pulse. Such pathological conditions signify cold syndrome of internal asthenia.

#### 1.3.3.1.3 Fever without cold

Fever without cold means that the patient only has fever and does not feel cold or, on the contrary, dislikes heat. Such a problem usually pertains to internal heat syndrome caused by exuberance of yang or asthenia of yin. According to the degree, time and features, fever can be further divided into high fever, tidal fever and mild fever.

**High fever**: High fever means that the patient suffers from serious high fever hard to be relieved with the symptoms of aversion to heat instead of to cold. It is usually caused by wind-cold invading into the interior and transforming into heat, or by transmission of wind-heat into the interior, struggle between pathogenic factors and healthy qi and internal exuberance of yang-heat, the steaming of which manifests externally. High fever is usually seen at the qi phase stage of exogenous febrile disease, pertaining to internal sthenia-heat syndrome, usually accompanied by flushed cheeks, profuse sweating, dysphoria, thirst and preference for cold drinks.

（1）新病恶寒：多因感受寒邪较重，直中脏腑，阳气被遏，机体失于温煦所致。如患者突然恶寒，四肢不温，伴脘腹冷痛，或咳喘痰鸣者，属里实寒证。

（2）久病畏寒：多因阳气虚衰，形体失于温煦所致。患者经常畏寒肢冷，得温可缓，舌淡嫩，脉沉迟无力等，为里虚寒证。

### 3. 但热不寒

但热不寒是指患者只发热，不觉寒冷，或反恶热。多属阳盛或阴虚的里热证。根据发热的轻重、时间、特点等不同，可分为壮热、潮热、微热三种类型。

（1）壮热：患者高热不退，不恶寒，反恶热，称为壮热。多因风寒入里化热，或风热内传，邪正相争，阳热内盛，蒸达于外所致。多见于外感温热病的气分阶段，属里实热证。常兼面赤、汗多、烦躁、口渴喜饮冷等症。

**Tidal fever**: Tidal fever is marked by regular occurrence or regular worsening. According to its cause and pathogenesis, it can be further divided into the following categories.

Yangming afternoon fever: It is marked by continuous fever and severity in the afternoon (3-5 o'clock in the afternoon) when qi in yangming meridian is superabundant, accompanied by constipation and unpressable abdominal hardness and pain due to invasion of pathogenic heat into yangming, retention of dry-heat in stomach and intestines as well as obstruction of intestinal qi.

Damp-warm tidal fever: Damp-warm tidal fever is marked by fever, worsening in the afternoon or evening and dull fever (that means that it does not feel feverish when the hand touches on the skin at first, but after a while the hand feels scorching hot), usually accompanied by epigastric and abdominal fullness and oppression, nausea and vomiting, heavy sensation of the head and body, loose stool and diarrhea as well as thick and greasy tongue fur, often caused by retention of damp-heat in the middle energizer, stagnation of dampness and latency of heat and failure of heat to get out of the body as well as stagnation of dampness and steaming of heat.

Yin-asthenia tidal fever: It is marked by fever in the afternoon or evening and feverish sensation over the five centers (palms, soles and chest) or steaming fever in the bones), usually accompanied by flushed cheeks, night sweating, dry mouth and throat as well as reddish tongue with scanty fluid, often caused by consumption of yin fluid, failure of yin to control yang and endogenous asthenia-heat.

Besides, one of its major symptoms is worsening of fever in the night due to invasion of heat into nutrient phase

（2）潮热：发热如潮汐之有定时，即按时发热，或按时热更甚，称为潮热。根据其病因病机的不同，有阳明潮热、湿温潮热、阴虚潮热等。

① 阳明潮热：又称为日晡潮热。发热不退，以日晡时（下午3～5时）阳明经气旺时热势更甚为特点，兼见大便秘结、腹满硬痛拒按等症，为邪热内犯阳明，胃肠燥热内结，腑气不通所致。

② 湿温潮热：发热，午后或夜间热盛，以身热不扬（肌肤初扪之不觉很热，但扪之稍久即感灼手）为特点，常兼脘腹痞闷、恶心呕吐、头身困重、大便溏泄、舌苔厚腻等症，为湿热遏阻中焦，湿遏热伏，热难透达，湿郁热蒸所致。

③ 阴虚潮热：午后或夜间发热，以五心烦热或骨蒸发热为特点，常兼颧红、盗汗、口咽干燥、舌红少津等症，为阴液亏损，阴不制阳，虚热内生所致。

此外，温病热入营分，灼伤营阴，身热夜甚是其主要症

and consumption of nutrient yin in febrile disease.

**Mild fever**: Mild fever, also known as low fever, means that the fever is slight or indistinct or subjective sensation of fever with normal temperature. Mild fever is marked by longer duration. The cause and disease involved are complicated. For example, internal heat due to yin asthenia leads to prolonged low fever; prolonged mild fever, also known as fever due to qi asthenia, is usually caused by asthenia of spleen qi, sinking of gastrosplenic qi and failure of lucid yang to rise which stagnate into heat; mild fever may be caused by emotional upsets and failure of the liver to disperse and convey, leading to fever due to qi stagnation.

#### 1.3.3.1.4 Alternate cold and fever

Alternate cold and fever means that aversion to cold and fever occur alternately due to struggle between healthy qi and pathogenic factors, signifying development and abatement of cold and fever. Irregular alternate cold and fever is seen in shaoyang disease pertaining to semi-internal and semi-external syndrome due to struggle between healthy qi and pathogenic factors. The predomination of pathogenic factors leads to aversion to cold, while the predomination of the healthy qi leads to fever. If pathogenic factors and healthy qi predominate alternately, it leads to alternate cold and fever. Regular cold and fever, once a day or once two and three days, accompanied by severe headache, thirst and profuse sweating, pertains to malaria. When pathogenic factors invades the body, they stay in the semi-internal and semi-external region. When they get inside, they struggle with yin; and when they get out, they struggle with yang. That is why chills and high fever appear alternately and continually.

状之一。

（3）微热：又称为低热。是指轻度发热，热势不甚明显，或仅自觉发热而体温并不升高。微热大多发病时间较长。病因与病证较复杂，如阴虚内热，多为长期低热；脾气虚弱，中气下陷，清阳不升，郁而为热，亦可致长期微热，称为气虚发热；情志不舒，肝失疏泄，气郁化热，亦可表现为时有微热，称为气郁发热。

4. 寒热往来

寒热往来是指恶寒与发热交替发作，是邪正相争，互为进退的表现。若寒热往来，发无定时，可见于少阳病，属半表半里证，因邪正相争，邪胜则恶寒，正胜则发热，邪正互胜，所以恶寒与发热交替发作。若寒热往来，发有定时，每日发作一次，或二三日发作一次，并兼有头痛剧烈、口渴、多汗等症，属疟疾病。由于疟邪侵入人体，伏藏于表里之间，入与阴争则寒，出与阳争则热，故寒战与高热交替出现，休作有时。

### 1.3.3.2 Inquiry of sweating

Sweating is transformed from body fluid by yangqi and excretes from the sweat pores. Normally sweat functions to regulate yingqi and weiqi and moisten the skin. Under pathological conditions, sweating becomes abnormal due to the invasion of pathogenic factors and imbalance between yin and yang inside the body. Inquiry of sweating can enable one to understand the nature of the pathogenic factors and the conditions of yin and yang inside the body. Inquiry of sweating includes hidrosis and anhidrosis as well as time, region and quantity of sweating.

#### 1.3.3.2.1 Anhidrosis

Anhidrosis when there should be sweating is usually caused by exogenous cold or insufficiency of yin blood and body fluid or asthenia of yangqi.

**Anhidrosis in external syndrome:** This condition is often seen in external sthenia syndrome due to exogenous cold. Since cold tends to stagnate and contract, the muscular interstices become tense and the sweat pores are closed up, preventing sweating from excreting. The usual symptoms are serious aversion to cold, mild fever and floating and tense pulse, etc.

**Anhidrosis in internal syndrome:** This condition is usually seen in blood asthenia syndrome and yang asthenia syndrome due to insufficiency of body fluid. If it is accompanied by such symptoms like dry skin, dry mouth, dry feces, it is usually caused by depletion of body fluid due to exhaustion of the sweat source; if it is accompanied by pale complexion and lips, whitish pale tongue, it is usually caused by insufficiency of yin blood and exhaustion of sweat source; if it is accompanied by aversion to cold and cold limbs, it is usually caused by insufficiency of yangqi and hypofunction to transform qi.

### （二）问汗

阳气蒸化津液从玄府出于体表而成为汗。正常的出汗有调和营卫、滋润皮肤等作用。疾病过程中汗出异常，与病邪的侵扰和机体的阴阳失调等密切相关。询问患者有无汗出异常的情况，可以了解病邪的性质及人体的阴阳盛衰。询问时，应注意了解患者有汗无汗，出汗的时间、部位、多少等情况。

**1．无汗**

当汗出而无汗，多因外感寒邪，或阴血、津液不足，或阳气亏虚所致。

（1）表证无汗：多见于外感寒邪所致的表实证。因寒性收引凝滞，腠理致密，玄府闭塞，因而无汗。常兼恶寒重发热轻、脉浮紧等。

（2）里证无汗：多见于津液不足证、血虚证、阳虚证。若兼见皮肤干燥、口干咽燥、大便干结，多属津液亏虚，汗液生化无源；若兼见面、唇淡白无华，舌质淡白，多因阴血不足，汗液乏源；若兼畏寒肢冷，则因阳气亏虚，蒸化无力所致。

### 1.3.3.2.2 Hidrosis

Sweating can be caused by exogenous cold attack, or wind-heat invading the superficies, or exuberance of endogenous heat, or endogenous heat due to yin asthenia, or weakness of weiqi due to qi asthenia, or excretion of body fluid due to sudden loss of yangqi.

**Hidrosis in external syndrome**: This condition is usually seen in external asthenia syndrome due to exogenous wind attack, or external heat syndrome due to exogenous wind-heat and diseases due to weakness of weiqi complicated by exogenous wind attack. Wind tends to open and leak, while heat tends to rise and disperse. Attacked by wind and heat, the muscular interstices become loose and sweat excretes. Sweat tends to excrete if weiqi is weak and the muscular interstices are loose. If accompanied by fever, aversion to wind and floating and slow pulse, it is external asthenia syndrome; if accompanied by high fever, light aversion to cold, sore-throat and floating and rapid pulse, it is external heat syndrome.

**Hidrosis in internal syndrome**: This condition is usually seen in exuberance of endogenous heat syndrome, endogenous heat syndrome due to yin asthenia, weakness of weiqi due to qi asthenia and sudden loss of yangqi.

Spontaneous sweating: Spontaneous sweating refers to constant sweating, especially after physical movement, often seen in qi asthenia syndrome and yang asthenia syndrome. Since asthenia of yangqi fails to protect the superficies, the sweat pores will become loose and body fluid will excrete. That is why sweat is constant. Since physical movement further consumes yangqi, sweating becomes more serious.

Night sweating: Night sweating refers to sweating occurring when the patient falls asleep but stopping after

### 2. 有汗

若外感风邪，或风热犯表，或里热炽盛，或阴虚内热，或气虚卫表不固，或阳气暴脱，津液外泄，均可导致不同程度的出汗。

（1）表证有汗：多见于外感风邪所致的中风表虚证，或外感风热所致的表热证，以及卫阳不固、复感风邪的病证。风性开泄，热性升散，风热袭表，可致腠理疏松而汗出；如卫阳素虚，肌表不固，则更易汗出。若兼发热恶风、脉浮缓，则为中风表虚证，若兼见发热重恶寒轻、咽痛、脉浮数者，则为表热证。

（2）里证有汗：多见于里热炽盛证、阴虚内热证、气虚卫表不固证、阳气暴脱证。

① 自汗：经常汗出不止，活动之后更甚者，称为自汗。常见于气虚、阳虚证。因阳气虚弱，不能固护肌表，玄府不密，津液外泄，则经常汗出不止。每当活动更加耗伤阳气，因而汗出更甚。

② 盗汗：入睡之后汗出，醒后则汗止，称为盗汗。常见

the patient wakes up. It is usually seen in endogenous heat syndrome due to yin asthenia, or asthenia syndrome of both qi and yin. It is caused by endogenous heat due to yin asthenia. When people fall asleep, yangqi enters into the body, the muscular interstices become loose and asthenic heat steams the body fluid to excrete. That is why sweating occurs during sleep. After people wake up, yangqi returns to the superficies, the muscular interstices become tense. Under this condition, endogenous heat with yin asthenia cannot steam the body fluid to excrete. That is why sweating stops after people wake up. Asthenia of both qi and yin usually lead to both spontaneous sweating and night sweating.

Profuse sweating: Profuse sweating is either asthenic or sthenic. Profuse sweating with high fever, flushed complexion, thirst, preference for cold drinks and full large pulse is seen in sthenic heat syndrome due to exuberance of endogenous heat which drives body fluid to excrete. If profuse sweat occurs in patients with prolonged illness accompanied by symptoms like pale complexion, cold limbs and indistinct pulse, it is yang exhaustion syndrome due to sudden loss of yang which leads body fluid to excrete.

Sweating following shivering: Sweating following shivering is usually seen during the course of exogenous febrile disease, marking the turning point of conflict between healthy qi and pathogenic factors and the development of pathological conditions. If fever abates, pulse calms down and the body turns cool after sweating, it is a sign that pathogenic factors are being expelled; if there are restlessness and rapid pulse after sweating, it is a critical sign of domination of pathogenic factors and decline of healthy qi.

Head sweating: Head sweating means that sweat only

于阴虚内热证，或气阴两虚证。由于阴虚内热所致。因入睡之时，卫阳入里，肌表不固，虚热蒸津外泄，故睡时汗出；醒后卫阳复归于表，肌表固密，虽阴虚内热，也不能蒸津外出，故醒后汗止。若气阴两虚，常自汗、盗汗并见。

③ 大汗：即津液大泄，汗出量多。大汗有虚实之分：若汗出量多、壮热面赤、口渴喜冷饮、脉洪大，属实热证，因里热亢盛，蒸迫津液外泄所致。若久病重病患者突然冷汗淋漓、面色苍白、四肢厥冷、脉微欲绝者，属亡阳证，因阳气暴脱，津失依附而外泄。

④ 战汗：先恶寒战栗，几经挣扎，而后汗出者，称为战汗。战汗多见于外感热病过程中，是邪正相争，病情发展的转折点。若汗出热退，脉静身凉，是邪去正安的表现；若汗出而仍烦躁不安，脉来疾急，是邪胜正衰的危候。

⑤ 头汗：指汗出仅见于

appears over the head. The causes of head sweating are various, including exuberant heat in the upper energizer which drives body fluid to excrete in the upper, often accompanied by reddish complexion and thirst; accumulation of damp heat in the middle energizer in which the stagnation of dampness and steaming of heat drive the body fluid to excrete in the upper, often accompanied by abdominal fullness, heaviness of the head and body; prolonged and serious disease with primordial qi on the verge to exhaust in which asthenic yang floats upward and the body fluid excretes in the upper together with yang, often accompanied by pale complexion and cold limbs. Besides, exuberance of yangqi due to extravagant intake of pungent food or hot soup and drinking of wine may drive heat to steam in the upper and lead to head sweating. But head sweating in this case is not pathological.

Hemihidrosis: Hemihidrosis means sweating appears over half of the body, either the upper or the lower, the left side or the right side. The location of disease is on the part of the body without sweat. This problem is usually seen in apoplexy, flaccidity and hemiplegia, often caused by wind phlegm or stagnant phlegm and obstruction of the meridians by wind dampness which prevent weiqi and yingqi from flowing as well as qi from normal circulation.

Sweating over palms and soles: If it is accompanied by dry mouth and throat, restless feverish sensation over the palms, soles and chest as well as thin and rapid pulse, it is usually caused by steaming of stagnant heat in the yin meridians; if it is accompanied by restless thirst, preference for cold drinks, brownish urine, constipation and full and rapid pulse, it is usually caused by exuberant heat in the yangming meridian; if it is accompanied by heaviness of the head and body, dull fever and yellowish greasy fur,

头项部。导致头汗的原因有：上焦热盛，逼津上泄，常兼满面通红、口渴等；中焦湿热蕴结，湿郁热蒸，逼津上泄，常兼脘腹痞闷、头身困重等；久病重病，元气将脱，虚阳上浮，津随阳泄，常兼面色苍白、四肢厥冷等。此外，在进食辛辣或热汤及饮酒时，阳气旺盛，热蒸于上，亦可出现头汗，不属病候。

⑥ 半身汗：是指身体一半出汗，另一半无汗，或见于左侧，或见于右侧，或见于上半身，或见于下半身。其病变的部位是无汗的半身。多见于中风病、痿证及截瘫病人。多因风痰或瘀痰、风湿之邪阻滞经络，营卫不得周流，气血失于和利所致。

⑦ 手足心汗：伴口咽干燥、五心烦热、脉细数者，多为阴经郁热薰蒸所致；伴烦渴饮冷、尿赤便秘、脉洪数者，多属阳明热盛之故；伴头身困重、身热不扬、苔黄腻者，多属中焦湿热郁蒸所致。

it is usually caused by steaming of damp heat in the middle energizer.

Chest sweating: Chest sweating is usually of asthenia syndrome. If it is accompanied by lassitude, anorexia, palpitation and insomnia, it is usually caused by simultaneous asthenia of the heart and spleen; if it is accompanied by palpitation, dysphoria, insomnia, dreaminess and aching waist and knees, it is usually due to imbalance between the heart and the kidney.

Besides, it is also necessary to know the temperature and colour of sweating. Generally speaking, cold sweating is due to decline of yangqi, while feverish sweating is due to exogenous wind heat or steaming of endogenous heat. Yellowish sweating is often due to interaction of wind, dampness and heat.

### 1.3.3.3 Inquiry of pain

Pain is a commonly encountered subjective symptom in clinical treatment. Pain may appear at any part of the body. It may be caused by sthenia, such as invasion of exogenous pathogenic factors, or qi stagnation and blood stasis, or stagnation of phlegm, or retention of food, or parasitic infestation which obstruct the meridians, prevent qi and blood from normal circulation and consequently bring about pain. It may also be caused by asthenia, such as insufficiency of qi and blood, or consumption of yin essence which deprives the viscera and meridians from nutrition and cause pain.

Inquiry of pain includes such aspects like the location, nature, degree and time of pain as well as personal aversion and preference.

#### 1.3.3.3.1 Inquiry of the pain location

This can enable one to understand which viscus or meridian the pain is located.

⑧心胸汗：多属虚证。若兼神疲倦怠、纳呆食少、心悸失眠等，多属心脾两虚；兼心悸心烦、失眠多梦、腰膝酸软等，多属心肾不交。

此外，还需了解汗的冷热、颜色。一般而言，冷汗多因阳气虚衰所致，热汗多由外感风热或内热蒸迫所致。黄汗多因风湿热邪交蒸而成。

### （三）问疼痛

疼痛是临床上常见的自觉症状。可发生于机体的各个部位。其形成有因实致痛的，如感受外邪，或气滞血瘀，或痰浊凝滞，或食滞、虫积等阻滞脏腑经络，闭塞气机，使气血运行不畅，"不通则痛"；也有因虚致痛的，如气血不足，或阴精亏损，使脏腑经络失养，"不荣而痛"。

问疼痛，应注意询问疼痛的部位、性质、程度、时间、喜恶等。

#### 1. 问疼痛的部位

询问疼痛的部位，可了解病变所在的脏腑经络，对诊断有重要意义。

**Headache**: The three yang meridians of both the hand and foot are directly connected with the head, the liver meridian also extends to the head, the other yin meridians are indirectly connected with the head. The location of pain over the head can enable one to decide which meridian and which viscus are involved. For example, if neck is involved in headache, it is a problem related to the taiyang meridian; if pain appears on both sides of the head, it is a problem related to the shaoyang meridian and also connected with the gallbladder and triple energizer; if pain appears over the forehead and supraorbital bone, it is a problem related to the stomach and intestines; if pain appears over the vertex, it is a problem related to the jueyin meridian and connected with the liver. The causes of headache are various. Headache of sthenia syndrome is usually caused by such factors like attack by exogenous wind, cold, summer-heat, dampness, pathogenic fire as well as obstruction or disturbance of the upper orifices by phlegm and blood stasis. Headache of asthenia syndrome is usually due to insufficiency of qi and blood and depletion of essence and marrow which fail to nourish the head. The causes and the types of headache should be analyzed according to the nature of headache and the accompanied symptoms.

**Chest pain**: The lung is located in the chest, so chest pain is usually seen in heart and lung problems. The precordial pain or pain involving the inner side of the arm indicates that the location of the pain is in the heart due to asthenia of heart yang and qi as well as stagnation of qi and blood; distress and puncturing pain over the precordium is usually due to blood stasis in the heart vessels. Pain over the chest means that the location of pain is in the lung due to exogenous pathogenic factors invading the lung or retention of phlegm and fluid in the lung which prevent

（1）头痛：手、足三阳经直接与头部联系，足厥阴经上行于头，其他阴经也多间接与头部联系。根据头痛的部位，可确定病在何经，与何脏腑相关。如头痛连项，属太阳经；两侧头痛，属少阳经，与胆和三焦相关；前额连眉棱骨痛，属阳明经，与胃和肠相关；巅顶痛，属厥阴经，与肝相关。引起头痛的原因甚多，如外感风、寒、暑、湿、火邪，以及痰浊、瘀血阻滞或上扰清窍所致的头痛，多属实证；气血不足，精髓亏少，不能上荣于头，致使脑海空虚所致的头痛，多属虚证。应结合头痛的性质及兼症，分析病因，辨明虚实。

（2）胸痛：胸部为心肺所居，故胸痛多见于心肺的病变。胸前虚里部位作痛或痛引内臂，病位在心，多因心阳气虚，气血瘀阻所致；虚里部位憋闷，痛如针刺，多为血瘀心脉。胸膺部位作痛，病在肺，多因外邪犯肺或痰饮伏肺，气机不畅所致；胸痛而咳吐脓血腥臭痰，多为肺痈，因

qi from smooth flowing; chest pain with expectoration of foul sputum mingled with pus and blood indicates lung abscess due to exuberance of pathogenic heat in the lung which stagnates qi and blood and putrefies blood to cause abscess.

**Hypochondriac pain**: The liver and gallbladder are located in the hypochondrium. The liver and gallbladder meridians circulate to the sides. Therefore, hypochondriac pain is often related to liver and gallbladder disorders. For example, hypochondriac pain is often seen in such disorders like liver depression and qi stagnation, damp heat in the liver and gallbladder, exuberant heat in the liver and gallbladder and retention of fluid in the hypochondrium, etc.

**Epigastric pain**: Epigastrium refers to the part below the xiphoid process where the stomach is located. Epigastric pain is usually caused by failure of the stomach to descend food and stagnant flow of qi due to cold, heat, retention of food in the stomach and qi stagnation, etc. Stagnation leads to pain. If pain becomes worsened after intake of food, it is a sthenia syndrome; if pain becomes alleviated after intake of food, it is an asthenia syndrome.

**Abdominal pain**: Abdomen may be further divided into large abdomen, small abdomen and lower abdomen. The part between the epigastrium and the navel is large abdomen; the part between the navel and the margin of pubic region is the small abdomen where the kidney, bladder, intestines and uterus are located; the two sides of the small abdomen are lateral part of small abdomen where the liver meridian penetrates. Besides, pain over the lateral parts of the small abdomen is also related to the large intestine disorder. The causes of abdominal pain are various. Sthenia syndrome of abdominal pain is usually caused by cold stagnation, heat retention, qi obstruction,

邪热壅肺，气血壅滞，腐而为脓。

（3）胁痛：肝胆居于胁部，肝胆两经循行于胁，所以，胁痛多与肝胆病变有关。如肝郁气滞、肝胆湿热、肝胆火盛，以及悬饮等病证，常会出现胁痛。

（4）脘痛：脘，指上腹部，在剑突下，是胃所在的部位，故又称胃脘。脘痛常因寒、热、食积、气滞等原因，引起胃失和降，气机不畅，不通则痛。进食后痛势加剧的，多属实证；进食后痛势缓解的，多属虚证。

（5）腹痛：腹部的范围较广，可分为大腹、小腹、少腹三部分。脘下脐上为大腹，属脾胃；脐以下至耻骨毛际以上为小腹，属肾、膀胱、大小肠、胞宫；小腹两侧为少腹，是足厥阴肝经所过之处。此外，少腹痛也与大肠病变有关。导致腹痛的原因很多，如寒凝、热结、气滞、血瘀、食积、虫积等所致者，多属实证；气虚、血虚、阳虚等所致者，多属虚证。

blood stasis, retention of food and parasitic infestation, while asthenia syndrome of abdominal pain is usually caused by asthenia of qi, blood and yang, etc. In the examination of patients with abdominal pain, inquiry should be done together with pulse taking in order to exactly locate the region of pain and decide the viscera involved and differentiate the cause and nature of the problem.

**Backache**: Backache with inability to stretch or bend the back is often caused by impairment of the governor vessel; backache involving the neck is usually caused by retention of wind cold in the taiyang meridian; aching pain of the shoulder and back is usually caused by obstruction of wind and dampness which obstruct the meridians.

**Lumbago**: Pain over the spine or over the waist and sacrum is often caused by obstruction of cold and dampness, or obstruction of the meridians by blood stasis, or asthenia of the kidney. Lumbago involving the lower limbs is often caused by retention of cold dampness in the meridians which stagnates qi and blood. Stiff and painful loins due to falling or sprain marked by immobility and inflexibility is usually caused by obstruction of blood stasis. Dull pain over the sides of waist with slow onset is usually due to asthenia of the kidney.

**Pain of the limbs**: Pain of the limbs is usually caused by invasion of wind, cold and dampness, or by accumulation of damp heat which obstructs the circulation of qi and blood. Pain of the limbs may result from weakness of the stomach and the spleen which fail to transport cereal nutrients to the four limbs. Pain over the heel or aching pain over the legs and knees is usually due to asthenia of the kidney, often seen in the aged and weak people.

**General pain**: General pain in the new disease is usually of sthenia syndrome due to attack by pathogenic wind, cold and dampness. General pain in prolonged

对于腹痛患者,应当问诊与按诊密切结合,以查明腹痛的确切部位,判断病变所在的脏腑,了解引起腹痛的原因,辨清病证的性质。

(6)背痛:背痛不可俯仰,多因督脉损伤所致;背痛连及项部,多因风寒之邪客于太阳经脉而致;肩背酸痛,多为风湿阻滞,经气不利所致。

(7)腰痛:腰脊或腰骶部疼痛,多属寒湿痹病,或为瘀血阻络,或由肾虚所致。腰痛连及下肢,多属寒湿客于经脉,气血阻滞;跌仆闪挫后,腰部强直疼痛,固定不移,转侧俯仰不利,多属瘀血阻滞;起病缓慢,腰痛以两侧为主,隐隐作痛,多属肾虚。

(8)四肢痛:多因风寒湿邪侵袭,或因湿热蕴结,阻滞气血运行所致;亦有由于脾胃虚损,水谷精微不能达于四肢而作痛者;独见于足跟或胫膝酸痛,则属肾虚,多见于年老体衰者。

(9)周身疼痛:新病周身疼痛,多属实证,以感受风寒湿邪居多;久病卧床不起而周

disease is of asthenia syndrome due to deficiency of qi and blood which fails to nourish the body.

#### 1.3.3.3.2　Inquiry of the nature of pain

The nature of pain varies due to the cause and pathogenesis. So the inquiry of the nature of pain is helpful for differentiating the cause and pathogenesis of disease. Generally speaking, pain in new disease is serious, constant and unpalpable. Since it is caused by sthenic pathogenic factors, it is of sthenia syndrome. While pain in chronic disease is mild, intermittent and palpable. Since it is caused by asthenic pathogenic factors, it is of asthenia syndrome.

**Distending pain**: Pain accompanied by distension is caused by qi stagnation. If distending pain appears now and then over the chest, hypochondrium, epigastrium and abdomen, it is caused by qi stagnation. However, distending pain of the head and eyes is usually seen in hyperactivity of liver yang or upflaming of liver fire.

**Stabbing pain**: Stabbing pain is a sign of blood stasis, usually appearing over the chest, hypochondrium, epigastrium and abdomen due to blood stasis.

**Wandering pain**: Wandering pain means that the pain is not fixed and is migratory. Wandering pain of joints is usually seen in obstructive disease due to wind and dampness attack. Wandering pain over the chest, hypochondrium, epigastrium and abdomen is often caused by qi stagnation.

**Fixed pain**: Fixed pain over the chest, hypochondrium, epigastrium and abdomen is often caused by blood stasis. While fixed pain of the limbs and joints is usually seen in the obstructive disease caused by cold and dampness.

**Cold pain**: Cold pain means that the pain is

身作痛，多属虚证，因气血亏虚，形体失其荣养所致。

**2．问疼痛的性质**

由于导致疼痛的病因病机不同，因而疼痛的性质特点各异，故询问疼痛的性质特点，可辨疼痛的病因与病机。一般而言，凡新病疼痛，痛势较剧，持续不解，痛而拒按，为因实致痛，属实证；凡久病疼痛，痛势较轻，时痛时止，痛而喜按，为因虚致痛，属虚证。

（1）胀痛：是指疼痛且胀的感觉，是气滞作痛的特点。如胸、胁、脘、腹等处胀痛，时发时止，多属气滞之证。但是，头目胀痛，多见于肝阳上亢或肝火上炎的病证。

（2）刺痛：是指疼痛如针刺之状，是瘀血疼痛的特点之一。刺痛常见于胸、胁、脘、腹等处，均为血瘀所致。

（3）走窜痛：是指疼痛部位游走不定，或走窜攻痛。肢体关节疼痛而游走不定，多见于风湿痹病。胸胁脘腹部走窜攻痛，多因气滞所致。

（4）固定痛：是指痛处固定不移。胸、胁、脘、腹等处固定作痛，多属血瘀。肢体关节疼痛，固定不移，多为寒湿痹病。

（5）冷痛：是指疼痛且有

accompanied by cold sensation and preference for warmth, aggravated by cold and alleviated by warmth. Serious and unpalpable cold pain is caused by sthenic cold which obstructs the meridians; while mild cold pain with preference for warmth is caused by asthenic cold due to insufficient yangqi which fails to warm the body.

**Scorching pain:** Scorching pain refers to pain with burning sensation, preference for cold and aversion to heat. Serious and unpalpable scorching pain is of sthenic heat syndrome, usually caused by invasion of pathogenic fire into the meridians; mild scorching pain with preference for palpation is of asthenic heat syndrome, often caused by exuberant fire due to yin asthenia which impairs the viscera and meridians.

**Colic pain:** Colic pain means sharp pain, often caused by substantial pathogenic factors obstructing the activity of qi or coagulation of pathogenic cold obstructing qi activity. The examples are "angina pectoris" due to obstruction of the heart vessels, small abdominal or lumbar colic pain due to obstruction of the urinary duct by calculus, colic pain of the epigastrium and abdomen due to invasion of pathogenic cold into the stomach and intestines.

**Dull pain:** Dull pain means that the pain is not sharp and tolerable, but constant. Dull pain often appears over the head, chest, hypochondrium, epigastrium and abdomen due to consumption of essence and blood, or insufficiency of yangqi and endogenous exuberance of yin cold which deprives the body of warmth.

**Heavy pain:** heavy pain usually appears over the head, limbs and loins due to pathogenic dampness preventing qi from flowing. However, heavy pain of the head may also be caused by hyperactivity of liver yang and accumulation of qi and blood in the upper.

**Dragging pain:** Dragging pain usually involves other

冷感而喜暖，遇寒则甚，得温痛减。痛势较剧而拒按，多属实寒，因寒邪阻络所致；痛势较缓而喜按，多属虚寒，因阳气不足，失于温煦而致。

（6）灼痛：是指疼痛且有灼热之感，喜冷恶热。痛势较剧而拒按，多属实热证，常因火邪窜络所致；痛势较缓而喜按，多属虚热证，常因阴虚火旺，脏腑、经络失润所致。

（7）绞痛：是指疼痛剧烈如刀绞。多因有形实邪阻闭气机，或寒邪凝闭气机所致。如心脉痹阻引起的"真心痛"，结石阻塞尿路引起的小腹或腰部绞痛，寒邪内侵胃肠所致的脘腹绞痛等。

（8）隐痛：是指疼痛不甚剧烈，尚可忍耐，但绵绵不休。常见于头、胸、胁、脘、腹等部位，多由精血亏损，或阳气不足，阴寒内盛，机体失却充养温煦所致。

（9）重痛：是指疼痛并有沉重之感。常见于头部、四肢、腰等部位，多因湿邪困阻气机而致。但头部重痛亦可因肝阳上亢，气血上壅所致。

（10）掣痛：是指抽掣牵

parts of the body due to malnutrition of the meridians or obstruction of the meridians. Since the liver governs the tendons, dragging pain is often caused by liver disorder.

**Vacuous pain**: Vacuous pain usually appears over the head or small abdomen, often caused by consumption of qi, blood, essence and marrow as well as malnutrition of the viscera and meridians.

### 1.3.3.4 Inquiry of sleep

Sleep is in close relation with the circulation of weiqi and the conditions of yin and yang. Sleep is also, to a certain degree, in relation with the conditions of qi and blood as well as the functions of the heart and kidney. Inquiry of whether the sleep time is long or short, whether the sleep is easy or difficult and whether there is dream or not is helpful for understanding whether yin, yang, qi and blood are predominant or declined and whether the functions of the heart and kidney are strong or weak.

#### 1.3.3.4.1 Insomnia

Insomnia is characterized by difficulty in sleeping, or easiness to wake up and difficulty in falling asleep again, or shallow sleep or easiness to be disturbed in sleep, or even inability to sleep all night, usually accompanied by frequent dreaming. The pathogenesis of insomnia is the failure of yang to enter into yin and failure of spirit to maintain calm. The causes of insomnia are various and the nature of insomnia is either asthenic or sthenic. Asthenic syndrome of insomnia is usually caused by depletion of blood or exuberance of fire due to yin asthenia and malnutrition of heart spirit; while sthenic syndrome of insomnia is caused by exuberance of phlegmatic heat inside, or retention of food and disturbance of the heart spirit. If insomnia is accompanied by palpitation, dysphoria and

扯而痛，由一处而连及他处。也常称为引痛、彻痛。多因经脉失养或阻滞不通所致。由于肝主筋，所以掣痛多与肝病有关。

（11）空痛：是指疼痛且有空虚之感。一般多见于头部或小腹部，多由气血精髓亏虚，脏腑、经络失养所致。

### （四）问睡眠

睡眠与人体卫气的循行和阴阳的盛衰密切相关，同时，与气血的盛衰以及心、肾功能也有一定关系。通过询问睡眠时间的长短、入睡难易、有无多梦等情况，可了解阴阳气血的盛衰和心、肾等脏腑功能的强弱。

#### 1. 失眠

失眠又称不寐，或不得眠。以经常不易入睡，或睡而易醒不能再睡，或睡而不酣，时易惊醒，甚至彻夜不眠为特点，且常并见多梦。失眠的病机是阳不入阴，神不守舍。引起失眠的原因很多，概括起来其性质有虚实之分，虚证多由营血亏虚或阴虚火旺，心神失养所致；实证则因痰热内盛或食积内停，心神被扰所致。若失眠兼见心悸、心烦、舌红少苔者，为心阴不足；若不易入睡兼见心悸、腰膝酸软者，为

reddish tongue with scanty fur, it is caused by insufficiency of heart yin; if difficulty in sleeping is accompanied by palpitation and aching flaccidity of the loins and knees, it is caused by imbalance between the heart and the kidney; if easiness to wake up is accompanied by palpitation, reduced appetite, pale tongue and weak pulse, it is caused by asthenia of both the heart and the spleen; if insomnia is accompanied by profuse sputum and yellowish greasy fur, it is caused by phlegmatic heat disturbing the heart; if disturbed sleep is accompanied by dizziness, timidity, nausea and bitter taste in the mouth, it is caused by gallbladder depression and phlegm disturbance.

#### 1.3.3.4.2 Dreaminess

The cause and pathogenesis of dreaminess are almost the same as that of insomnia. Dreaminess and insomnia usually appear at the same time and can be treated with the same kind of drugs. Therefore, diagnosis of dreaminess can be made according to that of insomnia.

#### 1.3.3.4.3 Somnolence

Somnolence refers to sleepiness in both daytime and night. Somnolence is often seen in diseases of yang asthenia and yin predomination as well as internal exuberance of phlegmatic dampness. For example, somnolence accompanied by lassitude, heaviness of head and eyes, oppression and fullness of the chest and heaviness of the limbs is usually caused by internal exuberance of phlegmatic dampness and failure of lucid yang to rise; postcibal somnolence accompanied by spiritual lassitude, reduced appetite and indigestion is often due to insufficiency of gastrosplenic qi and failure of the spleen to transform and transport; spiritual lassitude and somnolence following serious disease are signs of healthy qi failing to be restored.

心肾不交；若睡后易醒兼见心悸、食少、舌淡、脉弱者，为心脾两虚；若失眠兼见痰多、舌苔黄腻者，为痰热扰心；若睡眠时时惊醒，兼见眩晕、胆怯、恶心、口苦者，为胆郁痰扰。

2. 多梦

多梦的病因病机与失眠大致相似，两者亦常常并见，治疗用药也类同。因此，诊断时可参考失眠，不再赘述。

3. 嗜睡

嗜睡是指患者不论昼夜，睡意很浓，经常不自主地入睡，或称多寐，多眠睡。嗜睡多见于阳虚阴盛、痰湿内盛的病证。如困倦嗜睡，伴头目昏沉、胸闷脘痞、肢体困重，多因痰湿内盛，清阳不升所致；饭后嗜睡，兼神疲倦怠、食少纳呆，多由中气不足，脾失健运所致；大病之后精神疲乏而嗜睡，是正气未复的表现。

Besides, the condition of extreme spiritual lassitude and half-sleep and half-waking is known as "tendency to sleep" caused by asthenia of heart and kidney yang and internal exuberance of yin cold. High fever and lethargy in exogenous febrile disease are signs of invasion of heat into the pericardium. Lethargy with snore and rale of sputum in the patient with apoplexy is caused by phlegm and stasis confusing the mind. This morbid state is actually coma.

### 1.3.3.5 Inquiry of diet and partiality

Inquiry of diet and partiality includes the inquiry of thirst, drinking of water, intake of food and partiality. The doctors should pay attention to inquiry of thirst, quantity of drinking of water, preference for cold or hot drinks, appetite, quantity of the intake of food, partiality and aversion of food, abnormal taste and odor in the mouth. Inquiry of diet can enable one to understand whether the disease is of heat or cold, or of asthenia or sthenia, whether the functions of the spleen, stomach, liver and the gallbladder are strong or weak, whether the body fluid is sufficient or insufficient and whether the distribution of the body fluid is normal or abnormal. Such information is very important in clinical diagnosis.

#### 1.3.3.5.1 Thirst and drinking of water

Thirst means the desire for water and drinking water means the quantity of water being drunk. Generally speaking, the patient with thirst likes to drink water and the patient without thirst does not want to drink water. But it is not always the case. In clinical diagnosis, doctors should try to inquire the characteristics of thirst and the accompanied symptoms. Whether there is thirst or not and whether the water drunk is more or less are the signs of the conditions of body fluid and its distribution.

**No thirst but desire for drinking of water**: This

此外,精神极度疲惫,似睡而非睡者,称"但欲寐",属心肾阳虚,阴寒内盛。外感热病出现高热昏睡,是热入心包之象;中风病人出现昏睡而有鼾声痰鸣者,为痰瘀蒙蔽心神,应属昏迷。

### (五)问饮食口味

问饮食口味包括对口渴、饮水、进食、口味等情况的询问。应注意询问有无口渴、饮水多少、喜冷喜热、有无食欲、食量的多少、食物的喜恶、口中有无异味感和气味等。询问饮食口味情况,可以了解病证的寒热虚实,脾胃肝胆等脏腑功能的盛衰,体内津液的盈亏及输布是否正常,对临床诊断有重要作用。

**1. 口渴与饮水**

口渴是指口干渴的感觉,饮水是指饮水量的多少,口渴与饮水,是密切相关的,一般口渴者多喜饮,口不渴者不欲饮,但有时也不尽然。临床注意询问口渴特点及其兼症。口渴与否,以及饮水量的多少,是体内津液的盛衰和输布状况的反映。

(1)口不渴饮:口不渴饮

condition indicates that the body fluid is not consumed, usually seen in cold syndrome, dampness syndrome or syndrome without evident dryness and heat.

**Thirst with desire to drink water:** This condition is a sign of the consumption of body fluid, often seen in dryness syndrome, heat syndrome; also seen in diseases marked by non-consumption of body fluid, dysfunction in qi transformation and failure of body fluid to flow to the upper part of the body. Extreme thirst with preference for cold drinks accompanied by reddish complexion, sweating and surging and rapid pulse is usually caused by exuberance of internal heat and serious consumption of body fluid; thirst with much drinking of water, accompanied by profuse urination, polyphagia and frequent hunger and gradual emaciation, is consumptive disease usually caused by excretion of fluid from the lower resulting from failure of kidney to transform body fluid due to asthenia; thirst with preference for hot drinks but without much drinking of water is usually due to internal retention of phlegmatic fluid, or asthenia of yangqi and failure of body fluid to flow to the upper part of the body; thirst without much drinking of water accompanied by dull fever, heaviness of body and head and oppression in the epigastrium is usually caused by internal stagnation of damp heat, failure of body fluid to transform qi and to flow to the upper part of the body; thirst without much drinking of water accompanied by worsened fever at night and crimson tongue is yingfen syndrome in seasonal febrile disease due to invasion of pathogenic factors into yingfen which steams ying yin to flow to the upper, leading to less thirst and less drinking of water; dry mouth with desire to gargle but not to drink water, accompanied by purplish ecchymosis on the tongue, is usually caused by internal retention of blood stasis, failure of qi to transform body fluid and failure of

为津液未伤，多见于寒证、湿证，或无明显燥热的病证。

（2）口渴欲饮：口渴欲饮，一般为津液损伤的表现，多见于燥证、热证；亦可见于津液未伤，气化不利，津不上承的病证。大渴喜冷饮，兼面赤、汗出、脉洪数，多属里热炽盛，津液大伤；口渴多饮，小便量多，多食易饥，体渐消瘦，为消渴病，多由肾虚水不化津而下泄所致；渴喜热饮，饮水不多，多为痰饮内停，或阳气虚弱，水津不能上承所致；口渴而不多饮，兼身热不扬、头身困重、脘闷，多因湿热内阻，津液气化不利，不能上承所致；口渴饮水不多，兼身热夜甚、舌红绛，为温病营分证，因邪入营分，蒸腾营阴上承，故口不甚渴而饮水不多；口干，但欲漱水不欲咽，兼见舌有紫斑，多因瘀血内阻，气不化津，津不上承所致。

body fluid to flow to the upper.

#### 1.3.3.5.2 Appetite and repast

Appetite refers to the demand for food and enjoyable sensation of taking food. Repast refers to the actual amount of food being taken. Inquiry of appetite and repast is significant in understanding the conditions of the spleen and stomach and the prognosis of disease.

**Reduced appetite**: The meaning of reduced appetite includes anorexia, poor appetite and indigestion which are similar to each other but are not totally the same. Reduced appetite in new disease is a sign of healthy qi fighting against pathogenic factors, indicating mild morbid condition and favourable prognosis. Reduced appetite in prolonged disease accompanied by spiritual lassitude, sallow complexion, pale tongue and weak pulse is usually caused by weakness of the stomach and spleen to transport and transform. Reduced appetite and indigestion accompanied by heaviness of head and body, distending oppression of the epigastrium and abdomen as well as yellowish greasy fur is often caused by failure of the spleen to transform and transport due to dampness encumbering the spleen.

**Anorexia**: Anorexia means aversion to food or to the smell of food, often due to retention of food in the stomach, accumulation of damp heat in the liver, gallbladder, spleen and stomach. Anorexia accompanied by acid regurgitation, distending fullness of the epigastrium and abdomen is usually caused by indigestion due to retention of food in the stomach and intestines. Disliking oil and greasy food accompanied by chest oppression, vomiting and distending fullness of the epigastrium and abdomen is often caused by indigestion due to retention of food in the stomach. Disliking greasy and rich diet accompanied by distending pain of the hypochondrium and bitter taste in

### 2. 食欲与食量

食欲是指进食的要求和对进食的欣快感觉，食量是指实际的进食量。询问患者的食欲与食量，对于判断脾胃功能的强弱以及疾病的预后转归，有重要意义。

（1）食欲减退：包括不欲食、纳少、纳呆，三者含义虽很相似，但又不能完全等同。新病食欲减退，一般是正气抗邪的保护性反应，病情较轻，预后良好。久病食欲减退，兼神疲倦怠、面色萎黄、舌淡脉虚，多属脾胃虚弱，运化无力。食少纳呆，伴头身困重、脘腹胀闷、舌苔黄腻，多属湿盛困脾，脾运不健。

（2）厌食：或称为恶食。是指厌恶食物，或恶闻食味。多为食积内停，或肝胆、脾胃湿热内蕴的病证。厌食，兼嗳气酸腐、脘腹胀满，多属食积停滞胃腑，受纳腐熟无权。厌食油腻，兼胸闷呕恶、脘腹胀满，多属脾胃湿热；厌食油腻厚味，伴胁肋胀痛、口苦，多属肝胆湿热内蕴。孕妇若有厌食反应，多因妊娠后冲脉之气上逆，影响胃之和降，一般属

the mouth is frequently caused by internal accumulation of damp heat in the liver and gallbladder. Anorexia in the gravida is due to upward adverse flow of qi in the thoroughfare vessel which prevents the stomach qi from descending. This is a normal phenomenon. However, serious morning sickness is a commonly encountered disease seen in the course of pregnancy.

**Polyphagia and frequent eating**: Polyphagia and frequent eating refers to hyperorexia and hunger not long after eating, usually caused by exuberance of stomach fire and fast digestion. Polyphagia and frequent eating with emaciation is often seen in consumptive disease.

**Excessive eating and frequent hunger with loose stool**: This condition indicates strong function of the stomach and weak function of the spleen. Strong function of the stomach causes fast digestion which leads to excessive eating and frequent hunger; while weakness of the spleen prevents it from performing normal transportation and transformation, therefore leading to loose stool.

**Hunger without desire to eat**: This means that the patient feels hungry, but has no desire to eat or just eats a little food. It is usually due to insufficiency of gastric yin and internal disturbance of asthenic fire. Internal disturbance of asthenic fire leads to easiness to feel hunger; while failure of asthenic yin to moisten the stomach leads to hypofunction of the stomach to digest food. That is why there is no desire to eat.

Besides, during the course of a disease, restoration of appetite and increase of appetite are the signs of gradual restoration of gastric qi and tendency of healing. While gradual anorexia and decrease of appetite are the signs that the functions of the stomach and the spleen gradually become weak, suggesting aggravation of disease. Sudden

正常现象。但严重者为妊娠恶阻,是妊娠期常见的疾病。

(3)消谷善饥:或称多食易饥。是指食欲过于旺盛,食后不久即感饥饿,进食量多,是胃火炽盛,腐熟太过所致。若消谷善饥,形体反见消瘦,多见于消渴病。

(4)多食易饥,大便溏泄:为胃强脾弱。胃强腐熟功能过亢,故多食易饥;脾弱则运化失职,故大便溏泄。

(5)饥不欲食:是指患者虽有饥饿感,但不欲食,或进食不多。多因胃阴不足,虚火内扰所致。虚火内扰则易于饥饿,阴虚胃失濡润,受纳腐熟水谷功能减退,故不欲食。

此外,在疾病过程中,食欲恢复,食量渐增,是胃气渐复,疾病向愈之兆。若食欲逐渐不振,食量渐减,是脾胃功能逐渐衰弱的表现,提示病情加重。久病或重病患者,原本

increase of appetite or even crapulence in the patients suffering from prolonged illness or serious disease with anorexia or even inability to eat is known as "exhaustion of the gastrosplenic qi".

#### 1.3.3.5.3 Taste

Taste refers to the sense in the mouth. Abnormal taste in the mouth may reflect the disorders of the spleen and stomach as well as other viscera.

**Bland taste in the mouth**: Bland taste means hypogeusesthesia due to asthenia of gastrosplenic qi or seen in cold syndrome.

**Bitter taste in the mouth**: This condition is usually seen in syndromes due to exuberance of liver and gallbladder fire and upward adverse flow of gallbladder qi.

**Sweet taste in the mouth**: Sweet and sticky sensation in the mouth is usually caused by damp heat resulting from excessive intake of rich and sweet food; or by accumulation of exogenous damp heat in the spleen and stomach, the confliction of which with the cereal qi steams the mouth. Sweet taste in the mouth with thin fur and drooling is often caused by failure of the spleen to transport due to asthenia.

**Sour taste in the mouth**: Sour taste in the mouth, or acid regurgitation, is usually caused by stagnation of liver qi attacking the stomach which leads to disharmony between the liver and the stomach and failure of the gastric qi to descend.

**Sour and putrid taste in the mouth**: Sour and putrid taste in the mouth is usually caused by failure of the stomach and the spleen to digest, transport and transform, or by retention of food which putrefies and leads to acid regurgitation.

**Puckery taste in the mouth**: Puckery taste in the mouth usually appears simultaneously with dryness of the

食少无味，甚至不能食，如突然欲食或暴食，称为"除中"，是脾胃之气将绝的征象。

### 3. 口味

口味是指口中的味觉。口味异常可反映脾胃及其他脏腑的病变。

（1）口淡：即味觉减退，口中淡而无味。多为脾胃气虚证，或见于寒证。

（2）口苦：即自觉口中有苦味。多见于肝胆火旺，胆气上逆所致。

（3）口甜：即自觉口中有甜味。口中甜而粘腻不爽；多因过食肥甘，滋生湿热；或外感湿热，蕴结于脾胃，与谷气相搏，上蒸于口所致。口甜，舌苔薄净，口中流涎，多因脾虚失运所致。

（4）口中泛酸：即自觉口中有酸味，或口泛酸水。多由肝气郁结，横逆犯胃，肝胃不和，胃失和降，而致泛吐酸水。

（5）口中酸馊：即自觉口中有酸馊味或酸腐味。多由胃脾腐熟运化失职，或食滞内停，化腐生酸，上泛于口所致。

（6）口涩：即口有涩味，如食生柿子的感觉，常与舌燥

tongue, usually caused by dryness and heat consuming body fluid, or by predominant yang heat in the viscera and upward adverse flow of qi and fire.

**Salty taste in the mouth:** Salty taste in the mouth is usually due to asthenia of the kidney and upward flow of cold water.

**Sticky and greasy taste in the mouth:** Sticky and greasy taste in the mouth is usually accompanied by thick and greasy tongue fur, often caused by retention and stagnation of phlegm and damp turbidity. Sticky and greasy taste in the mouth with sweetness is usually due to damp heat in the spleen and stomach; sticky and greasy taste in the mouth with bitterness is often due to damp heat in the liver and gallbladder; sticky and greasy taste in the mouth accompanied by chest oppression, epigastric fullness and profuse and sticky sputum is due to internal accumulation of damp phlegm.

### 1.3.3.6 Inquiry of urination and defecation

Defecation, though directly governed by the large intestine, is closely related to the functions of the spleen and the stomach to digest, transport and transform, the functions of the liver to convey and disperse, the functions of mingmen (vital gate) to warm and the functions of the lung to cleanse and descend. Urination, though directly governed by the bladder, is in close relation with the function of the kidney to transform qi, the functions of the spleen to transport, transform and distribute, the functions of the lung to cleanse and descend as well as the functions of the triple energizer to regulate water passage. So the inquiry of urination and defecation not only is a way to directly understand the digestive function of the body and metabolism of fluid, but also is an important evidence to determine whether the disease is cold or heat and asthenia or sthenia.

同时出现。多因燥热伤津,或脏腑阳热偏盛,气火上逆所致。

（7）口咸：即自觉口中有咸味。多与肾虚及寒水上泛有关。

（8）口粘腻：即口中粘腻不爽。常伴舌苔厚腻。多由痰饮、湿浊停滞所致。口粘腻而甜,多为脾胃湿热；口粘腻而苦,多属肝胆湿热。口中粘腻,伴胸闷脘痞,痰多而粘,则为痰湿内蕴。

### （六）问二便

大便的排泄,虽直接由大肠所司,但与脾胃的腐熟运化、肝的疏泄、命门的温煦、肺气的肃降等有密切关系。小便的排泄,虽直接由膀胱所主,亦与肾的气化、脾的运化转输、肺的肃降和三焦的通调等功能有关。故询问大小便状况,不仅可直接了解机体消化功能、水液代谢的情况,亦是判断疾病寒热虚实的重要依据。

Inquiry of urination and defecation includes the nature, colour, odor, time, quantity, frequency, sensation and the accompanied symptoms of urination and defecation. The following is detailed discussion on the nature, frequency and quantity of urine and stool as well as the sensation in urination and defecation.

### 1.3.3.6.1 Defecation

Normally a person defecates once a day and the stool is marked by normal shape, no dryness, proper dampness, smooth discharge, yellow colour without pus, mucus and indigested food.

**Abnormal frequency of defecation:**

Constipation: Constipation means difficulty in defecation or prolonged defecation or even no defecation in several days due to dry feces. Constipation is usually caused by retention of heat in the intestines, or consumption of body fluid, or insufficiency of yin blood which fails to moisten the intestines and causes excessive dryness in the intestines. Sometimes constipation also results from failure of asthenic qi to propel, or from obstruction of the intestines due to cold coagulation due to yang asthenia. Constipation, accompanied by abdominal fullness, distending pain and unpalpable pain, fever and yellowish dry fur, is due to heat retention in the intestines which prevents qi in the fu organ to flow; constipation, accompanied by cold pain in the abdomen, cold extremities, pale tongue with whitish fur and deep and slow pulse, is due to failure of asthenic yang to transport and internal exuberance of yin cold which stagnate the intestinal qi; constipation, accompanied by shortness of breath, spiritual lassitude, pale tongue and weak pulse, is usually due to qi asthenia; constipation, accompanied by pale complexion, lips and tongue, dizziness and palpitation, is usually due to blood asthenia; constipation, accompanied by dry mouth, red

问二便应注意询问大小便的性状、颜色、气味、时间、量的多少、排便次数、排便时的感觉以及兼有症状。这里着重介绍二便的性状、次数、便量、排便感等内容。

### 1. 大便

正常人一般每日大便一次，成形不燥，干湿适中，排便通畅，多呈黄色，便内无脓血、粘液及未消化的食物等。

（1）便次异常：

① 便秘：是指大便燥结难解，排便间隔时间延长，甚则多日不排便。多因热结肠道，或津液亏少，或阴血不足，肠失濡润，以致肠道燥化太过；亦有由于气虚推动无力，或阳虚寒凝，以致肠道气机滞塞。若大便秘结，腹满胀痛拒按，发热，舌苔焦黄，为热结肠道，腑气不通；便秘，腹中冷痛，手足不温，舌淡苔白，脉沉迟，为阳虚不运，阴寒内盛，凝滞肠道气机；便秘，短气，神疲乏力，舌淡脉虚，多属气虚；便秘，面、唇、舌淡白，眩晕心悸，多为血虚；便秘，口咽干燥，颧红，舌红少苔，多为阴虚津亏。

cheeks and reddish tongue with scanty fur, is usually due to consumption of body fluid resulting from yin asthenia.

Diarrhea: Diarrhea refers to loose, water-like and frequent discharge of stool, usually due to improper diet, exogenous pathogenic factors, insufficiency of yangqi in the body and emotional disorders which lead to failure of the spleen to transform and failure of the small intestine to separate lucidity from turbidity, resulting in direct downward flow of water and failure of the large intestine to transmit. Generally speaking, acute diarrhea in new disease is usually of sthenia syndrome; slow diarrhea in prolonged disease is often asthenia syndrome. Diarrhea, marked by fulminant discharge, yellowish chyle, abdominal pain and scorching heat sensation of the anus, is usually due to internal accumulation of damp heat in the intestines; clear loose stool mingled with water and feces, accompanied by abdominal pain, borborygmus and whitish greasy tongue fur, is caused by internal invasion of cold dampness which encumbers the spleen yang to separate lucidity from turbidity; diarrhea following abdominal pain, marked by putrid and foul odor like decayed eggs, alleviation of pain after diarrhea and acid regurgitation is usually due to retention of food which damages the spleen and stomach and leads to failure of the intestines to transmit; loose stool following dry feces, accompanied by abdominal distension, reduced appetite, worsened distension after meal and lassitude, is often caused by asthenia of splenic qi and failure of the spleen to transport and transform; diarrhea following abdominal pain before dawn, marked by loose stool with indigested food, is called morning diarrhea, usually resulting from decline of fire in mingmen (vital gate) and internal accumulation of yin cold and damp turbidity; diarrhea following abdominal pain and often worsened by emotional upsets is frequently caused by

② 泄泻：是指便质稀薄，甚至便稀如水样，便次增多。多因内伤饮食、感受外邪、机体阳气不足、情志失调等原因，导致脾失健运，小肠不能分别清浊，水液直趋于下，大肠传导失常所致。一般来说，新病泻急者，多属实证；病久泄缓者，多属虚证。若暴注下泄，泻下黄糜，腹痛，肛门灼热，多属肠腑湿热内蕴；大便清稀，水粪相杂，腹痛肠鸣，舌苔白腻，为寒湿内犯，脾阳被困，清浊不分；腹痛则泻，泻下腐臭如败卵，泻后痛减，嗳腐吞酸，多属食积内停，脾胃被伤，肠失传导；大便先干后稀，腹胀纳少，食后胀甚，倦怠乏力，多属脾气虚弱，运化无力；每于黎明前腹痛作泻，大便稀溏，完谷不化，称五更泻，多由肾虚命门火衰，阴寒湿浊内积所致；腹痛便泻，每因情志不遂而加重，多属肝脾不调。

imbalance between the liver and the spleen.

**Abnormal texture of stool**: Besides dryness and looseness, the texture of stool is also marked by indigested food, looseness complicated by dryness, feces with pus and blood and hematochezia, etc. Stool with indigested food is usually due to asthenia cold in the spleen and stomach or kidney asthenia and decline of fire in the vital gate. Occasional dry and loose stool is called looseness complicated by dryness usually caused by liver depression and spleen asthenia as well as imbalance between the liver and the spleen; loose stool following dry feces in defecation is often due to weakness of the spleen and the stomach; stool mingled with pus, blood and mucus is known as pus and blood stool, usually seen in dysentery due to accumulation of damp heat in the intestines which damages the meridians and coagulates qi and blood into pus blood; blood in stool is known as hematochezia which is divided into distal bleeding marked by bleeding following stool with purplish blood and proximal bleeding marked by bleeding preceding stool with fresh blood; loose stool with black colour like pitch is usually due to damage of the stomach collateral and retention of blood stasis.

**Abnormal sensation in defecation**: Scorching sensation of anus is often caused by downward migration of damp heat or invasion of stagnant heat in the large intestine into the rectum, usually seen in diarrhea due to heat or dysentery due to damp heat. Abdominal pain with frequent desire to defecate, prolapsing sensation of the anus and obstructive defecation is called tenesmus, often caused by internal retention of damp heat and obstruction of intestinal qi seen in dysentery. Difficult and astringent sensation in defecation accompanied by abdominal pain, distension and frequent flatus is caused by liver qi attacking the spleen and obstruction of intestinal qi; incontinence

（2）便质异常：便质异常除干燥、稀薄之外，还有完谷不化、溏结不调、脓血便、便血等。大便中经常夹有较多未消化的食物，称为完谷不化，多属脾胃虚寒或肾虚命门火衰。大便时干时稀，称为溏结不调，多因肝郁脾虚，肝脾不调所致；若大便先干后溏，多属脾胃虚弱。大便中夹有脓血粘液，称为脓血便，多见于痢疾，因湿热积滞交阻于肠，脉络受损，气血瘀滞而化为脓血所致。大便出血，称为便血，先便后血，便血紫暗，则为远血；先血后便，便血鲜红，则为近血。大便稀溏，色黑，状如柏油，多为胃络损伤，瘀血留滞。

（3）排便感觉异常：肛门灼热，多因大肠湿热下注，或大肠郁热下迫直肠所致，常见于热泻或湿热痢。腹痛窘迫，时时欲便，肛门重坠，便出不爽，称为里急后重，多因湿热内阻，肠道气滞所致，常见于痢疾。排便不畅，有滞涩难尽之感，称为排便不爽，兼腹痛、腹胀、矢气频频，为肝气犯脾，肠道气滞；大便不能控制，滑出不禁，甚则便出而不自

of stool is usually due to asthenia of the spleen and the kidney failing to control the anus, often seen in patients with weakness due to prolonged illness and senility or chronic diarrhea. Fulminant diarrhea in new disease or spontaneous defecation with coma is also due to failure of the anus to control, but is not necessarily caused by weakness of the spleen and kidney. Prolapsing sensation of the anus or even prolapse of the anus is known as qi prolapse of the anus which often occurs after overstrain or becomes worsened after defecation, usually due to prolapse of the gastrosplenic qi and seen in patients with chronic diarrhea or prolonged dysentery.

#### 1.3.3.6.2 Urination

Normally a person urinates 3 - 5 times in the daytime and 0 - 1 time in the night, and the volume of urine discharged in a day and a night is 1,200 - 2,000 ml. The frequency and volume of urine are affected by such factors like drinking of water, body temperature, sweating and age.

Urine is transformed from body fluid. The inquiry of urine is helpful for understanding the conditions of body fluid and qi transforming functions of the concerned viscera.

**Abnormal volume of urine**: Clear and profuse urine is usually due to asthenic cold syndrome. Profuse urine is also an important evidence in diagnosing other diseases, such as polyuria in diabetes marked by emaciation, polydipsia and polyphagia. Reduced urine is often caused by exuberant heat consuming body fluid, or sweating, vomiting and diarrhea which over consume body fluid and weakens the transformation source. Polyuria may also be caused by dysfunction of the lung, spleen and kidney as well as improper transformation of qi.

**Abnormal frequency of urine**: Frequent urination

means increased times of urination and frequent desire to urinate. Frequent urination marked by brownish scanty and urgent urine is usually due to damp heat in the lower energizer and failure of the bladder to transform qi; frequent urination with profuse discharge, clear colour and aggravation in the night is due to asthenic cold in the lower energizer resulting from insufficiency of the kidney yang, weakness of kidney qi and failure of the bladder to control. Obstructive urination with dripping discharge is known as retention of urine; blockage of urine is called obstruction in urination; the conditions of both are collectively called retention of urine. The retention of urine due to downward migration of damp heat or blood stasis and obstruction by calculus is of sthenia syndrome; while retention of urine due to insufficiency of kidney yang, improper transformation of qi or insufficiency of kidney yin and deficiency of body fluid is of asthenia syndrome.

**Abnormal sensation in urination**: Obstructive urination with pain, often accompanied by urgency and scorching heat, is often due to accumulation of damp heat in the bladder and improper function of the bladder to transform qi, usually seen in stranguria. Dripping urination is usually due to asthenia of kidney qi and failure of the kidney to manage closure and opening, often seen in old and weak patients with prolonged illness. Inability to control urine and spontaneous discharge of urine is called incontinence of urine, usually due to insufficiency of kidney qi and weakness of kidney function. If coma is accompanied by incontinence of urine, it is a critical pathological condition. Spontaneous urination during sleep is called enuresis, usually caused by insufficiency of kidney qi and failure of the bladder to control urine.

### 1.3.3.7 Inquiry of the head and face

Many of the symptoms appearing on the head and

face are also the manifestations of diseases of the whole body. The following is a brief discussion.

#### 1.3.3.7.1 Vertigo

Vertigo means that the patient subjectively feels that his or her body or the things in sight are swirling. Vertigo may be caused by up-flaming of liver fire, hyperactivity of liver yang, encumbrance and stagnation of phlegmatic dampness, insufficiency of qi and blood as well as deficiency of kidney essence. Vertigo, accompanied by distension, flushed cheeks and red eyes, dysphoria, susceptibility to anger, hypochondriac pain and bitter taste in the mouth, is due to up-flaming of liver fire; vertigo, accompanied by distending pain, tinnitus and aching flaccidity of loins and knees, is usually caused by hyperactivity of liver yang; vertigo, accompanied by head heaviness like being bound, chest oppression, nausea and heaviness of limbs, is often caused by internal retention of phlegmatic dampness and failure of lucid yang to rise; vertigo, accompanied by lassitude, shortness of breath, lethargy to speak, pale complexion, light colour of tongue and aggravation after overstrain, is due to qi asthenia and blood deficiency which fail to nourish the upper part; vertigo, accompanied by vacuity sensation, tinnitus, amnesia and aching flaccidity of the loins and knees, is frequently caused by asthenia of kidney essence.

#### 1.3.3.7.2 Tinnitus

Tinnitus refers to noise in the ears like chirping of a cicada or tidal sound. Fulminant tinnitus like the noise made by frog or tide, which cannot be reduced by pressure, is of sthenia syndrome due to exuberant liver and gallbladder fire to disturb the upper orifices; low and gradual tinnitus like chirping of a cicada,

也是全身疾病的表现。现择要介绍如下。

**1. 头晕**

是指自觉头部有晕眩感，病重者感觉自身或景物旋转，站立不稳。肝火上炎、肝阳上亢、痰湿困滞、气血不足、肾精亏虚等，均可导致头晕。若头晕而胀，面红目赤，烦躁易怒，胁痛口苦，多为肝火上炎；头晕胀痛，耳鸣，腰膝酸软，多为肝阳上亢；头晕且昏沉，如物裹缠，胸闷呕恶，肢体困重，多为痰湿内阻，清阳不升；头晕乏力，气短懒言，面白舌淡，每因劳累而加重，为气虚血少，不能上荣；头晕而空，耳鸣健忘，腰膝酸软，为肾精亏虚。

**2. 耳鸣**

是指自觉耳内鸣响，如闻蝉鸣，或如潮声。若突发耳鸣，声大如蛙聒，或如潮声，按之鸣声不减，属实证，多因肝胆火盛，上扰清窍所致；耳鸣渐起，声音细小，如闻蝉鸣，按

which can be reduced or stop by pressure, is of asthenia syndrome due to asthenia of liver and kidney yin and hyperactivity of liver yang, or deficiency of kidney essence and insufficiency of brain which fails to nourish the ears.

#### 1.3.3.7.3 Deafness and diplacusis

Deafness means hypoacusis or even anakusis. The condition of hypoacusis, unclear hearing and hearing of repeated voice is called diplacusis. Sudden deafness and diplacusis are of sthenia syndrome due to accumulation of adverse rise of fire from the liver and gallbladder in the ears, or due to phlegmatic turbidity and pathogenic wind obstructing the ears; deafness and diplacusis in prolonged disease are usually of asthenia syndrome due to failure of essence to replenish the upper orifices resulting from asthenia.

#### 1.3.3.7.4 Dizziness

Dizziness means swirling of things like sailing on a boat or flying of flies before the eyes. Dizziness and vertigo usually appear simultaneously. Dizziness caused by pathogenic wind and fire attacking the upper orifices or phlegmatic dampness confusing the upper orifices is of sthenia syndrome; dizziness due to prolapse of gastrosplenic qi and failure of lucid yang to rise, or due to insufficiency of the kidney and liver, deficiency of essence and blood as well as malnutrition of eyes, is of asthenia syndrome.

#### 1.3.3.7.5 Ocular itching

Ocular itching means itching sensation in the eyelid, canthus or pupil of the eyes. Ocular itching can be eased by light rubbing in mild case. However, it is unbearable in severe case which is usually of sthenia syndrome. Ocular itching like insects creeping with photophobia, tearing and scorching pain is caused by wind fire in the liver meridian

之鸣声减轻或暂止,属虚证,多因肝肾阴虚,肝阳上亢所致,或肾虚精亏,髓海不充,耳失所养而成。

**3. 耳聋、重听**

耳聋是指听力减退,甚至听觉丧失,不闻外声,亦称耳闭。若听力减退,听音不清,声音重复,则称为重听。耳聋、重听骤发,多属实证,常因肝胆火逆,上壅于耳,或痰浊上蒙,风邪上袭,闭塞耳窍所致;久病逐渐出现耳聋、重听,多属虚证,多因精气虚衰,不能上充清窍所致。

**4. 目眩**

是指视物旋转动荡,如乘舟车,或眼前如有蚊蝇飞动之感。目眩与头晕常相兼而作,称为眩晕。因风火上扰清窍,或痰湿上蒙清窍所致的,属实证;因中气下陷,清阳不升,或肝肾不足,精血亏虚,目窍失于充养所致的,属虚证。

**5. 目痒**

是指眼睑、眦内或目珠有痒感,轻者揉拭则止,重者极痒难忍。目痒甚者,多属实证。如两目痒如虫行,畏光流泪,并有灼热之感,是由肝经风火上扰所致。两目微痒而

disturbing the upper part. Mild itching and dryness of eyes is often due to malnutrition of the eyes caused by insufficiency of liver blood or asthenia of liver and kidney yin.

#### 1.3.3.7.6 Ocular pain

Ocular pain refers to pain of one or double eyes which is usually of sthenia syndrome. Unbearable ocular pain, accompanied by red eyes, bitter taste in the mouth, irritability and susceptibility to anger is usually caused by up-flaming of liver fire. Red and swelling pain of eyes with photophobia and ocular excreta is a sign of wind heat disturbing the upper, usually seen in fulminant conjunctivitis or epidemic conjunctivitis.

#### 1.3.3.7.7 Blurred vision, night blindness and diplopia

These three morbid conditions of eyes are of the signs of hypoacusis. Though characteristically different, they share the same cause and pathogenesis, usually caused by asthenia of the liver and kidney, insufficiency of essence and blood and malnutrition of eyes, often seen in the patients with chronic disease or the aged and weak people.

#### 1.3.3.7.8 Pain and numbness of the tongue

Pain of the tongue is usually due to exuberance of fire in the liver, heart and stomach that affects the tongue. Numbness of the tongue is caused either by blood asthenia, yin asthenia and malnutrition of the tongue, or by stagnation of phlegm in the tongue collaterals.

干涩,多是肝血不足或肝肾阴虚,目失所养所致。

#### 6．目痛

是指单目或两目疼痛。目痛多属实证。目痛难忍,兼面红目赤,口苦,烦躁易怒,为肝火上炎所致。目赤肿痛,羞明眵多,是风热上扰之象,多为暴发火眼或天行赤眼。

#### 7．目昏、雀盲、歧视

视物昏暗不明,模糊不清,称为目昏。白昼视力正常,每至黄昏视物不清,如雀之盲,称雀目、夜盲。歧视是指视一物成两物而不清。目昏、雀盲、歧视三者均为视力减退的病变,各有特点,其病因、病机基本相同,多因肝肾亏虚,精血不足,目失濡养所致。常见于久病或年老、体弱之人。

#### 8．舌痛、舌麻

舌痛多因心、肝、胃火热炽盛,上炎于舌所致。舌麻可由血虚、阴虚,舌体失养所致,亦可由痰阻舌络而成。

Besides, headache is also a commonly encountered symptom involving the head and face which is discussed in the part of inquiry of pain.

### 1.3.3.8 Inquiry of chest and abdomen

The chest and abdomen are the regions where viscera are located. The disorder of the viscera may bring about various symptoms over the chest and abdomen. The following is a brief discussion.

#### 1.3.3.8.1 Chest oppression

Chest oppression is a subjective sensation of discomfort and fullness in the chest, usually due to inhibited circulation of qi in the heart, lung and liver. Chest oppresioon with cough and profuse sputum is caused by internal retention of phlegmatic dampness and obstruction of pulmonary qi; chest oppression with palpitation and shortness of breath is usually caused by asthenia of heart and pulmonary qi and inaction of chest yang; chest oppression with frequent sighing is often due to emotional upsets and stagnation of liver qi.

#### 1.3.3.8.2 Palpitation

Palpitation refers to subjective feeling of quick heart beating and throbbing, usually a sign of the disorder of the heart or the heart spirit. If palpitation is caused by fright or palpitation accompanied by anxiety, it is called fright palpitation, indicating mild pathological condition. If the heart is beating rapidly from the chest to the navel with longer duration, it is called severe palpitation, indicating serious pathological condition and the further development of palpitation and fright palpitation. Fright disturbs qi, that is why the heart spirit is in disharmony; asthenia of blood leads to the malnutrition of the heart; yin asthenia leads to exuberance of fire which disturbs the heart spirit; asthenia of the heart qi and yang deprives the heart of

此外，头痛也是头面部常见症状，详见"问疼痛"。

### （八）问胸腹症状

胸腹是脏腑所居之处。内脏发生病变，可出现多种胸腹部的症状，现择要介绍如下。

#### 1. 胸闷

是指自觉胸中痞闷不舒。多因心、肺、肝等脏气机不畅所致。胸闷，喘咳痰多，多属痰湿内阻，肺气壅滞；胸闷，心悸气短，多属心肺气虚，胸阳不振；胸闷，喜太息，则多由情志不遂，肝气郁滞所致。

#### 2. 心悸、惊悸、怔忡

心悸是指经常自觉心跳、心慌、悸动不安，甚至不能自主。多是心神或心脏病变的反映。若因受惊而致心悸不已，或心悸易惊，恐惧不安，时发时止，病情较轻，称为惊悸。若心跳剧烈，上至心胸，下至脐腹，持续时间较长，病情较重，则称为怔忡，常是心悸、惊悸的进一步发展。惊则气乱，心神不安；营血亏虚，心神失养；阴虚火旺，内扰心神；心气阳虚，心失温养；脾肾阳虚，水

warmth and nutrition; asthenia of spleen and kidney yang results in hydraulic qi invading the heart; obstruction of the heart vessels prevents blood from free circulation. These conditions all may cause palpitation, fright palpitation and severe palpitation, which should be analyzed according to the characteristics of palpitation and the accompanied symptoms.

#### 1.3.3.8.3 Hypochondriac distension

Hypochondriac distension refers to distension and discomfort over one side or both sides of hypochondrium, usually seen in disorders of the liver and gallbladder. Hypochondriac distension with susceptibility to anger is usually due to emotional upsets and stagnation of liver qi; hypochondriac distension with bitter taste in the mouth and yellowish greasy tongue fur is usually caused by damp heat in the liver and gallbladder.

#### 1.3.3.8.4 Epigastric distress

Epigastric mass refers to subjective feeling of oppression and discomfort in the epigastrium, usually seen in disorders of the spleen and stomach. Epigastric mass with acid regurgitation is often due to retention of food in the stomach; epigastric oppression with reduced appetite and loose stool is usually caused by weakness of the spleen and stomach.

#### 1.3.3.8.5 Abdominal distension

Abdominal distension refers to subjective sensation of distension and discomfort in the abdomen, usually due to weakness of the spleen and stomach, internal retention of sthenic heat, mingling of qi, blood and fluid. Palpable abdominal distension is of asthenia syndrome due to weakness of the spleen and stomach which fail to perform the normal functions of transportation and transformation; unpalpable abdominal distension is of sthenia syndrome

气凌心；心脉痹阻，血行不畅等，均可导致心悸，或惊悸、怔忡。应根据心悸的轻重、特点和兼症具体分析。

3. 胁胀

是指自觉胁的一侧或两侧胀满不舒。多见于肝胆病变。胁胀易怒，多为情志不舒，肝气郁结；胁胀口苦，舌苔黄腻，多属肝胆湿热。

4. 脘痞

是指自觉胃脘部痞闷不舒。多见于脾胃病变。脘痞，嗳腐吞酸，多为食积停胃。脘痞，食少便溏，多属脾胃虚弱。

5. 腹胀

是指自觉腹部胀闷不舒，如物支撑。脾胃虚弱，食积胃肠，实热内结，气、血、水互积，均可以导致腹胀。腹胀喜按属虚，多因脾胃虚弱，失于健运所致；腹胀拒按属实，多因食积胃肠，或实热内结，阻塞气机而引起。鼓胀患者出现

due to retention of food in the stomach and intestines or internal retention of sthenic heat which obstructs the circulation of qi. Tympanites with abdominal distension accompanied by bulgy veins on the abdominal wall may be caused by various factors, such as qi stagnation, retention of dampness and blood stasis in the abdomen.

#### 1.3.3.8.6 Borborygmus

Borborygmus may be caused by asthenia of splenic qi, asthenia of splenic yang, internal exuberance of cold dampness, disharmony of the liver and spleen, internal retention of fluid and disharmony of qi activity in the intestines. Borborygmus with diarrhea, continuous abdominal pain and preference for warmth and pressure is caused by asthenia of splenic yang; borborygmus with abdominal prolpase sensation is caused by prolapse of gastrosplenic qi; borborygmus with thunderous noise, accompanied by abdominal cold pain, preference for warmth, cold body and limbs, is usually caused by invasion of exogenous cold and dampness; borborygmus with gurgling noise is caused by retention of fluid in the intestines.

Chest pain, hypochondriac pain, epigastric pain and abdominal pain are the commonly encountered symptoms over the chest and abdomen, which is discussed in detail in the part of inquiry of pain. Besides, attention should be paid to the inquiry of other subjective symptoms, such as nausea, heartburn and dysphoria, etc.

### 1.3.3.9 Inquiry of the symptoms over the loins, back and four limbs

Symptoms over the loins, back and four limbs can be seen in the regional disorders of the loins, back and four limbs, but also seen in the disorders of the viscera. The inquiry of such symptoms should be done together with the inquiry of other symptoms.

腹胀,可伴见腹壁青筋暴露,则因多种原因导致腹内气滞、湿阻、血瘀而成。

#### 6. 肠鸣

肠鸣可因脾气虚、脾阳虚、寒湿内盛、肝脾不调、水饮内停,肠腑气机不和所致。肠鸣泄泻,腹痛缠绵,喜温喜按,属脾阳虚;肠鸣腹部坠胀,为中虚气陷所致;肠鸣雷响,腹冷痛喜温,形寒肢冷,多为外受寒湿所致;肠鸣辘辘有声,为水饮流溢肠腑。

胸痛、胁痛、脘痛、腹痛等也是胸腹部的常见症状,详见"问疼痛"。此外,如恶心、嘈杂、心烦等,都是病人的自觉症状,也应注意询问。

### (九)问腰背四肢症状

腰背四肢的症状,既可见于腰背四肢局部病变,往往也是内脏病变的表现,应结合其他兼症具体分析。

#### 1.3.3.9.1 Cold sensation in the back
This condition is often caused by exogenous wind and cold or predomination of yin due to yang asthenia or internal retention of phlegm and fluid.

#### 1.3.3.9.2 Aching loins
Aching loins refers to continuous discomfort and aching sensation in the waist, usually caused by kidney asthenia, or by obstruction of wind and dampness, or by sprain due to overstrain.

#### 1.3.3.9.3 Heaviness of the body
Heaviness of the body refers to the heavy, aching and lethargic sensation of the body, usually accompanied by dropsy, often caused by failure of the lung to disperse and descend, failure of the triple energizer to dredge water passage, or failure of the spleen to transport and transform, or failure of the kidney to govern water, giving rise to retention of fluid in the muscles. Heaviness of the body with spiritual lassitude and dyspnea is usually caused by failure of the spleen to transform due to asthenia, encumbrance of the spleen by dampness and obstruction of yangqi.

#### 1.3.3.9.4 Numbness of the four limbs
Numbness of the four limbs refers to hypoesthesia or disappearance of the sense of muscles on the four limbs, usually caused by asthenia of qi and blood, or by internal disturbance of liver wind, or by damp phlegm and obstruction of the meridians and vessels by blood stagnation.

### 1.3.3.10 Inquiry of symptoms in andropathy
Symptoms in andropathy are also related to the diseases of the whole body. The following are some examples.

#### 1.3.3.10.1 Impotence
Impotence refers to inability to erect penis or weak erection of penis, usually due to insufficiency of

1. 背冷
是指自觉背部冷凉。多因外感风寒,或阳虚阴盛,或痰饮内伏所致。

2. 腰酸
是指腰部酸楚不适,绵绵不已。多因肾虚,或风湿痹阻,或劳损等所致。

3. 身重
是指身体有沉重酸困的感觉。身重伴有浮肿,多因肺失宣降,通调失职,或脾失健运,或肾不主水,水泛肌肤所致。身重困倦,神疲气短,多见于脾虚失运,脾为湿困,阳气被遏所致。

4. 四肢麻木
是指四肢肌肤感觉减退,甚至消失。亦称不仁。多因气血亏虚,或肝风内动,或湿痰、瘀血阻络所致。

(十)问男科症状
男科症状往往也与全身疾病有关。现举例介绍如下。

1. 阳痿
是指阴茎萎软不举,或举而不坚。多因肾阳不足,肾精

kidney yang, deficiency of kidney essence, asthenia of both the heart and the spleen, spreading of damp heat as well as liver depression and qi stagnation. Impotence, accompanied by aching weakness of the loins and knees, aversion to cold and cold limbs, is frequently caused by asthenia of kidney yang; impotence, accompanied by dizziness, tinnitus, amnesia and aching loins, is often caused by deficiency of kidney essence; impotence, accompanied by palpitation, shortness of breath, spontaneous sweating, spiritual lassitude and abdominal distension with reduced appetite, is usually due to asthenia of both the heart and the spleen; impotence, accompanied by dampness or itching and pain of the scrotum, is usually due to downward migration of damp heat; impotence, accompanied by restlessness, susceptibility to anger and depression, is often caused by depression of liver qi.

#### 1.3.3.10.2 Seminal emission

Seminal emission refers to frequent loss of sperm not caused by coitus. Seminal emission in dreams is called nocturnal emission; seminal emission without dream or even in conscious state is called spontaneous emission. Seminal emission is usually caused by yin asthenia and exuberant fire, hyperactivity of the kidney fire, or by weakness of kidney qi, or by invasion of damp heat, etc. Seminal emission, accompanied by easiness to erect, hectic fever and night sweating as well as aching weakness of the loins and knees, is usually caused by deficiency of kidney yin and hyperactivity of kidney fire; seminal emission, accompanied by aversion to cold, cold limbs and aching cold of loins and knees, is usually caused by decline of kidney yang and weakness of kidney qi; seminal emission, accompanied by dripping and painful urination and pudendal itching, is frequently due to invasion of damp heat.

亏虚，心脾两虚，湿热浸淫，肝郁气滞等所致。阳痿，伴腰膝酸软、畏寒肢冷，多属肾阳虚；伴眩晕耳鸣、健忘、腰酸，多属肾精亏虚；伴心悸气短、自汗神疲、食少腹胀，多属心脾两虚；伴阴囊潮湿或瘙痒、疼痛，多属湿热下注；伴烦躁易怒、郁闷不乐，多属肝气郁结。

**2. 遗精**

是指不因性生活而精液频繁遗泄。其中有梦而遗精，称为梦遗；无梦而遗精，甚至清醒时而遗精，称为滑泄。遗精多属阴虚火旺，相火妄动，亦有因肾气不固，或湿热浸淫等所致。遗精兼见阳强易举，潮热盗汗，腰膝酸软，多属肾阴亏虚，相火妄动；兼畏寒肢冷，腰膝酸冷，多属肾阳虚衰，肾气不固；兼小便淋漓涩痛，阴部瘙痒，则属湿热浸淫。

### 1.3.3.10.3 Immature ejaculation

It is usually caused by deficiency of kidney yang, weakness of kidneyqi, or abundancy of fire due to yin deficiency or stagnancy of liver qi. If it is complicated by aversion to cold, cold and aching sensation in the waist and knees, it frequently results from deficiency of kidney yang. If complicated by liability to erection, hectic fever, night sweating, ache and weakness of the waist and knees, it is usually caused by kidney yin deficiency and abnormal activity of xianghuo. If complicated by dribbing and painful urination and pudendal pruritus, it is often caused by spreading of damp-heat.

### 1.3.3.11 Inquiry of symptoms in gynecology

Physiologically, women are characterized by menstruation, leukorrhea, pregnancy and delivery of baby. Abnormal conditions of menstruation and leukorrhea are the commonly encountered diseases in women, which are also the signs of diseases of the whole body. Therefore, attention should be paid to menstruation, leukorrhea, pregnancy and delivery of baby in diagnosing diseases in women. The following is a brief introduction to the inquiry of menstruation and leukorrhea.

### 1.3.3.11.1 Inquiry of menstruation

Menstruation refers to regular uterine bleeding in women of childbearing age. Menstruation normally occurs once a month. Inquiry of menstruation includes the cycle, duration, quantity, colour, nature and accompanied symptoms of menstruation. If necessary, inquiry of menstruation should also include the date of the last menstruation, menarche or age of menopause.

**Abnormal menstrual cycle:** Normally menstruation occurs once every 28 days and lasts for 3 – 5 days. If

### 3. 早泄

是指在性生活过程中，精液过早泄出，以致不能进行正常的性生活。多因肾阳虚弱，肾气不固，或阴虚火旺，或肝郁气滞等所致。早泄兼畏寒肢冷、腰膝酸冷，多属肾阳虚衰，肾气不固；兼见阳强易举、潮热盗汗、腰膝酸软，多属肾阴亏虚，相火妄动；兼小便淋漓涩痛、阴部瘙痒，则属湿热浸淫。

### （十一）问妇科症状

妇女有月经、带下、妊娠、产育等生理特点。月经、带下等方面的异常，既是妇科的常见疾病，往往也是全身病变的反映。因此对妇女的问诊，还应注意月经、带下、妊娠、产育等情况。这里主要介绍问月经、问带下的主要内容。

### 1. 问月经

月经是指育龄妇女周期性的子宫出血。一般每月一次，信而有期。询问妇女月经情况，应注意了解月经周期、行经天数、经量、经色、经质及伴随症状。必要时须询问末次月经日期，初潮或停经年龄。

（1）经期异常：正常月经约28天行经一次，行经期一

menstruation occurs 8-9 days in advance, it is called advanced menstruation, usually due to qi asthenia and weakness of the thoroughfare and conception vessels, or due to yang exuberance and blood heat, liver depression and blood heat as well as yin asthenia and exuberant fire which disturb the thoroughfare and conception vessels and uterus. Menstruation occurs 8-9 days later than usual is called delayed menstruation, usually caused by asthenia of blood, or by decline of yangqi and lack of warmth and nourishment which deprive the uterus of having regular sufficient blood, or by qi stagnation and blood stasis which prevent blood and qi from free circulation in the thoroughfare and conception vessels, or by coagulation of cold and blood stasis which obstruct the thoroughfare and conception vessels.

**Abnormal amount of menstrual blood**: The menstrual blood discharged in healthy women is 50-100 ml, which may vary due to constitutional and age factors. Evident increase of menstrual blood with normal menstrual cycle is called polymenorrhea, usually caused by bleeding due to blood heat and damage of the thoroughfare and conception vessels, or by qi asthenia, weakness of the thoroughfare and conception vessels to control blood, or by blood stagnation in the uterus collateral and bleeding due to collateral impairment. Normal menstrual cycle with evident reduction of menstrual blood or even scanty menstruation is called oligomenorrhea, usually caused by deficiency of blood and insufficient blood in the uterus, or by asthenia of kidney qi, insufficiency of essence and blood and insufficient blood in the uterus, or by cold coagulation, blood stasis or obstruction of phlegmatic dampness.

**Abnormal colour and texture of menstrual blood**: The normal colour of menstrual blood is marked by red colour, proper in density and mixture of blood clot. Pale and thin menstrual blood is a sign of deficiency of blood. Brownish and thick menstrual blood indicates exuberant heat in blood. Purplish menstrual blood with blood clot accompanied by lower abdominal pain is caused by cold coagulation and blood stasis.

**Profuse and sudden uterine bleeding**: This morbid condition refers to irregular uterine bleeding, not in menstruation, or continuous uterine bleeding. Sudden and profuse uterine bleeding is called uterine burst of bleeding; gradual uterine bleeding with moderate amount of blood is called uterine leakage. Though different in occurrence, uterine burst and uterine leakage of blood usually appear simultaneously, usually caused by heat impairing the thoroughfare and conception vessels and driving blood to extravasate, or by asthenia of the spleen and kidney qi, weakness of the thoroughfare and conception vessels which fail to control menstrual blood, or by blood stagnation in the thoroughfare and conception vessels and extravasation of blood.

**Amenorrhea**: Amenorrhea refers to stoppage of menstruation for over three months without pregnancy at the age of menstruation or not during lactation in women. It is usually caused by qi asthenia and blood deficiency and vacuity of the thoroughfare vessel, or by asthenia of liver and kidney yin, failure of essence to transform blood and malnutrition of the thoroughfare and conception vessels, or by qi stagnation and blood stasis, or by cold coagulation and retention of phlegm as well as obstruction of the uterine vessels.

**Dysmenorrhea**: Dysmenorrhea refers to regular lower abdominal pain, during menstruation or before and after menstruation, or pain involving the waist and sacrum, or even unbearable pain. Regular lower abdominal distending pain or sharp pain during or before menstruation

为血少不荣。经色深红质稠，为血热内炽。经色紫暗，夹有血块，兼小腹冷痛，属寒凝血瘀。

（4）崩漏：不在行经期间，不规则阴道出血，或持续下血，淋漓不止者，称为崩漏。来势急，出血量多的称崩；来势缓，出血量少的称漏，或称漏下。崩与漏虽有缓急之分，但又常互相转化，相兼出现，故统称为崩漏。多因热伤冲任，迫血妄行；或脾肾气虚，冲任不固，不能约制经血；或瘀阻冲任，血不归经所致。

（5）闭经：在行经年龄，若停经超过3个月而又未受孕，或不在哺乳期月经不来潮，称为闭经。多因气虚血亏，血海空虚所致；或肝肾阴虚，精不化血，冲任失养；或气滞血瘀，或寒凝痰阻，胞脉不通而致。

（6）痛经：正值经期或行经前后，出现周期性小腹疼痛，或痛引腰骶，甚至剧痛不能忍受，称为痛经，又称经行腹痛。经前或经期小腹胀痛

is usually caused by qi stagnation and blood stasis; lower abdominal pain alleviated with warmth is often due to cold coagulation or yang asthenia; lower abdominal dull pain during or after menstruation is frequently brought about by asthenia of both qi and blood and malnutrition of the uterus.

#### 1.3.3.11.2 Inquiry of leukorrhea

Leukorrhea is a kind of milky, odorless and scanty vaginal excreta which can lubricate vagina. Inquiry of leukorrhea includes the quantity, colour, texture and odor of leukorrhea. If leukorrhea is profuse and dripping, or coloured and varying in texture, or foul in smell, it is a disease of leukorrhagia; whitish, thin and dripping leukorrhea is usually due to asthenia of spleen and kidney yang and downward migration of cold dampness; yellowish, sticky and foul leukorrhea is known as yellow leukorrhea due to downward migration of damp heat; whitish leukorrhea mingled with blood is called bloody and whitish leukorrhea, often causedy by stagnation of heat in the liver meridian, or by downward migration of damp heat.

### 1.3.3.12 Inquiry of symptoms in pediatrics

The infantile viscera are delicate, vigorous and fast in development. Under pathological conditions, they are characterized by quick onset, variability and susceptibility to both asthenia and sthenia. So, apart from the usual aspects included in inquiry, the inquiry of symptoms in pediatrics should be done according to the infantile physiological features.

Since diseases in the newborn (from the date of birth to one month after birth) are usually due to congenital factors or delivery conditions, inquiry should be emphasized on such aspects like the health condition of the mother

或刺痛,多属气滞血瘀。小腹冷痛,得温则减轻者,多属寒凝或阳虚。经期或经后小腹隐痛,多属气血两虚,胞脉失养所致。

**2. 问带下**

带下是指妇女阴道内的一种少量乳白色、无臭的分泌物,具有濡润前阴的作用。问带下,应注意带下的量、色、质和气味等情况。若带下过多,淋漓不断,或有色、质的改变,或有臭气,即为带下病。带下色白量多,质稀如涕,淋漓不绝,为白带,多属脾肾阳虚,寒湿下注。带下色黄,质粘臭秽,为黄带,多属湿热下注。白带中混有血液,赤白杂见,为赤白带,多因肝经郁热,或湿热下注所致。

**(十二)问儿科症状**

小儿脏腑娇嫩,生机蓬勃,发育迅速。一旦患病,具有发病较快,变化较多,易虚易实的特点,因此,问小儿病除一般问诊内容外,还需注意结合小儿的生理病理特点。

新生儿(出生后至1个月)的疾病多与先天因素或分娩情况有关,故应着重询问其母妊娠期及产育期的营养健

during pregnancy and delivery periods, the contraction of diseases, the drugs taken, whether there was dystocia and immature delivery.

Because infants (one month to 3 years old) develop fast physically and need much more nutrition than adults, while the functions of the infantile spleen and stomach are weak, improper feeding tends to lead to malnutrition, diarrhea, five kinds of flaccidity and five kinds of retardation. So the inquiry in pediatrics should emphasize the feeding, sitting, crawling, standing, walking, eruption of tooth and learning to speak so as to understand the postnatal nutrition and development of infants.

At 6 months to 5 years of age, infantile immunity obtained from the mother's body gradually disappears while the postnatal immunity has not fully developed. During this period, infants are susceptible to varicella and measles. Preventive inoculation can help infants reinforce their insistence against diseases and reduce contraction of diseases. The contraction of some epidemic diseases, such as measles, can develop immunity all life. Close contact with patients suffering from epidemic diseases, such as varicella, erysipelas and liver disease, may result in infection and contraction of the disease in infants. Therefore, the aspects of inquiry mentioned above can be used as important evidences in making diagnosis.

Since the infantile viscera are delicate and weak in resisting against diseases and regulating functions, they are very easy to be affected by changes of weather and environment and are likely to be attacked by six exogenous pathogenic factors, thus developing such symptoms like fever, aversion to cold, cough and sore-throat, etc. The infantile spleen and stomach are weak in digestion and are liable to dyspepsia, leading to such symptoms like vomiting and diarrhea. Since the infantile primordial spirit is

康状况,有何疾病,曾服何药,分娩时是否难产、早产等,以了解小儿的先天情况。

婴幼儿(1个月至3周岁)发育较快,需要的营养远较成人为多,而脾胃功能又较弱,如喂养不当,易患营养不良、腹泻以及五软、五迟等病。故应重点询问喂养方法及坐、爬、立、走、出牙、学语的情况,从而了解小儿后天营养状况和生长发育情况。

小儿6个月至5周岁之间,从母体获得的先天免疫力逐渐消失,而后天的免疫功能尚未形成,故易患水痘、麻疹等急性传染病。预防接种可帮助小儿增强抗病能力,以减少感染发病。患过某些传染病,如麻疹,常可获得终身免疫力,而不会再患此病。若密切接触传染病患者,如水痘、丹痧及某些肝病等,常可引起小儿感染发病。因此,询问上述情况,可作为诊断的重要依据。

小儿脏腑娇嫩,抗病力弱,调节功能低下,易受气候及环境影响,感受六淫之邪而患外感病,出现发热、恶寒、咳嗽、咽痛等症。小儿脾胃薄弱,消化力差,极易伤食,出现呕吐、泄泻等。婴幼儿元神稚嫩,易受惊吓,而见哭闹、惊叫等症。

not sufficiently developed, infants are very easy to be frighted, causing crying and frightened shouting.

Pediatrics was called dumb department in the ancient times. Direct inquiry of the infants is not only difficult, but also inaccurate. So the inquiry in the pediatrics should be done with the parents, or by inspection, olfaction and listening. The following is a brief introduction to the main points.

**Infantile crying**: Infantile crying refers to incessant crying in the daytime and night, or sudden crying with fright, even with changes of the facial expression, usually caused by asthenic cold in the spleen meridian, accumulation of heat in the heart meridian, weakness of the heart function and retention of food, etc.

**Five kinds of infantile stiffness**: Infantile stiffness refers to stiffness of the head and neck, hands, feet, chest and waist as well as muscles, usually due to congenital defects, coagulation of cold and wind as well as predominant liver subjugating the spleen.

**Five kinds of infantile retardation**: Five kinds of infantile retardation refer to retardation in standing, walking, growth of hair, eruption of teeth and speech, usually caused by congenital defects, asthenia of kidney essence, or postnatal malnutrition and weakness of the spleen and stomach, etc.

**Five kinds of infantile flaccidity**: Five kinds of infantile flaccidity refers to the flaccidity of head and neck, mouth, hands, feet and muscles, often resulting from congenital defects or postnatal malnutrition, or improper feeding after illness and asthenia of qi and blood.

### 1.3.4 Inquiry of anamnesis

Anamnesis, also known as history of past illness,

儿科古称"哑科"。直接向患儿询问其患病后的症状，不仅较困难，而且也不一定准确。常常依靠间接询问其亲属，或借助于望诊、闻诊。现将儿科常见症状择要介绍如下。

1. 小儿啼哭

是指小儿昼夜啼哭不休，或突然惊叫啼哭，甚则面色变异。多因脾经虚寒，心经积热，心虚禀弱，伤食积滞等所致。

2. 小儿五硬

是指小儿头项硬、手硬、足硬、胸腰硬、肌肉硬，难以屈伸。多因先天禀赋不足，风寒凝结，肝旺乘脾所致。

3. 小儿五迟

是指小儿立迟、行迟、发迟、齿迟、语迟等生长发育迟缓的表现。多因先天禀赋不足，肾元亏损，或后天失调，脾胃虚弱所致。

4. 小儿五软

是指小儿头项软、口软、手软、足软、肌肉软。多因先天不足或后天喂养失当，或病后失调，气血虚弱所致。

## 四、问既往史

既往史又称过去病史，主

mainly includes the constitution of the patient and previous contraction of diseases.

#### 1.3.4.1 Inquiry of past physique

The past physique of the patient may be relevant to the present illness. For example, if the physique is usually strong, the disease is often sthenic; if the physique is usually weak, the disease is often asthenic; if yin is often in asthenia, the disease is usually of heat syndrome due to the susceptibility to the invasion of pathogenic febrile and dry factors; if yang is often in asthenia, the disease is usually of cold syndrome due to susceptibility to the invasion of cold and dampness.

#### 1.3.4.2 Inquiry of previous illness

Inquiry of previous illness includes the category, relapse, present treatment, present manifestations and relation with the present illness.

Besides, inquiry of previous illness should also includes contraction of dysentery, malaria, diphtheria and measles, inoculation, allergy and operation.

### 1.3.5 Inquiry of family history

Inquiry of family history includes the health of the parents, brothers and sisters, spouse and children who are living together with the patient. If necessary, inquiry of family history should also include the cause of the death of the directly-related family members. Because some hereditary diseases are closely related to ties of blood; some epidemic diseases, such as pulmonary tuberculosis are caused by contact in daily life.

要包括患者平素体质状况,以及过去曾患疾病的情况。

#### (一)问既往体质状况

患者的以往体质状况,可能与其现在所患疾病有一定关系,故需注意询问。如素体健壮,病多实证;素体虚弱,病多虚证;素体阴虚,易感温燥之邪,病多热证;素体阳虚,易受寒湿之邪,病多寒证。

#### (二)问既往患病情况

问既往患病情况,需注意询问患者过去曾患何种其他疾病,是否复发过,现在是否痊愈,现在还有何病状表现,与现在所患疾病有无联系等。

此外,是否患过如痢疾、疟疾、白喉、麻疹等传染病,是否接受过何种预防接种,有无药物或其他物品的过敏史,作过何种手术治疗等,都应加以询问。

### 五、问家族史

问家族史包括询问与患者长期生活相处的父母、兄弟姐妹、配偶、子女等及接触密切的人的健康和患病情况,必要时还需询问直系亲属的死亡原因。这是由于某些遗传性疾病,常与血缘关系密切;有些传染病,如肺痨等,与生

## 1.4 Pulse-taking and palpation

Pulse-taking means that the doctor use his or her hand to palpate, feel and press certain part of the patient's body to diagnose disease, including taking pulse and palpation.

### 1.4.1 Pulse-taking

Pulse-taking means that the doctor uses his or her hand to press certain part of the patient's pulse to examine the conditions of the pulse and diagnose disease.

The pulse conditions are closely related to the viscera and qi and blood. The heart is connected with the vessels; the heart qi propels blood to circulate in the vessels all through the body, that is, from viscera to all the limbs and joints of the body. Such an incessant circulation leads to the pulsation of the vessels. Besides, the heart exerts certain effect on the production of blood. The lung governs qi and "connects with all vessels". The distribution of pulmonary qi helps the heart propel blood. The spleen and the stomach are "the source of qi and blood"; the spleen direct blood to circulate in the vessels. The liver governs conveyance and coursing, regulating the activity of qi through the body and promoting blood circulation; the liver also stores blood and regulates the flow of blood. The kidney stores essence; the kidney essence, qi, yin and yang constitute the source of yin and yang in the other viscera. Since essence can transform into blood, the exuberance of kidney essence ensures sufficiency of blood in

活接触有关。

## 第四节 切诊

切诊,是医者用手在患者体表的一定部位进行触、摸、按、压,以了解病情的一种诊察方法。包括脉诊和按诊两部分。

### 一、脉诊

脉诊是医者用手指触按患者一定部位的脉搏,以体察脉象、了解病情的一种诊病方法。

脉象的形成与诸脏腑、气血的功能密切相关。心脏与血脉紧密相连;心气心阳推动血液通过脉管而布运全身,内入五脏六腑,外至四肢百骸,运行不息,并导致脉搏的跳动。另外,心对于血液的生成具有一定的作用。肺主气,"肺朝百脉",肺气的敷布是心对血液推动作用的辅助。脾胃为"气血生化之源";脾又主统血,血液在脉管内流行不致逸出脉外,有赖脾气的统摄。肝主疏泄,对于全身气机的调畅起着重要的作用,并促进血液营运不休;肝又主藏血,能调节血流量。肾藏精,肾中精、气、阴、阳是人体各脏腑

1 Diagnostic methods

the body.

The vessels are the organs to hold blood and the pathways for qi and blood to circulate. The conditions and circulation of qi and blood as well as the tension, elasticity and thickness of the vessels directly influence the states of pulse.

Besides, the functional activities of all viscera as well as the conditions and circulation of qi, blood and body fluid in them all can directly or indirectly affect the states of pulse. When pathogenic factors invade the body and cause dysfunction of the viscera, qi, blood and body fluid, the conditions of pulse will change accordingly. Therefore, examination of pulse can help diagnosis of diseases.

### 1.4.1.1 Regions and methods for taking pulse
#### 1.4.1.1.1 Regions for taking pulse

Cunkou is the usual region selected to take pulse. Cunkou, also known as "qikou" (opening of qi) or "maikou" (opening of pulse), refers to pulsation of radial artery on the wrist.

Cunkou is located on the pulsation of the lung meridian where qi and blood in the lung meridian flows by. Besides, qi and blood from all viscera circulates through the lung and converges over cunkou. The lung meridian starts from the middle energizer and converges with the spleen meridian. Since the spleen and the stomach are the sources of qi and blood and function as postnatal base of life, cunkou can reflect the conditions of the gastric qi. On the other hand, the lung meridian is the meridian from where all the other meridians begin and end their circulation, because the circulation of qi and blood in all the twelve meridians starts from and ends at the lung meridian, finally converging over cunkou. That is why

阴、阳的根本；且精可以化生血，肾精充足，则血有所充。

脉为血之府，是气血运行的通道。气血的盛衰和运行状况，脉管的紧张度、弹性、粗细等，直接对脉象产生影响。

因此，人体各脏腑功能活动及气、血、津液的盛衰和运行状况，都可以直接或间接地对脉象产生影响。当致病因素作用于人体，引起脏腑、气、血、津液的功能失常，脉象亦随之发生改变。故通过诊脉可以诊察疾病。

### （一）诊脉的部位与方法
#### 1. 诊脉的部位

现在通行的是诊寸口。寸口又称"气口"或"脉口"，即手腕后桡动脉搏动处。

寸口位于手太阴肺经的脉动应手之处，是肺经气血流通之处，同时，全身脏腑气血循行都要流经肺而大会于寸口；手太阴肺经起于中焦，与足太阴脾经相通，而脾胃为气血生化之源，后天之本，故寸口可以反映胃气的强弱。另外，肺经为十二经之始终，十二经气血循环流注起于肺经又终止于肺经，复会于寸口。所以，全身脏腑、气血、经络的盛衰，功能的强弱，都可以反

cunkou can reflect the conditions of all viscera, qi, blood and meridians in the body.

Pulse over cunkou is divided into three parts: cun, guan and chi. The part slightly below the styloid process of radius is guan pulse, the part anterior the guan pulse is the cun pulse, and the part posterior the guan pulse is the chi pulse (see Fig. 3). Both hands have three divisions of pulse, i.e. cun pulse, guan pulse and chi pulse. So altogether there are six divisions of pulse.

映于寸口。

寸口诊法将寸口脉分为寸、关、尺三部。以掌后高骨（桡骨茎突）稍内下方的部位为"关"，关前（腕端）为"寸"，关后（肘端）为"尺"（见图3）。左右两手各有寸、关、尺三部，共六部脉。

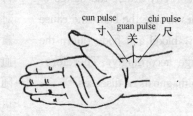

Fig. 3  Divisions of pulse over cunkou
图3  寸口脉寸关尺部位图

Clinically the correspondence of cunkou pulse and the viscera is decided according to the description in Neijing (Canon of Medicine), that is the upper pulse (cun pulse) corresponds to the upper part of the body and the lower pulse (chi pulse) corresponds to the lower part of the body:

The left cun pulse and the corresponding viscera: the heart and tanzhong (the part between the breasts).

The right cun pulse and the corresponding viscera: the lung and the thorax.

The left guan pulse and the corresponding viscera: the liver and the gallbladder.

The right guan pulse and the corresponding viscera: the spleen and the stomach.

The chi pulse and the corresponding viscera: the kidney and the lower abdomen.

关于寸口脉三部分候脏腑，目前临床所用多根据《内经》"上竟上"、"下竟下"的原则，即上（寸脉）以候上（身躯上部），下（尺脉）以候下（身躯下部），具体内容如下：

左寸候：心与膻中；

右寸候：肺与胸中。

左关候：肝与胆；

右关候：脾与胃。

左尺候：肾与小腹；

The right chi pulse and the corresponding viscera: the kidney and the lower abdomen.

Such a theory about the relationship between the cunkou pulse and the corresponding viscera is significant in clinical diagnosis. However, the application should be flexible and based on the synthetic analysis of the data obtained from the four diagnostic methods.

#### 1.4.1.1.2 The methods for taking pulse

The following points should be borne in mind in taking pulse.

**Time**: Early morning is the ideal time for taking pulse because the conditions of the pulse are not affected by food and other activities. However, this requirement is difficult to fill in clinical practice. To ensure accurate pulse taking, the patient should rest for a while to tranquilize the heart and breath before the taking of pulse. The pulse should be taken at least for one minute each time in order to correctly examine the conditions of the pulse.

**Normal and calm breath**: Normal and calm breath means that the doctor keeps his or her own breath quiet to examine the pulse of the patient and calculate the beat of the pulse according to his or her own cycle of exhalation and inhalation. Healthy people breathe 16 - 18 times one minute under normal conditions. And the pulse beats 4 - 5 times in a cycle of exhalation and inhalation, about 60 - 90 beats per minute.

**Posture**: The patient sits erect or lies in supination and the forearms stretches out naturally to the level of the heart. The wrist is put straight, the palm turns over and the fingers are relaxed to extend the cunkou region and enable qi and blood to flow freely.

**Arrangement of fingers**: The three fingers of the

右尺候：肾与小腹。

这种寸口脉三部分候脏腑的理论具有一定的临床参考价值，但临床运用时切不可机械刻板，必须四诊合参，综合分析，才能得出比较正确的诊断。

**2. 切脉的方法**

切脉的方法，主要应掌握以下几点。

（1）时间：清晨，脉象尚未受饮食、活动等因素的影响，是诊脉的理想时间。但是，临床上一般很难做到。只是要求患者在诊脉前休息片刻，使之心静气宁，也可以诊得较准确的脉象。每次诊脉时间至少在1分钟以上，以准确体察脉象。

（2）平息：诊脉时医者要调匀自己的呼吸，静心凝神，体察脉象，并以自己的一呼一吸的时间来计算患者的脉率。正常人平静状态下呼吸每分钟16～18次，每次呼吸脉动4次，间或5次，即一息四五至，约60～90次/分钟。

（3）姿势：患者正坐或仰卧，前臂自然平展，与心脏同一水平。直腕、仰掌，手指放松，使寸口部充分伸展，气血流畅。

（4）布指：医者三指平

doctor are put at the same level and slightly arched to press the pulse with the belly of the fingers. The middle finger presses on the guan pulse, the index finger presses on the region anterior the guan pulse (distal to the heart region), the ring finger on the chi pulse posterior to the guan pulse (proximal to the heart region). The arrangement of the fingers is made according to the conditions of the patient's arm. In diagnosing diseases in children, "one finger is used to press just the guan pulse". It is unnecessary to divide the pulse into three parts in this case.

**General pressure and single pressure**: General pressure means to press the pulse with three fingers to distinguish the conditions of cun, guan and chi pulses on both hands. Single pressure means to examine the pulse on one hand with just one finger to differentiate the states of cun, guan and chi pulses. Clinically these two methods are used according to the pathological conditions in question.

**Lifting, pressing and searching**: Lifting, pressing and searching refer to flexible pressure of pulse in order to distinguish the conditions of pulse. Light pressure means "lifting"; heavy pressure means "pressing"; and mobile moderate pressure means "searching" which is used to look for the most obvious region of the pulse. In the procedure of diagnosis, doctors should pay attention to the use of these three methods to distinguish the variations of pulse.

**Examining the conditions of pulse**: The conditions of the pulse refers to the sensation of pulse felt by the fingers. The examination of pulse conditions means to distinguish the features of pulse according to the position of pulse, the rhythm of pulse, the shape of pulse and the

齐,手指略呈弓形,以指目按脉脊。中指定关,食指在关前（远心端）定寸,无名指在关后（近心端）定尺,布指的疏密需与患者手臂长短相适应。小儿可采用"一指定关法"而不细分三部。

（5）总按与单按：总按是三指同时切脉,从总体上辨别寸、关、尺三部和左右两手的脉象。单按是用一个手指诊察一部脉象,分别了解寸、关、尺各部的脉象。临床上可根据需要,总按与单按结合运用。

（6）举按寻：这是诊脉时运用指力的轻重和挪移,以探求脉象的手法。用轻指力诊脉为"举",又称"浮取"或"轻取";用重指力诊脉为"按",又称"沉取"或"重按";用力适中,不轻不重,或左右推寻挪移,以寻找脉象应指最明显的部位,为"寻"。诊脉时必须注意体会举、按、寻不同指力下的脉象变化。

（7）体察脉象：脉象是指脉动应指的形象。体察脉象就是分别从脉位（脉搏显现部位的浮沉和长短）、至数（脉搏频率的快慢和节律）、形态（脉

strength of pulse.

搏的幅度、充盈度、紧张度、流利度)、气势(脉搏应指的强弱)等方面辨别脉动应指的指感特征。

### 1.4.1.2 Normal pulse

Normal pulse refers to the pulse conditions of the healthy people.

#### 1.4.1.2.1 The shape of the normal pulse

The normal pulse is neither floating nor sunken, neither fast nor slow, sensible with moderate pressure, usually beating 4 - 5 times in a cycle of breath (about 60 - 90 beats per minute), gentle in sensation, powerful in rebounding, moderate in size, regular in beating and varying with physical activities and environmental changes.

#### 1.4.1.2.2 The characteristics of the normal pulse

The normal pulse is marked by gastric qi, spirit and root. Gastric qi means that the pulse is located at the middle, neither floating nor sunken, regular in beating, moderate in size, gentle in sensation and floating. Spirit means that the pulse is soft, powerful and rhythmic. Root means that the chi pulse is powerful and constantly beating under heavy pressure.

Gastric qi, spirit and root are three basic features of the normal pulse which complement each other and cannot be separated. Simultaneous appearance of the three reflects strong functions of the viscera and sufficiency of qi and blood.

(二) 常脉

常脉是指人体在健康状况下的脉象,又称为平脉。

1. 常脉的形象

不浮不沉,中取即得,不快不慢,一息四五至(60~90次/分钟),从容和缓,应指有力,不大不小,节律均匀无歇止,并随生理活动和外在环境的变化而有一定的变化。

2. 常脉的特点

常脉具有胃、神、根三个特点。有胃,即脉有胃气。是指脉位居中,不浮不沉;脉律调匀,不快不慢;脉力充盈,不大不小;脉势和缓,从容流利。其中最主要的是和缓、从容、流利。有神,是指脉象应指柔和有力,节律整齐。有根,是指脉象尺部沉取有力,应指不绝。

总之,胃、神、根是从不同侧面强调正常脉象的特点,三者相互补充而不能截然分开。若三者兼备,则反映机体脏腑功能强健,气血充盈。

#### 1.4.1.2.3 Main factors to affect the normal pulse

The normal pulse may vary with physiological and psychological factors in the human body and the environmental factors outside.

**Age, sex and building of the body:** The pulse is usually small and fast in children, smooth and slippery in young people, taut and hard in old people, moderate and powerful in men, soft and thin in women, slippery and fast in gravida, sunken and thin or soft and thin in obese people, floating and large in lean people, long in tall people and short in small people.

**Daily life and psychological factors:** The pulse appears slippery, fast and powerful after movement, eating and drinking of wine, weak with hunger, taut in anger and irregular in fright.

**Seasonal, alternation of day and night and geographical factors:** The pulse appears slightly taut in spring, slightly full in summer, slightly floating in autumn and slightly sunken in winter; slightly floating and powerful in the daytime and slightly sunken, thin and slow in night; sunken and energetic among the people in the north and soft among the people in the south.

Besides, the changes of the anatomic position of the radial artery may shift the pulse normally at the cunkou region to the dorsum of the hand from the chi region, known as oblique flying pulse. The pulse, shifted to the back of the cunkou region, is called ectopic radial pulse.

All the factors above mentioned may affect the conditions of the pulse. However, if the pulse still keeps gastric qi, spirit and root, it is still the normal pulse.

### 3. 影响常脉的主要因素

在人体内外环境各种因素的影响下,常脉可以出现一定范围内的变化。

(1)年龄、性别、形体等因素:如儿童脉多小数,青年脉多平滑,老人脉多弦硬;男子脉多缓而有力,女子脉多濡细而略数,妊妇脉多滑数;肥胖者脉沉细或濡细,消瘦者脉较浮大,身材高大者脉位较长,身材矮小者脉位较短。

(2)生活起居、精神状态等因素:如运动、饱餐、酒后脉多滑数有力,饥饿时脉多软弱;怒时脉弦,惊时脉动无序。

(3)四季气候、昼夜、地理环境等因素:如春季脉微弦,夏季脉微钩(洪),秋季脉微毛(浮),冬季脉微石(沉);昼日脉偏浮而有力,夜间脉偏沉而细缓;北方人脉多沉实,南方人脉多软弱。

此外,由于桡动脉解剖位置的变异,寸口不见脉象搏动,而由尺部斜向手背,称为斜飞脉;若脉象搏动出现于寸口的背侧,则称为反关脉。

上述各种因素都可能导致脉象出现相应的变化,但只要有胃、有神、有根,均属常脉范围,临床应与病脉相鉴别。

### 1.4.1.3 Morbid pulse

The pulse in a morbid condition is called morbid pulse, in which the manifestations of pulse conditions are either the changes of the position of the pulse, or the difference in rhythm, or variation in morphology, or changes in strength. Sometimes morbid pulse may show difference in various aspects, such as the position, rhythm and strength of the pulse. The following is a specific discussion:

#### 1.4.1.3.1 Floating pulse

Features: Sensible under light pressure, weak and constant beating under heavy pressure. Floating pulse is marked by superficial beating.

Clinical significance: Floating pulse Indicates external syndrome, floating and powerful pulse signifying external sthenia syndrome while floating and weak pulse manifesting external asthenia syndrome. Floating pulse can also be seen in internal asthenia syndrome due to consumption of essence and blood in chronic disease and external floating of asthenic yang.

#### 1.4.1.3.2 Scattered pulse

Features: Rootless, arrhythmic and disappearing under pressure.

Clinical significance: Indicating depletion of primordial qi, visceral essence at the verge to exhaust and external floating of asthenic yang.

#### 1.4.1.3.3 Hollow pulse

Features: Floating, large and hollow like the leaf of scallion.

## （三）病脉

在疾病过程中出现的异常脉象,即为病脉。在病脉中,有些脉象主要表现为脉位的变化,或表现出至数的不同,或表现为形态各异,或是脉的气势强弱不同；有些脉象则在位、数、形、势等方面同时具有多个方面的变化。现将常见病脉分别介绍如下：

**1. 浮脉**

脉象特征:轻取即得,按之稍弱而不空。浮脉以脉动显现部位浅表为特点。

临床意义:多主表证,浮而有力为表实,浮而无力为表虚。亦可见于久病精血亏虚,虚阳外越的里虚证。

**2. 散脉**

脉象特征:浮散无根,至数不清,按之消失。散脉以脉位浮取应指,稍按则无,脉势软弱,脉律不齐,至数模糊不清为特点。

临床意义:主元气耗散,脏腑精气将绝,虚阳外越。

**3. 芤脉**

脉象特征:浮大中空,如按葱管。芤脉以脉位浮,脉形大而势软,按之空豁为特点。

Clinical significance: Indicating loss of blood and impairment of yin.

#### 1.4.1.3.4　Sunken pulse
Features: Sensible only under heavy pressure.

Clinical significance: Indicating internal syndrome. Sunken and powerful pulse signifies sthenia internal syndrome, while sunken and weak pulse shows asthenic internal syndrome.

#### 1.4.1.3.5　Slow pulse
Features: No more than 4 beats in a cycle of breath (<60/min).

Clinical significance: Indicating cold syndrome. Slow and powerful pulse signifies sthenia cold syndrome, while slow and weak pulse shows asthenic cold syndrome. Such a pulse condition is also seen in internal sthenia heat syndrome due to internal accumulation of pathogenic heat. Athletes with slow pulse are in a normal condition.

#### 1.4.1.3.6　Moderate pulse
Features: The pulse is moderate and powerful, beating 4 times in a cycle of breath; or moderate and sluggish, beating 4 times in a cycle of breath (60 - 70/min).

Clinical significance: Indicating damp disease and weakness of the stomach and spleen.

#### 1.4.1.3.7　Fast pulse
Features: The pulse beats over 5 - 6 times in a cycle of breath (90 - 110/min).

Clinical significance: Indicating heat syndrome. Fast and powerful pulse signifies sthenia heat syndrome, while fast and weak pulse shows asthenic heat syndrome. Such a pulse condition is also seen in the syndrome due to external floating of asthenic yang.

临床意义：主失血,伤阴。

**4．沉脉**

脉象特征：轻取不应,重按始得。沉脉以脉动显现部位较深沉为特点。

临床意义：主里证。沉而有力为里实,沉而无力为里虚。

**5．迟脉**

脉象特征：脉来迟慢,一息脉动不足四至(<60次/分钟)。

临床意义：主寒证。迟而有力为实寒,迟而无力为虚寒。亦可见于邪热结聚的里实热证。运动员或青壮年锻炼有素者出现迟脉属生理现象,应予以鉴别。

**6．缓脉**

脉象特征：脉来和缓有力,一息四至；或脉来缓怠,一息四至(60～70次/分钟)。

临床意义：主湿病,脾胃虚弱。

**7．数脉**

脉象特征：脉来快数,一息五六至(90～110次/分钟)。

临床意义：主热证。有力为实热,无力为虚热。亦可见于虚阳外越证。

#### 1.4.1.3.8 Swift pulse

Features: The pulse beats over 7 times in a cycle of breath (≥140/min).

Clinical significance: Indicating loss of control of hyperactive yang, declination of kidney yin and near depletion of primordial qi.

#### 1.4.1.3.9 Weak pulse

Features: Weak pulse is marked by weak beating of the pulse at all the cun, guan and chi regions.

Clinical significance: Indicating asthenia syndrome, usually seen in asthenia of both qi and blood, especially in qi asthenia.

#### 1.4.1.3.10 Powerful pulse

Features: Powerful pulse is marked by powerful sensation of pulse beating at cun, guan and chi regions under superficial, moderate and heavy pressure.

#### 1.4.1.3.11 Slippery pulse

Features: The pulse is beating freely and smoothly like the movement of beads of an abacus.

Clinical significance: Indicating retention of phlegm and fluid, dyspepsia and sthenia heat. Such a pulse condition is also seen among young and strong people and gravida.

#### 1.4.1.3.12 Astringent pulse

Features: The pulse is beating in an inhibited way like scraping a piece of bamboo.

8. 疾脉

脉象特征：脉来急疾，一息七至以上(≥140次/分钟)。

临床意义：主阳亢无制，真阴垂绝，元气将脱。

9. 虚脉

脉象特征：三部脉举之无力，按之空豁，是无力脉的总称。虚脉以寸、关、尺三部，浮、中、沉三候均应指势弱，鼓动无力为特点。

临床意义：主虚证。多见于气血两虚，尤以气虚为主。

10. 实脉

脉象特征：三部脉举按皆充实有力，是有力脉的总称。实脉以寸、关、尺三部，浮、中、沉三候均应指势强，鼓动有力为特点。

临床意义：主实证。

11. 滑脉

脉象特征：往来流利，应指圆滑，如盘走珠。滑脉以脉搏形态应指圆滑，往来之间有一种回旋前进的感觉为特点。

临床意义：主痰饮，食滞，实热。亦可见于青壮年或妇人妊娠。

12. 涩脉

脉象特征：往来艰涩不畅，如轻刀刮竹。涩脉以脉力

Clinical significance: Astringent and powerful pulse indicates qi stagnation and blood stasis; astringent and weak pulse signifies lack of essence and insufficiency of blood.

#### 1.4.1.3.13 Full pulse

Features: Full pulse is marked by wide size and full content, beating like roaring waves and sensibility under light pressure and surges as well as sudden flowing and ebbing.

Clinical significance: Indicating exuberant internal heat.

#### 1.4.1.3.14 Thin pulse

Features: The pulse is as thin as a thread, weak and quite sensible under pressure.

Clinical significance: Indicating asthenia of both qi and blood, various overstrain and diseases due to pathogenic dampness.

#### 1.4.1.3.15 Soft pulse

Features: Soft pulse is superficial and thin as well as sensible and weak under light pressure.

Clinical significance: Indicating insufficiency of qi and blood, and dampness syndrome.

#### 1.4.1.3.16 Feeble pulse

Features: Feeble pulse is deep and thin as well as sensible and weak under heavy pressure.

Clinical significance: Indicating declination of both qi and blood.

与节律都不均匀为特点。

临床意义：涩而有力主气滞，血瘀；涩而无力主精伤，血少。

### 13．洪脉

脉象特征：脉体宽大，充实有力，滔滔满指，如波涛汹涌，来盛去衰。洪脉以脉形宽大，轻取可得，按之势不减，充实有力，大起大落为特点。

临床意义：主里热炽盛。

### 14．细脉

脉象特征：脉体细小如线，软弱无力，应指明显。细脉以脉形细小，脉势软弱，但应指明显为特点。

临床意义：主气血两虚，诸虚劳损；又主湿邪为病。

### 15．濡脉

脉象特征：浮而细软。濡脉以脉位浮浅，轻取即得，脉形细小，应指软弱少力为特点。

临床意义：主气血不足，湿证。

### 16．弱脉

脉象特征：极软而沉细。弱脉以脉位深沉，重按始得，脉形细小，应指软弱无力为特点。

临床意义：气血俱衰。

#### 1.4.1.3.17  Indistinct pulse

Features: Indistinct pulse is very thin and soft, almost insensible under pressure.

Clinical significance: Indicating extreme deficiency of qi and blood as well as declination of yangqi.

#### 1.4.1.3.18  Taut pulse

Features: Taut pulse appears straight, energetic and hard like the feeling of pressing the string of a violin.

Clinical significance: Indicating disorders of the liver and gallbladder, pain syndrome and retention of phlegm and fluid.

#### 1.4.1.3.19  Tense pulse

Features: Tense pulse appears like the pulling of a rope and flicks the finger when pressed.

Clinical significance: Indicating cold syndrome, pain syndrome and retention of food.

#### 1.4.1.3.20  Rapid and intermittent pulse

Features: Rapid and intermittent pulse beats fast with occasional and irregular intermittence.

Clinical significance: Fast and powerful pulse indicates hyperactivity of yang heat, qi stagnation, blood stasis and retention of phlegm and food; fast and weak pulse signifies weakness of visceral qi and insufficiency of blood.

#### 1.4.1.3.21  Slow and intermittent pulse

Features: The pulse beats slow with occasional and

17. 微脉

脉象特征：极细极软,按之欲绝,若有若无。微脉以脉形极为细小,脉力极为软弱,应指极不明显为特点。

临床意义：主气血大虚,阳气衰微。

18. 弦脉

脉象特征：端直以长,挺然指下,如按琴弦。弦脉以脉形挺直,脉势较强而硬为特点。

临床意义：主肝胆病,痛证,痰饮。

19. 紧脉

脉象特征：脉来紧张,如牵绳转索,按之弹指。紧脉以指感比弦脉更为紧张有力为特点。

临床意义：主寒证,痛证,宿食内阻。

20. 促脉

脉象特征：脉来急数,时有中止,止无定数。促脉以脉率较快,并有不规则的歇止为特点。

临床意义：促而有力主阳热亢盛,气滞,血瘀,痰食停滞;促而无力主脏气虚弱,阴血虚少。

21. 结脉

脉象特征：脉来迟缓,时

irregular intermittence.

Clinical significance: Slow, intermittent and powerful pulse indicates predominance of yin, qi stagnation, retention of phlegm and blood stasis; while slow, intermittent and weak pulse signifies declination of qi and blood.

#### 1.4.1.3.22 Slow-intermittent-regular pulse

Features: The pulse beats slowly with regular and longer intermittence.

Clinical significance: Indicating declination of visceral qi and asthenia of primordial qi.

#### 1.4.1.3.23 Long pulse

Features: The pulse surpasses the range of cun, guan and chi regions.

Clinical significance: Indicating yang syndrome, heat syndrome and sthenia syndrome.

#### 1.4.1.3.24 Short pulse

Features: The pulse appears shorter than the normal content of cun, guan and chi regions.

Clinical significance: Indicating qi disorders. Short and powerful pulse indicates qi stagnation; while short and weak pulse signifies qi asthenia.

The development of diseases is complicated and may be caused by various pathogenic factors, leading to the variations of the functions of yin and yang, qi and blood and viscera as well as the states of the conflict between the healthy qi and pathogenic factors. Therefore, the pulse conditions mentioned above do not exist in a single form in the clinical practice. Usually two or more pulse

有中止,止无定数。结脉以脉率缓慢,并有不规则的歇止为特点。

临床意义:结而有力主阴盛气结,痰阻,血瘀;结而无力主气血虚衰。

### 22. 代脉

脉象特征:脉来缓弱,时有中止,止有定数,良久方来。代脉以脉率缓慢,脉力较弱,并有较规则的歇止,且歇止时间较长为特点。

临床意义:主脏气衰微,元气虚损。

### 23. 长脉

脉象特征:脉体长,应指范围超过寸、关、尺三部。

临床意义:主阳证,热证,实证。

### 24. 短脉

脉象特征:脉体短,应指范围不足本位,多现于关部,而寸、尺常不能满部。

临床意义:主气病。短而有力为气郁,短而无力为气虚。

疾病的过程是错综复杂的,可以由多种致病因素相兼为患,机体本身的阴阳、气血、脏腑功能亦有差异,邪正斗争的形势亦不断发生变化。因此,上述诸病脉在临床上往往不是单独存在,而是两种或两

conditions appear at the same time. Such a pulse condition called combined pulse. The conditions of pulse may appear at the same time, unless they are contrary in nature, so as to comprehensively reflect the pathological changes in the body.

Generally speaking, the disease indicated by the combined pulse is the synthesis of the diseases indicated by the pulse conditions appearing simultaneously in a case. For example, floating pulse indicates external syndrome and fast pulse signifies heat syndrome, so floating and fast pulse shows external heat syndrome; floating pulse indicates external syndrome and tense pulse signifies cold syndrome, so floating and tense pulse manifests external cold syndrome; taut pulse indicates disorder of the liver and gallbladder and fast pulse signifies heat syndrome, so taut and fast pulse manifests liver depression transforming into fire or damp heat in the liver and gallbladder, etc.

On the whole, all related factors should be taken into consideration in differentiating pulse for making correct clinical diagnosis.

## 1.4.2 Palpation

Palpation means to use fingers or palms to feel or press certain regions of the patient's body to understand whether the local regions are cold or warm, dry or moist and soft or hard as well as whether there are tenderness, lump or other abnormal changes. Palpation can not only help understand the location, nature and severity of disease, but also help make manifestations of some diseases objective, further complementing the data obtained from inspection, olfaction and listening and inquiry as well as

种以上的脉象同时出现。这种数种脉象同见的脉，称为相兼脉。只要不是性质完全相反的脉象一般都可以相兼出现，从而能较全面地反映出内在的病机变化。

一般来说，相兼脉的主病，就是构成该脉象的各种脉象主病的综合。如：浮脉主表证，数脉主热证，浮数脉即主表热证；浮脉主表证，紧脉主寒证，浮紧脉即主表寒证；弦脉主肝胆病，数脉主热证，弦数脉即主肝郁化火，或肝胆湿热等。

总之，辨脉时务必体察脉象诸方面的变化，并将各种变化因素作为临床诊断的辨证依据。

## 二、按诊

按诊是医者用手指或手掌直接触摸或按压患者体表的某些部位，以了解局部冷热、润燥、软硬、压痛、肿块或其他异常变化的一种诊病方法。通过按诊不仅可以进一步探明疾病的部位、性质和程度，同时也使一些病证表现进一步客观化，是对望、闻、问诊

providing necessary evidence for analyzing pathological conditions and judging the nature of diseases.

### 1.4.2.1 Methods for palpation
#### 1.4.2.1.1 Postures

The postures for palpation is selected according to the aim and regions for palpation. The usual posture used is sitting or supination.

When the patient is seated, the doctor stands or sits in front of the patient, holding the patient with the left hand and palpating local regions of the patient with the right hand. The usual techniques for palpation is to palpate skin, hands and feet as well as acupoints. If the patient is asked to lie in supination with the relaxation of the whole body and natural stretching or bending the legs, the doctor stands at the right side of the patient and palpates the patient with the right hand or both hands. Such a way of palpation is often used to press chest and abdomen.

#### 1.4.2.1.2 Techniques for palpation

The usual techniques used are palpation, feeling, pressing and tapping, etc.

Palpation: To use fingers or palm to feel the forehead, four limbs, chest and abdomen skin to understand whether the local skin is cold or feverish and moist or dry.

Feeling: To use fingers or palm to feel the chest, abdomen and four limbs of the patient to see if there are superficial pain and lumps as well as the shape and size of the lumps.

Slight pressure: To use hand slightly press the chest, abdomen, four limbs and lumps to know the boundary, texture and movement of the lumps as well as the degree and nature of local swelling.

所得资料的补充和完善,为全面分析病情、判断疾病提供重要的依据。

（一）按诊的方法
1. 按诊的体位

应根据按诊的目的和检查部位的不同而采取不同的体位。一般患者取坐位或仰卧位。

患者取坐位时,医者面对患者而坐或站,用左手稍扶患者身体,右手触摸按压局部。多用于按皮肤、手足、腧穴等部位。患者取仰卧位时,应全身放松,两腿自然伸直或屈起双膝,医者立于患者右侧,用右手或双手按诊。多用于按胸腹等部位。

2. 按诊的手法

一般有触、摸、按、压、叩等手法。

触：用手指或手掌轻触患者的额、四肢、胸腹等部位的皮肤,以了解局部肌肤的寒热、润燥等情况。

摸：用手指或手掌抚摸患者的胸腹、四肢等处,以了解机体浅表部位有无疼痛、肿块,以及肿块的形态、大小等。

按：以手稍用力按胸腹、四肢及肿块部位等处,以了解肿块的界限、质地、活动程度、局部肿胀的程度、性质等。

Heavy pressure: To press heavily the morbid region to detect whether there is pain in the deep layer and whether there is suppuration, etc.

Tapping: To use hand to tap certain regions of the patient to produce tapping sound and waving sensation or vibration to decide the nature and degree of pathological changes. Tapping is either direct or indirect. Direct tapping means that the doctor uses his or her hand to directly tap the superficial regions of the patient; indirect tapping means that the doctor puts his or her left palm over the surface of the patient's body and uses his or her right fist to tap the left hand dorsum. While tapping, the doctor asks the patient about the sensation to decide the location and degree of disease.

The methods mentioned above emphasize on different aspects in performing palpation. However, they are used in combination. The usual order is palpating and feeling first, then pressing and finally tapping, which are performed from light degree to the heavy, from the superficial to the deep layer, from distal region to the proximal and from the upper part to the lower.

### 1.4.2.2 Pressing the chest and abdomen
#### 1.4.2.2.1 Pressing the chest

Pressing the chest is helpful for detecting the pathological changes of the heart, the lung and the precordium.

Bulgy chest with clear noise when tapped is seen in pneumatothorax. Pain of the chest under pressure and with dull noise when tapped is often seen in retention of fluid in the chest and diaphragm or accumulation of phlegmatic heat in the lung.

Precordium, located between the fourth and fifth

压：以手重压病变部位，以测知深部有无压痛，是否有脓等。

叩：是医者用手叩击患者的某些部位，使之震动产生叩击音、波动感或震动感，以此来确定病变的性质和程度的一种检查方法。叩击有直接叩击和间接叩击的区别。直接叩击是医者用手指直接叩击体表部位；间接叩击是医者用左手掌平贴在患者的体表，右手握成空拳叩击左手背。边叩边询问患者叩击部位的感觉，以推测病变部位和程度。

以上各法各有侧重，可以综合运用。一般是先触摸，后按压，再叩击，由轻到重，由浅入深，先远后近，先上后下地进行诊察。

### （二）按胸腹
#### 1. 按胸部

按胸部可以了解心肺及虚里的病变情况。

前胸高起，叩之膨膨然而音清的，可见于气胸；若按之胸痛，叩之音实的，常为饮停胸膈或痰热壅肺。

虚里位于左胸第四、五肋

ribs, below the nipple and slightly medial to the nipple, is the pulsation point of the apex of the heart where all the vessels converge. Pressing the precordium is helpful for detecting whether the thoracic qi is strong or weak, whether the disease is asthenic or sthenic and whether the prognosis is favourable or unfavourable. The pressing of precordium is especially useful when cunkou pulse is difficult to take in critical cases. Normally, the pulsation over the precordium is sensible and beating smoothly, moderately and rhythmically, indicating exuberance of heart qi, accumulation of thoracic qi in the chest and no signs of pathological changes. Weak and indistinct pulsation over the precordium suggests asthenia of the thoracic qi. Powerful pulsation over the precordium vibrating the clothes is hyperactivity of precordial beating, a sign of outburst of the thoracic qi.

#### 1.4.2.2.2 Pressing the hypochondrium

Pressing hypochondrium is helpful for detecting diseases related to the liver and gallbladder.

Distending pain of hypochondrium with sensible lumps below the sternum and evident tenderness is usually due to stagnation of liver qi and gallbladder qi or due to damp heat in the liver and gallbladder. Hypochondriac lumps with stabbing and unpalpable pain is often caused by depression of liver qi and blood stasis. Right hypochondriac lumps which is hard and uneven are due to accumulation of mass resulting from prolonged stagnation of qi or blood stasis, and cares should be taken to exclude liver cancer. Repeated relapse of malaria with hard and palpable lumps is called malaria with abdominal mass.

#### 1.4.2.2.3 Pressing epigastrium and abdomen

Pressing epigastrium and abdomen is helpful for detecting the disorders of the stomach, spleen, small intestine, large intestine, bladder and uterus, etc.

间，乳头下稍内侧，为心尖搏动处，为诸脉之所宗。诊虚里可测知宗气的强弱，疾病的虚实，预后的吉凶，尤其在危重证寸口脉难凭时，更具诊断价值。正常情况下，虚里搏动按之应手，动而不紧，缓而不急，节律均匀，是心气充盛，宗气积于胸中，无病的征象。若虚里搏动微弱不显的，是宗气内虚；若动而应衣为太过，是宗气外泄之象。

2. 按胁部

按胁部可以了解肝胆的疾病。

胁肋胀痛，剑突下右侧可触及痞块，压痛明显，多属肝胆气滞，或肝胆湿热；胁下肿块，刺痛拒按的，多属肝郁气滞血瘀；右胁下肿块质硬，按之表面凹凸不平的，则属癥积，因气结日久，血瘀日甚所致，应注意排除肝癌；疟疾反复发作，左胁下可触及痞块，按之硬，多为疟母。

3. 按脘腹

按脘腹可以诊察胃、脾、小肠、大肠、膀胱、胞宫等脏腑的病变。

Generally speaking, cold sensation of the skin when pressed with preference for warmth is usually of cold syndrome; feverish sensation of the skin when pressed with preference for cold is of heat syndrome; epigastric and abdominal pain with preference for pressure is of asthenia syndrome; and epigastric and abdominal pain with aversion to pressure is of sthenia syndrome.

Epigastric fullness with soft sensation and no pain when pressed is caused by weakness of the stomach; epigastric fullness with hard and painful sensation when pressed usually results from accumulation of sthenic pathogenic factors in the epigastrium. Distending epigastric pain with hard sensation and gurgling noise when pressed is due to retention of fluid in the stomach resulting from asthenia of the middle energizer qi and stagnation of qi.

Full sensation of the abdomen under pressure with tenderness is known as sthenic fullness due to qi stagnation, blood stasis or retention of fluid; soft sensation of the abdomen under pressure and without tenderness is known as asthenic fullness due to asthenia of yangqi or failure of transportation caused by qi asthenia.

Drum-like swelling of the abdomen with dull yellowish skin, visible veins over the abdominal wall and emaciation of the four limbs is called tympanites. Tympanites with fluid sensation when pressed and dull sound when tapped is called hydraulic tympanites; while tympanites with empty sensation when tapped is known as pneumotympanites.

Immobile abdominal lumps with fixed pain is unmovable mass due to blood stasis; mobile abdominal lumps with migratory pain is known as movable mass due to qi stagnation.

Unpalpable pain in right lower abdomen, with mass when pressing, is often seen in the intestinal abscess and

一般来说，脘腹部按之肌肤凉而喜温的，多属寒证；按之肌肤热而喜凉的，多属热证；脘腹痛而喜按的，多属虚证；脘腹痛而拒按的，多属实证。

脘部痞满，按之濡软而不痛的，多因胃腑虚弱所致；若按之较硬而疼痛的，多因实邪聚结胃脘所致。脘部胀痛，按之有形，推之辘辘有声的，多为中虚气滞，饮停于胃。

腹部按之饱满充实，压之痛的，为实满，多因气滞、血瘀，或水饮内停所致；按之虚软，无压痛的，为虚满，多因阳气亏虚，或气虚不运所致。

腹部胀大如鼓，肤色苍黄，腹壁脉络显露，四肢消瘦者，为鼓胀。其中，按之如囊裹水，叩之声音重浊的，为水臌；叩之如鼓空空然的，为气臌。

腹部肿块，推之不移，痛有定处的，为癥积，多属血瘀；推之可移，或痛无定处，聚散不定的，为瘕聚，多属气滞。

右少腹痛而拒按，按之有包块应手，常见于肠痈等病。

so on.

### 1.4.2.3 Palpation of the four limbs
#### 1.4.2.3.1 Detection of cold and heat

Feeling of cold and heat of the hands and feet is helpful for judging the states of diseases, such as cold and heat, asthenia and sthenia, internal and external aspects as well as favourable and unfavourable prognosis.

Generally speaking, cold sensation of hands and feet is usually of cold syndrome due to asthenia of yang and exuberance of cold; feverish sensation of hands and feet is often of heat syndrome due to predomination of yang and exuberance of heat. However, sometimes pathogenic heat deepens into the body and prevents yang from moving outward, leading to internal heat syndrome known as "deep heat and deep syncope", a critical sign of disease.

If the palms and soles are more feverish than the dorsa of hands and feet, it suggests fever due to internal impairment. If the forehead is more feverish than the palms, it is superficial fever. If the palms are more feverish than the forehead, it suggests internal heat.

#### 1.4.2.3.2 Palpating the skin from inner side of the elbow to the transverse lines on the wrist

It is helpful for judging the nature of disease according to its conditions of being tense or loose, slippery or astringent and cold or feverish.

If the skin is very feverish and the pulse is full, slippery, fast and powerful, it usually suggests fever in exogenous febrile disease; if the skin is cold and the pulse is thin and small, it indicates diarrhea and insufficiency of qi due to asthenia of yangqi and predomination of internal cold; if the skin is lubricant, it shows sufficiency of qi and blood; if the skin is as rough as scales of dry fish, it

(三) 按四肢
1. 察冷热

通过触摸患者手足部位的冷热,有助于判断疾病的寒热虚实以及表里、内外和顺逆。

一般来说,手足俱冷的,多是阳虚寒盛,属寒证;手足俱热的,多属阳盛热炽,属热证。但亦有热邪深伏,阳气内郁,不得外达,而致四肢厥冷的,即"热深厥深",是里热证。热证见手足热的,属顺候;热证反见手足逆冷的,属逆候,是病情严重的表现。

手足心热甚于手足背热的,多为内伤发热。额上热甚于手心热的,多为表热;手心热甚于额上热的,多为里热。

2. 按尺肤

尺肤是指肘部内侧至掌后横纹处的一段皮肤。根据其缓急、滑涩、寒热的情况,有助于判断疾病的性质。

尺肤热甚,脉象洪滑数盛的,多为外感热病发热;尺肤凉,脉象细小的,多为阳气亏虚,里寒偏盛的泄泻、少气;尺肤滑润的,多为气血充盛;尺肤粗糙如枯鱼之鳞,多为精血不足,或脾阳虚衰,水饮不化

suggests insufficiency of essence and blood or phlegm and fluid disorder due to failure of the spleen to transform fluid resulting from decline of splenic yang.

#### 1.4.2.3.3 Palpation of swelling and distension

Heavy pressure on swollen and distending skin with hands is helpful for differentiating edema and flatulence. If the fingers sink into the skin when the skin is pressed and the depression on the skin fails to rebound when the fingers are lifted, it is edema; if the depression on the skin produced by pressure rebounds when the fingers are lifted, it is flatulence.

### 1.4.2.4 Palpation of acupoints

Acupoints, the places where meridian qi converges and transmits, are the points that reflect visceral disorders on the surface of the body. Pressing certain acupoints, according to the changes and reaction of these acupoints, is helpful for diagnosing the disorders of certain viscera.

In pressing acupoints, cares should be taken to see if there are tenderness, nodules and sensitive response. For example, nodules over Feishu (BL 13) and tenderness over Zhongfu (LU 1) usually indicate lung disease; tenderness over Ganshu (BL 18) and Qimen (LR 14) shows liver disease; tenderness over Weishu (BL 21) and Zusanli (ST 36) suggests stomach disease; tenderness over Shangjuxu (ST 37) is usually a sign of intestinal abscess.

之痰饮病。

3. 诊肿胀

重手按压肌肤肿胀处，有助于辨别水肿和气胀。按之凹陷没指，举手不能即起的，是水肿；按之凹陷，举手即起的，是气胀。

（四）按腧穴

腧穴是脏腑经络之气汇聚转输之处，是内脏病变反映于体表的反应点。按压某些特定穴位，根据穴位处的变化和反应，有助于诊断某些内脏病证。

按腧穴应注意穴位处有无压痛、结节，以及其他敏感反应。如：肺俞穴有结节或中府穴有压痛，多为肺病；肝俞穴或期门穴有压痛，多为肝病；胃俞穴或足三里穴有压痛，多为胃病；上巨虚穴有压痛，多为肠痈的表现。

# 2 Differentiation of syndrome

Differentiation of syndrome means to analyzing and judging the data obtained from the four diagnostic methods so as to differentiate the nature of the disease and make clear the naming of the syndrome.

There are various methods for differentiating syndrome. This chapter mainly introduces syndrome differentiation with eight principles, syndrome differentiation of qi, blood and body fluid, syndrome differentiation of viscera and syndrome differentiation of six meridians as well as syndrome differentiation of wei, qi, ying and blood, among which the syndrome differentiation with eight principles is the leading one. Syndrome differentiation of qi, blood and body fluid as well as syndrome differentiation of viscera are mainly used to differentiate syndromes in miscellaneous diseases due to internal impairment, while syndrome differentiation of six meridians and syndrome differentiation of wei, qi, ying and blood are mainly used to differentiate syndromes in exogenous diseases. These methods for differentiating syndromes, though different characteristics and application, are interrelated and should be used synthetically in clinical practice.

## 2.1 Syndrome differentiation with eight principles

Syndrome differentiation with eight principles means

第二章 辨证

辨证，就是对四诊所获得病情资料进行分析、判断，从而识别疾病本质，并概括为具体证名的过程。

辨证的方法有多种，本章介绍八纲辨证、气血津液辨证、脏腑辨证、六经辨证、卫气营血辨证。其中，八纲辨证是各种辨证的纲领，气血津液辨证与脏腑辨证主要用于内伤杂病的辨证，六经辨证、卫气营血辨证主要用于外感病的辨证。各种辨证方法虽各有其不同的特点和适用范畴，但又互相联系，相辅相成，临床应综合运用。

第一节 八纲辨证

八纲辨证，即以阴、阳、

differentiating syndromes according to the principles of yin and yang, internal and external aspects, cold and heat as well as asthenia and sthenia.

The clinical manifestations of diseases, though complicated, can be analyzed with the eight principles according to the category, location and nature of disease as well as the conflict between the healthy qi and pathogenic factors. For this reason, the eight principles are the most basic ones to differentiate syndromes. Syndrome differentiation with eight principles is a method used to differentiate the common factors of diseases and is the leading one among all the methods for differentiating syndromes. It is therefore the essential one for differentiating syndromes and applicable for all clinical specialties for differentiating syndromes.

The eight principles concentrate on specific syndromes respectively. However, they are inseparable and not static. Among the eight principles, yin and yang are the general principles which can be used to generalize the other six principles, i.e. external, heat and sthenia are of yang; while internal, cold and asthenia are of yin. The syndromes of the eight principles are often complicated, transformable and intermingled. Sometimes there are false manifestations. Therefore, clinical differentiation of syndromes should concentrate both on the difference of the syndromes related to the eight principles respectively and on their close relationship so as to have a comprehensive cognition of the disease.

## 2.1.1 External and internal differentiation of syndromes

External and internal are two principles used to differentiate the location of diseases and the tendency of pathological changes.

表、里、寒、热、虚、实，作为辨证的纲领，对疾病进行辨证。

疾病的临床表现尽管错综复杂，但基本上都可以用八纲从疾病的类别和病位、病性、邪正盛衰等方面进行分析归纳。所以，八纲是最基本的证候分类的纲领，八纲辨证是分析疾病共性的辨证方法，是各种辨证的纲领，在诊断疾病过程中，有执简驭繁，提纲挈领的作用，适用于临床各科的辨证。

八纲各有其特定的证候，但它们之间不是孤立的、静止不变的。其中，阴阳是八纲中的总纲，可以概括其他六纲，即表、热、实证为阳；里、寒、虚证属阴。八纲证候常出现相兼、转化、夹杂，有时还会出现某些假象。因此，临床辨证时，既要注意八纲各自证候的区别，又要注意它们之间的密切关系，才能正确而全面地认识疾病。

## 一、表里辨证

表里，是辨别病变部位和病势趋向的两个纲领。

External and internal are two relative concepts. On the human body, the skin, hair, muscular interstices and shallow meridians and collaterals are external; while viscera, qi, blood and bone marrow are internal.

External and internal differentiation of syndromes is important to syndrome differentiation in exogenous diseases. This is because the disorder due to internal impairment starts from the interior and does not show the course of developing from the external to the internal. In this case there is no need to differentiate the external and internal. In exogenous disease, when the pathogenic factors often invade the human body, they first attack the superficies. In this case, the healthy qi fights against the pathogenic factors, giving rise to the formation of external syndrome. With the development of the pathological conditions, pathogenic factors transmit from the exterior into the interior and from the shallow layer into the deep layer to form internal syndrome. Therefore, external and internal syndrome differentiation is the most basic cognition of the developing stages of exogenous diseases. The external and internal syndrome differentiation enables doctors to understand conditions of pathogenic factors and the states and development of pathological changes so as to take proper and timely treatment.

#### 2.1.1.1 External syndrome

External syndrome refers to the symptoms appearing at the primary stage of exogenous diseases caused by invasion of six pathogenic factors into the body through skin, mouth and nose, marked by sudden onset, short duration and shallow location.

Clinical manifestations: The clinical manifestations are fever, aversion to cold (or aversion to wind), thin and white fur and floating pulse, accompanied by stuffy and running nose, sore-throat and cough.

表与里是相对而言,人体的皮毛、肌腠、浅表经络属表;脏腑、气血、骨髓属里。

表里辨证对外感病辨证有重要意义。这是因为内伤病多病起于里,一般没有由表入里的发展过程,勿需辨别表里。外感病,外邪侵袭人体,往往首先犯表,人体正气抗邪于表,形成表证。随着病情的发展,病邪由表入里,由浅入深,形成里证。所以,表里辨证是对外感病发展的阶段性的最基本的认识。通过表里辨证,可以了解病位的浅深、病情的轻重及病变发展的趋势,从而取得治疗的主动权。

(一) 表证

表证是指六淫之邪经皮毛、口鼻侵犯人体,而引起的外感病初期阶段所表现的证候。表证具有起病急、病程短、病位浅的特点。

临床表现:发热,恶寒(或恶风),舌苔薄白,脉浮,兼头身疼痛,鼻塞流涕,喉痒咽痛,咳嗽。

Analysis of the symptoms: Attack of pathogenic factors against the superficies and confliction between healthy qi and pathogenic factors lead to fever and aversion to wind and cold; stagnation of pathogenic factors in meridians prevents meridian qi from free flowing and results in pain; the lung governs skin and hair, the nose opens into the lung and the throat is the door of the lung, so attack of pathogenic factors against the surface of the body leads to dysfunction of the lung and causes stuffy and running nose, sore-throat and cough; the pathogenic factors retain in the superficies and have not damaged the interior, so the tongue fur is still thin and white without change; floating pulse is the sign of external confliction between the healthy qi and pathogenic factors.

### 2.1.1.2 Internal syndrome

Internal syndrome refers to the symptoms in disorders with deep location (such as disorders of viscera, qi and blood and bone marrow), usually seen at the middle and advanced stages of exogenous disease and the whole course of diseases due to internal impairment. Three conditions have contributed to the formation of internal syndrome: further development of exogenous disease due to interior transmission of pathogenic factors from the exterior and invasion of the viscera by the pathogenic factors; direct attack of the viscera by pathogenic factors; dysfunctions of the viscera and the imbalance between qi and blood due to impairment of the viscera caused by emotional upsets, improper diet and improper daily life.

Clinical manifestations: The clinical manifestations of internal syndrome are different due to different causes and location. Since syndrome is either cold or heat and asthenia or sthenia and since disease is due to the disorders of either qi or blood or body fluid, clinical manifestations of internal syndrome are various. However, the basic

证候分析：外邪袭表，邪正相争，故发热、恶风寒；邪郁经络，经气不畅，故头身疼痛；肺主皮毛，鼻为肺窍，咽喉为肺之门户，邪袭肌表，肺失宣肃，故鼻塞流涕、喉痒咽痛、咳嗽；病邪在表，未伤及里，故舌象尚无变化，仍为薄白苔。脉浮为邪正相争于表的征象。

### （二）里证

里证是指病变部位深入于里（脏腑、气血、骨髓）的一类证候。多见于外感病的中、后期和内伤病的全过程。里证的形成，主要有三种情况：一是外感病表证进一步发展，外邪内传入里，侵犯脏腑而致；二是外邪直接侵犯脏腑而形成；三是内伤七情、饮食、劳逸失度等因素，损伤脏腑，致使脏腑功能失调，气血不和而发病。

临床表现：里证既因病因不同，脏腑病位各异，而有不同的临床表现；又因证有寒热虚实之分，病属气血津液之异，故其临床表现繁多，但其基本特点是以脏腑功能失调

clinical manifestation is dysfunction of the viscera which will be discussed in the following sections. Here sthenic internal heat syndrome in exogenous disease is taken as an example to illustrate the clinical manifestations of internal syndrome. The basic manifestations are high fever, aversion to heat, restlessness, even coma with delirium, thirst with profuse drinking of water, scanty and brownish urine, retention of feces, reddish tongue with yellowish fur and fast and powerful pulse.

Analysis of symptoms: Exuberance of internal heat leads to high fever and aversion to heat; heat disturbing the heart spirit causes restlessness or even coma with delirium; consumption of body fluid by exuberant heat leads to thirst with profuse drinking of water, scanty brownish urine and retention of feces; reddish tongue with yellow fur and fast powerful pulse is the sign of exuberance of internal heat and confliction between healthy qi and pathogenic factors.

## Appendix: Half external and half internal syndrome

Half external and half internal syndrome refers to the symptoms appearing in exogenous disease at the stage marked by confliction of healthy qi and pathogenic factors between the exterior and interior phases, and is usually caused by transmission of pathogenic factors from the exterior to the interior but still lingering between the exterior and interior phases. The manifestations are alternation of cold and fever, oppression and distress over the chest and hypochondrium, dysphoria, susceptibility to belching, silence, anorexia, bitter taste in the mouth, dry throat, dizziness and taut pulse, etc. (see shaoyang syndrome in syndrome differentiation of six meridians).

### 2.1.2 Syndrome differentiation of cold and heat

Cold and heat are two principles used to differentiate

的症状为主要表现。具体内容见以下各节。现仅以外感病里实热证为例说明如下：壮热恶热，烦躁不宁，甚则神昏谵语，口渴引饮，小便短赤，大便秘结，舌红苔黄，脉数有力。

证候分析：里热炽盛，蒸腾于外，则壮热恶热；热扰心神，则烦躁不宁，甚则神昏谵语；热盛津伤，则口渴引饮、小便短赤、大便秘结。舌红苔黄，脉数有力，是热盛于里，邪正相争的征象。

附：半表半里证

半表半里证是指外感病中，邪正相争于表里之间所表现的证候。多因外邪由表内传，尚未入里，在于表里之间而形成。其表现为寒热往来，胸胁苦满，心烦喜呕，默默不欲饮食，口苦，咽干，目眩，脉弦等（详见六经辨证中的少阳病证）。

二、寒热辨证

寒热，是辨别疾病性质的

the nature of diseases.

Cold and heat nature of diseases are the reflection of the conditions of yin and yang in the body. Yin predomination or yang asthenia leads to cold syndrome; while yang predomination or yin asthenia leads to heat syndrome. Syndrome differentiation of cold and heat is helpful for understanding the nature of disease and providing evidence for selecting warming therapy or clearing therapy.

#### 2.1.2.1 Cold syndrome

Cold syndrome refers to symptoms caused by yang asthenia or yin predomination due to invasion of cold pathogenic factors or various other factors. This syndrome is usually caused by internal exuberance of cold due to invasion of cold pathogenic factors or excessive intake of cold food, or by consumption of yangqi due to internal impairment and chronic disease. Cold syndrome may be further divided into external cold syndrome, internal cold syndrome, asthenic cold syndrome and sthenic cold syndrome according to the causes and location of pathological changes.

Clinical manifestations: The clinical manifestations vary with different types of cold syndromes. The usual ones are aversion to cold or aversion to cold with preference for warmth, cold limbs and huddling up in sleeping, pale or light colored complexion, moist mouth without thirst, thin sputum, saliva and snivel, clear and profuse urine, loose stool, light colored tongue with whitish moist and slippery fur, slow or tense pulse.

Analysis of symptoms: Attack by pathogenic cold and stagnation of yangqi or insufficiency of yangqi to warm the body lead to aversion to cold or aversion to cold with preference for warmth, cold limbs, huddling up in sleeping, light colored or pale complexion; exuberant internal cold and non-consumption of body fluid account for moist mouth without thirst; failure of asthenic yang to warm and

两个纲领。

疾病性质的寒热是机体阴阳盛衰的反映。阴盛或阳虚的,表现为寒证;阳盛或阴虚的,多表现为热证。通过寒热辨证,可以了解病证的性质,为治疗上确定采用温法或清法提供依据。

#### （一）寒证

寒证,是指感受阴寒之邪,或多种原因导致机体阳虚,或阴盛所表现的证候。本证多因外感阴寒邪气,或过服生冷寒凉,致阴寒内盛;或内伤久病,耗伤阳气所形成。根据形成原因及病位的不同,寒证又可分为表寒、里寒、虚寒、实寒等。

临床表现:各类寒证的临床表现不尽一致,常见的有:恶寒或畏寒喜暖,肢冷蜷卧,面色㿠白或苍白,口润不渴,痰、涎、涕清稀,小便清长,大便稀溏,舌淡苔白而润滑,脉迟或紧等。

证候分析:感受寒邪,阳气被遏,或阳气不足,不能温养形体,则恶寒或畏寒喜暖,肢冷蜷卧,面色㿠白或苍白;阴寒内盛,津液未伤,则口润不渴;阳虚不能温化水液,以致痰、涎、涕、尿等排出物皆澄

transform fluid leads to clear sputum, snivel, saliva and urine; encumbrance of the spleen by pathogenic cold or asthenia of splenic yang causes loose stool. Light colored tongue with whitish slippery and moist fur and slow or tense pulse are the signs of yang asthenia and internal predominance of yin cold.

### 2.1.2.2 Heat syndrome

Heat syndrome refers to symptoms due to attack by yang heat or various other factors or yin asthenia. This syndrome is usually caused by invasion of exogenous yang heat, or by interior transmission of heat transforming from pathogenic cold, or by transformation of fire from emotional upsets, or by transformation of heat from improper diet, or by internal generation of asthenic fire resulting from excessive coitus, internal impairment due to overstrain, exhaustion of yin essence as well as yin asthenia and yang sthenia. Heat syndrome may be further divided into external heat syndrome, internal heat syndrome, asthenic heat syndrome and sthenic heat syndrome according to the cause and location of diseases.

Clinical manifestations: The manifestations vary with different types of syndromes. The usual symptoms are fever, aversion to heat with preference for cold, flushed complexion or flushed cheeks, thirst with preference for cold drinks, restlessness and insomnia, yellowish and sticky sputum and snivel, vomiting blood and epistaxis, scanty brownish urine, dry feces, reddish tongue with scanty moist and fast pulse, etc.

Analysis of symptoms: Predomination of yang heat or yin asthenia and yang sthenia leads to internal exuberance of asthenic heat and causes fever and aversion to heat with preference for cold; fire tends to flame up drives qi and blood to flow upwards, leading to flushed complexion or flushed cheeks; consumption of body fluid by exuberant

澈清冷；寒邪困脾，或脾阳亏虚，运化失健，则大便稀溏。舌淡苔白而润滑，脉迟或紧，为阳虚阴寒内盛的征象。

### （二）热证

热证，是指感受阳热之邪，或多种原因导致机体阳盛，或阴虚所表现的证候。本证多因外感阳热之邪，或寒邪化热入里；或七情过极，五志化火；或饮食不节，积蓄为热；或房事不节，劳倦内伤，劫夺阴精，阴虚阳亢，虚热内生所致。根据形成原因及病位的不同，热证又可分为表热、里热、虚热、实热等。

临床表现：各类热证表现不尽一致，常见的有：发热恶热喜冷，满面通红或颧赤，口渴喜冷饮，烦躁失眠，痰涕黄稠，吐血衄血，小便短赤，大便干结，舌红少津，脉数等。

证候分析：阳热偏盛，或阴虚阳亢，虚热内炽，则发热恶热喜冷；火性炎上，气血上壅，则见满面通红或颧赤；热盛伤津，或阴液亏虚，则口渴喜冷饮，小便短赤；热扰心神，

heat or deficiency of yin fluid gives rise to thirst with preference for cold drinks and scanty and brownish urine; heat disturbing the heart spirit results in restlessness and insomnia; body fluid scorched by heat causes yellowish and thick sputum and snivel; heat impairing blood vessels and driving blood to extravasate brings about hematemesis and epistaxis; consumption of body fluid by exuberant heat or deficiency of yin fluid deprives the intestines of lubrication and proper transmission and leads to dry feces; reddish tongue with scanty fluid and fast pulse are signs of exuberant heat impairing body fluid.

则烦躁不眠；津液被热煎熬，则痰涕黄稠；热伤血络，迫血妄行，则吐血衄血；热盛伤津，或阴液亏虚，肠失滋润，传导失司，则大便干结。舌红少津，脉数，为热盛津伤的征象。

### 2.1.3 Syndrome differentiation of asthenia and sthenia

Asthenia and sthenia are two principles to differentiate the conditions of healthy qi and pathogenic factors.

Asthenia refers to insufficiency of healthy qi, while sthenia refers to exuberance of pathogenic factors. Syndrome differentiation of asthenia and sthenia is helpful for understanding whether pathogenic factors are in predominance or decline so as to decide to select therapy for complementing asthenia and strengthening healthy qi or therapy for purging sthenia and eliminating pathogenic factors.

#### 2.1.3.1 Asthenia syndrome

Asthenia syndrome refers to symptoms marked by asthenia of healthy qi and non-predomination of pathogenic factors. The cause of asthenia syndrome is either congenital or postnatal, especially the postnatal one. The postnatal cause includes insufficiency of qi and blood production due to improper diet, impairment of visceral qi and blood due to emotional factors and overstrain, exhaustion of renal essence due to excessive coitus, or impairment of healthy qi due to chronic disease, etc.

Clinical manifestations: Healthy qi in the human

## 三、虚实辨证

虚实，是辨别邪正盛衰的两个纲领。

虚指正气不足，实指邪气盛实。通过虚实辨证，可以了解机体的邪正盛衰，为确定采用补虚扶正或泻实祛邪的治法提供依据。

### （一）虚证

虚证是指人体正气虚弱而邪气亦不盛所表现的证候。虚证的形成原因，有先天不足和后天失调两个方面，以后天失调为主。如饮食失调，气血生化不足；或七情劳倦，内伤脏腑气血；或房事过度，劫夺肾脏元真；或久病不愈，损伤正气等均可导致虚证。

临床表现：由于人体正气

body mainly includes yangqi, yin fluid, essence, blood and body fluid, all of which are closely related to the viscera. Therefore, asthenia syndrome is mainly marked by insufficiency of yangqi, yin fluid, essence, blood and body fluid as well as the decline of visceral functions. The clinical manifestations of asthenia syndrome vary with different types which will be explained in the following parts. Here the common symptoms are taken as example to analyze the clinical manifestations of asthenia syndrome. The common symptoms include fatigue, shortness of breath, no desire to speak, aversion to cold and cold limbs, spontaneous sweating, clear and profuse urine, loose stool, emaciation, feverish sensation over the five centers (palms, soles and chest), tidal fever, flushed cheeks, night sweating, pale or sallow complexion, dizziness, palpitation and insomnia, dry mouth and throat, thirst with desire to drink, dry skin, scanty urine and dry feces, tender tongue with thin fur or little fur and weak pulse, etc.

Analysis of symptoms: Fatigue, shortness of breath and no desire to speak are due to failure of asthenic yangqi to propel and nourish the body, leading to hypofunction of viscera and tissues; spontaneous sweating is caused by failure of deficiency of yangqi and failure of defensive qi to guard the superficies; clear and profuse urine and loose stool are due to failure of deficient yang to astringe, warm and transport; emaciation is due to failure of deficient yin to nourish the body; feverish sensation over the five centers, tidal fever and flushed cheeks are due to predominance of yang heat, internal generation of asthenic heat and yin asthenia failing to control yang; night sweating is due to asthenic heat driving body fluid to be excreted; pale or sallow complexion is due to blood asthenia failing to nourish the face; dizziness is due to blood asthenia failing to nourish the head and eyes; palpitation is due to

主要包括阳气、阴液、精、血、津液等,而其均与脏腑密切相关。因此,虚证主要表现为机体阳气、阴液、精、血、津液等不足,以及脏腑功能的衰退。各种虚证的临床表现极不一致,具体内容见以下各节。现仅以常见症状为例说明之。如疲倦乏力,气短懒言,畏寒肢冷,自汗,小便清长,大便稀溏;形体消瘦,五心烦热,潮热,颧红,盗汗;面色淡白无华或萎黄,头晕目眩,心悸失眠;口干咽燥,渴欲饮水,皮肤干燥或枯瘪,小便短少,大便干结等。舌质娇嫩,苔薄或苔少,脉虚等。

证候分析:阳气亏虚,推动和濡养功能减弱,致脏腑组织功能减退,则疲倦乏力,气短懒言;阳气亏虚,机体失于温煦,则畏寒肢冷;阳气亏虚,卫表不固,则自汗;阳虚失于固摄、温运,则小便清长,大便稀溏。阴虚不能濡养、滋润机体,则形体消瘦;阴虚不能制阳,阳热偏亢,虚热内生,则五心烦热,潮热,颧红;虚热迫津外泄,则盗汗。血虚不能上荣于面,则面色淡白无华或萎黄;血虚,头目失养,则头晕目眩;血虚,心失所养,则心悸;血虚,心神失养而不宁,则失

malnutrition of the heart; insomnia is due to blood asthenia failing to nourish heart spirit; dry mouth, desire to drink and dry skin are due to failure of deficient fluid to nourish and moisten the tissues and organs; scanty urine is due to deficiency of body fluid and insufficiency of body fluid production; dry feces is due to loss of lubrication in the large intestine; tender tongue, thin fur or little fur and weak pulse are signs of deficiency of healthy qi.

### 2.1.3.2 Sthenia syndrome

Sthenia syndrome refers to symptoms of predominant pathogenic factors and non-asthenic healthy qi. The cause of sthenia syndrome includes two factors: one is invasion of exogenous pathogenic factors into the body; the other is dysfunction of the viscera, leading to the accumulation of phlegm, fluid, dampness and blood stasis in the body.

Clinical manifestations: The clinical manifestations vary with different types of sthenia syndrome due to the difference of pathogenic factors and the invading and accumulating regions. For example, internal predominance of pathogenic cold manifests cold syndrome, while exuberance of pathogenic heat manifests sthenic heat syndrome. The internal sthenic syndromes due to internal exuberance of phlegm, fluid, dampness, blood stasis and retention of food also vary in clinical manifestations which will be discussed in the following sections. Here the common symptoms are taken as examples to show the characteristics of sthenia syndrome. The common symptoms include fever, restlessness, even coma with delirium, chest oppression, hoarse breath, exuberance of phlegm and drool, unpalpable pain of abdomen, retention of dry feces, or dysentery with blood and pus, tenesmus, inhibited urination, or painful stringuria, tough tongue, thick or greasy fur and sthenic pulse, etc.

眠。津液亏少，不能充养、滋润组织器官，则口干咽燥，渴欲饮水，皮肤干燥或枯瘪；津液亏少，化源不足，则小便短少；大肠失于滋润，则大便干结。舌质娇嫩，苔薄或苔少，脉虚，均为正气亏虚的征象。

### (二) 实证

实证是指邪气盛实而正气亦不虚所表现的证候。实证的成因可以概括为两个方面：一是外邪侵入人体；一是脏腑功能失调，以致痰饮、水湿、瘀血等病理产物停积于体内所致。

临床表现：由于致病邪气的性质及其所侵袭、停聚部位的不同，各种实证的临床表现极不一致，如寒邪内盛表现为实寒证，热邪炽盛表现为实热证；其他如痰饮、水湿、瘀血、食积等邪气内盛所致的里实证，其临床表现也各有特点，具体内容见以下各节。现仅以常见症状为例说明之。如发热，烦躁，甚至神昏谵语；胸闷，呼吸气粗，痰涎壅盛；腹胀痛拒按，大便秘结；或下利脓血，里急后重；小便不利，或淋沥涩痛等。舌质苍老，苔厚或腻，脉实等。

Analysis of symptoms: Fever is due to exuberant pathogenic factors, confliction between healthy qi and pathogenic factors and predomination of yang heat; restlessness is due to pathogenic heat disturbing the heart; coma with delirium is due to exuberant heat disturbing heart spirit or sthenic pathogenic factors confusing heart spirit; chest oppression, hoarse breath and profuse sputum with rale are due to retention of pathogenic factors in the lung which prevents the lung from dispersing and descending; retention of feces and unpalpable abdominal pain are due to accumulation of sthenic pathogenic factors in the stomach and intestines which prevents free flow of intestinal qi; dysentery with blood and pus and tenesmus are due to accumulation of damp heat in the large intestine which hinders the transportation of the large intestine; inhibited urination is due to retention of fluid and dampness and inhibited transformation of qi; painful stranguria is due to accumulation of damp heat in the bladder and inhibited transformation of qi in the bladder; tough tongue with thick or greasy fur and sthenic pulse are the signs of internal retention of pathogenic factors and confliction between healthy qi and pathogenic factors.

证候分析：邪气盛实，正气抗邪，阳热亢盛，则发热；邪热扰心，则烦躁；热盛扰乱心神或实邪蒙蔽心神，则神昏谵语；邪阻于肺，宣降失常，则胸闷，喘息气粗，痰盛者尚可见痰声辘辘；实邪积于胃肠，腑气不通，则大便秘结，腹胀痛拒按；湿热蕴结于大肠，大肠传导失司，可见下利脓血，里急后重；水湿内停，气化不行，则小便不利；湿热蕴结膀胱，膀胱气化不利，则致小便淋沥涩痛。舌质苍老，苔厚或腻，脉实，均为实邪内阻，正邪相争的征象。

### 2.1.4 Syndrome differentiation of yin and yang

Yin and yang are the principles for categorizing diseases and also the leading ones in the eight principles. Syndrome differentiation of yin and yang are used in two aspects: differentiating yin syndrome and yang syndrome; differentiating yin asthenia and yang asthenia as well as yin depletion and yang depletion.

#### 2.1.4.1 Yin syndrome and yang syndrome

Syndrome differentiation of yin and yang, based on the application of the conception that all things can be

### 四、阴阳辨证

阴阳，既是概括病证类别的两个纲领，又是八纲辨证的总纲。阴阳辨证具体应用于两个方面：一是辨别阴证和阳证；二是辨别阴虚和阳虚、亡阴和亡阳。

**（一）阴证和阳证**

从事物可分为阴阳两个方面的观点出发，阴阳辨证把

divided into two aspects known as yin and yang, generalizes diseases into two categories, i. e. yin syndrome and yang syndrome. External, heat and sthenia syndromes are of yang category; while internal, cold and asthenia syndromes are of yin category. Therefore, yin and yang are the leading ones in the eight principles and include the other six ones.

#### 2.1.4.1.1　Yin syndrome

Syndromes that correspond to the nature of "yin" are called yin syndromes. Internal syndrome, cold syndrome and asthenia syndrome are of yin category. However, yin syndrome usually refers to asthenia cold syndrome.

Clinical manifestations: Yin syndrome varies with different diseases. The usual symptoms are dull complexion, dispiritedness, fatigue, cold limbs, low voice, shortness of breath, bland taste in the mouth without thirst, clear and profuse urine, loose stool, pale and tender tongue, sunken and thin pulse, or sunken, slow and weak pulse, etc.

Analysis of symptoms: Yin signifies quietness and cold. Dispiritedness, fatigue, low voice and shortness of breath are signs of hypofunction of viscera; dull complexion, cold limbs, bland taste in the mouth without thirst, clear and profuse urine and loose stool are signs of insufficiency of yangqi and internal exuberance of yin cold; pale and tender tongue, sunken and thin pulse or sunken, slow and weak pulse are signs of asthenic cold syndrome.

#### 2.1.4.1.2　Yang syndrome

The syndromes that correspond to the nature of "yang" are of yang category. External syndrome, heat syndrome and sthenia syndrome are of yang category. However, usually yang syndrome refers to sthenic heat syndrome.

病证概括地分为阴证和阳证两大类,即表、热、实证属阳,里、寒、虚证属阴。所以,阴阳又是八纲辨证的总纲,它可以统括其他六纲。

**1. 阴证**

凡符合"阴"的一般属性的证候,称为阴证。里证、寒证、虚证都属于阴证的范畴,但习惯上阴证常指虚寒证。

临床表现:不同的疾病所表现的阴证不尽相同。一般常见的有:面色暗淡,精神委靡,倦怠乏力,形寒肢冷,语声低怯,气短,口淡不渴,小便清长,大便稀溏,舌淡胖嫩,脉沉细,或沉迟无力等。

证候分析:阴主静、主寒。精神委靡,倦怠乏力,语声低怯,气短,是气虚脏腑机能减退的表现;面色暗淡,形寒肢冷,口淡不渴,小便清长,大便稀溏,是阳气不足,阴寒内盛的表现。舌淡胖嫩,脉沉细,或沉迟无力,均为虚寒证的征象。

**2. 阳证**

凡符合"阳"的一般属性的证候,称为阳证。表证、热证、实证都属于阳证的范畴,但习惯上阳证常指实热证。

Clinical manifestations: Yang syndromes in diseases vary in manifestations. The usual symptoms are flushed complexion, fever with preference for cold, restlessness, high voice, hoarse breath, dyspnea with sputum rale, dry mouth with thirst and desire to drink, scanty brownish urine, retention of dry feces, deep reddish tongue with yellow and dry fur, powerful or full or slippery pulse, etc.

Analysis of symptoms: Yang governs movement and heat. Flushed complexion, fever with preference for cold, restlessness and high voice are signs of hyperfunction of the viscera; hoarse breath, dyspnea with sputum rale are the signs of retention of phlegm in the lung and failure of the lung to disperse and descend; dry mouth with thirst and desire to drink, scanty and brownish urine and retention of dry feces are signs of exuberant heat impairing body fluid; deep reddish tongue with yellow and dry fur and powerful or full or slippery pulse are signs of sthenic heat syndrome.

### 2.1.4.2　Yin asthenia syndrome and yang asthenia syndrome

#### 2.1.4.2.1　Yin asthenia syndrome

Yin asthenia syndrome refers to asthenic heat symptoms due to failure of yin to control yang resulting from deficiency of yin fluid.

Clinical manifestations: Emaciation, dry mouth and throat, dizziness, palpitation, insomnia, scanty tongue fur, thin pulse, or even feverish sensation over the five centers (palms, soles and chest), tidal fever, flushed cheeks, night sweating, deep reddish tongue with scanty fur and thin and fast pulse.

Analysis of symptoms: Emaciation, dry mouth and throat, dizziness, palpitation, insomnia, scanty tongue fur and thin pulse are due to malnutrition of the body,

临床表现：不同的疾病所表现的阳证不完全相同。一般常见的有：面色红赤，身热喜冷，烦躁，语声高亢，呼吸气粗，喘促痰鸣，口干渴饮，小便短赤，大便秘结，舌质红绛，苔黄而干，脉数有力，或洪大，或滑等。

证候分析：阳主动，主热。面色红赤，身热喜冷，烦躁，语声高亢，是热盛脏腑机能亢进的表现；呼吸气粗，喘促痰鸣，是痰湿阻肺，肺失宣降的表现；口干渴饮，小便短赤，大便秘结等是热盛伤津的表现。舌质红绛，苔黄而干，脉数有力，或洪大，或滑，均为实热证的征象。

### （二）阴虚证和阳虚证

#### 1. 阴虚证

阴虚证是指由于阴液亏损而导致阴不制阳所表现的虚热证候。

临床表现：形体消瘦，口咽干燥，头晕目眩，心悸，失眠，苔少，脉细，甚则五心烦热，潮热，颧红，盗汗，舌红绛少苔，脉细数。

证候分析：阴液亏损，形体脏腑组织失养，则形体消瘦，口燥咽干，头晕目眩，心

viscera and tissues; feverish sensation over the five centers, tidal fever, flushed cheeks, night sweating, reddish tongue with scanty fur as well as thin and fast pulse are due to interior generation of asthenic heat resulting from failure of asthenic yin to control yang.

### 2.1.4.2.2 Yang asthenia syndrome

Yang asthenia syndrome refers to asthenic cold symptoms due to failure of insufficient yangqi to control yin.

Clinical manifestations: Pale complexion, dispiritedness, fatigue, shortness of breath, no desire to speak, aversion to cold with cold limbs, spontaneous sweating, moist mouth without thirst, or thirst with preference for hot drinks, clear and profuse urine, loose stool, or scanty urine with edema, pale, bulgy and tender tongue, whitish slippery fur as well as slow, sunken and weak pulse, etc.

Analysis of symptoms: Failure of insufficiency of yangqi to propel and nourish leads to hypofunction of viscera and tissues, giving rise to such symptoms like pale complexion, dispiritedness, fatigue, shortness of breath and no desire to speak; deficiency of yangqi weakens the defensive qi, leading to spontaneous sweating; failure of deficient yangqi to control yin results in internal exuberance of yin cold, bringing about aversion to cold, cold limbs, bland taste in the mouth without thirst or thirst with preference for hot drinks; failure of asthenic yang to astringe and warm causes clear profuse urine and loose stool; scanty urine, swelling and distension are usually caused by failure of asthenic spleen and kidney yang to warm and transport which leads to internal retention of fluid and edema; pale, bulgy and tender tongue with whitish and slippery fur as well as sunken, slow and weak pulse are signs of internal exuberance of yin cold due to yang asthenia.

悸,失眠,苔少,脉细;阴虚不能制阳,致虚热内生,则出现五心烦热,潮热,颧红,盗汗,舌红绛少苔,脉细数等症。

### 2. 阳虚证

阳虚证是指由于阳气亏损而导致阳不制阴所表现的虚寒证候。

临床表现:面色㿠白,精神委靡,疲倦乏力,少气懒言,畏寒肢冷,自汗,口润不渴,或渴喜热饮,小便清长,大便稀溏,或尿少肿胀,舌淡胖嫩,苔白滑,脉沉迟无力。

证候分析:阳气不足,推动和濡养功能减弱,致脏腑组织机能减退,则面色㿠白,精神委靡,疲倦乏力,少气懒言;阳气亏虚,卫表不固,则自汗;阳气亏虚,阳不制阴,致阴寒内盛,则畏寒肢冷,口淡不渴,或渴喜热饮;阳虚失于固摄、温运,则小便清长,大便稀溏;若脾肾阳虚,温运无权,水湿内停,泛溢肌肤,则尿少肿胀。舌淡胖嫩,苔白滑,脉沉迟无力,为阳虚阴寒内盛的征象。

### 2.1.4.3 Yin depletion syndrome and yang depletion syndrome

#### 2.1.4.3.1 Yin depletion syndrome

Yin depletion syndrome refers to the critical conditions of severe exhaustion of yin fluid. This syndrome is usually caused by continuous high fever, profuse sweating and excessive vomiting and diarrhea in exogenous febrile diseases, or by massive bleeding, or by chronic disease in which profuse yin fluid is lost due to gradual consumption.

Clinical manifestations: Apart from the serious symptoms seen in the primary disease, there appear some other symptoms, including pyretic, salty and sticky sweating, fever over the body, warm limbs with aversion to heat, dry skin, flushed complexion, thirst with preference for cold drinks, restlessness, or even coma, scanty urine, reddish and dry tongue as well as thin, fast, swift and weak pulse, etc.

Analysis of the symptoms: Failure of exhausting yin fluid to control yang gives rise to internal exuberance of asthenic heat and drives fluid to be excreted, leading to feverish, salty and sticky sweating, feverish body and warm limbs with aversion to heat as well as flushed complexion; deficiency of yin fluid and loss of moisture lead to dry skin, thirst, preference for cold drinks and dry tongue; exhaustion of fluid causes scanty urine; heat disturbing heart spirit results in restlessness or even coma; reddish dry tongue as well as fast, swift and weak pulse are the signs of internal heat due to yin asthenia.

#### 2.1.4.3.2 Yang depletion syndrome

Yang depletion syndrome refers to critical symptoms due to declination of yangqi. This syndrome is usually caused by massive bleeding, profuse sweating, violent vomiting and diarrhea which lead to exhaustion of blood and loss of yang together with yin, or by sudden loss of

## （三）亡阴证和亡阳证

### 1. 亡阴证

亡阴证是指由于阴液严重亏损而欲竭所表现的危重证候。多因外感热病壮热不退、大汗、剧烈吐泻；或大量出血；或慢性病，阴液逐渐暗耗等，致阴液大量亡失而形成。

临床表现：除原发病的严重症状以外，尚可见汗热味咸而粘，身热肢温而恶热，肌肤干瘪，面色潮红，口渴喜冷饮，烦躁不安，甚则昏迷，小便极少，舌红而干，脉细数疾而按之无力。

证候分析：阴液欲竭，阴虚不能制阳，虚热内炽，迫津外泄，则汗热味咸而粘，身热肢温而恶热，面色潮红；阴液亏虚，失于濡润，则肌肤干瘪，口渴喜冷饮，舌干；津液耗竭，则小便极少；热扰心神，则烦躁不安，甚则昏迷。舌红而干，脉细数疾按之无力，为阴虚内热的征象。

### 2. 亡阳证

亡阳证是指由于阳气衰微而欲脱所表现的危重证候。多因大失血、大汗出、剧烈吐泻，致阴血消亡，阳随阴脱；或阴寒之邪极盛，侵袭人体，致

yangqi due to extreme exuberant cold attacking the body, or by chronic disease which gradually exhausts yangqi, or by retention of phlegm that obstructs the heart vessels, etc.

Clinical manifestations: Apart from severe symptoms in primary disease, there are still some other manifestations, such as profuse cold sweating, pale complexion, cold skin, cold limbs, bland taste in the mouth without thirst or with thirst and preference for hot drinks, weak breath, dispiritedness, or even unconsciousness, coma, pale and moist tongue as well as indistinct pulse.

Analysis of symptoms: Profuse cold sweating is due to depletion of yangqi that fails to astringe; pale complexion and pale tongue are due to decline of yangqi that fails to transport blood upwards; cold skin and limbs is due to decline of yangqi that fails to warm; bland taste in the mouth without thirst or with thirst and preference for hot drinks is due to internal exuberance of yin cold resulting from declination of yangqi; weak breath is due to loss of yangqi and asthenia of qi; dispiritedness and even unconsciousness and coma are due to declination of yangqi and loss of nutrition for spirit; indistinct pulse is due to depletion of yangqi that fails to warm and transport blood.

Both yin depletion syndrome and yang depletion syndrome may appear at the critical stage of diseases. Inaccurate differentiation of syndrome or delayed treatment will lead to separation of yin from yang and result in death. Since yin and yang in the human body depend on each other to exist, depletion of yin may lead to depletion of yang, and vice versa. In clinical practice, it is necessary to make clear whether yin depletion or yang depletion is primary for the benefit of timely treatment.

阳气暴伤；或慢性病，阳气渐伤致极；或瘀痰闭阻心脉等而形成。

临床表现：除原发病的严重症状以外，尚可见冷汗淋漓、面色苍白、肌肤凉、四肢冷、口淡不渴或渴喜热饮、呼吸微弱、精神委靡，甚则神志模糊、昏迷，舌淡而润，脉微欲绝。

证候分析：阳气虚脱，固摄无权，津液外泄，则冷汗淋漓；阳气虚衰，不能运血上荣，则面色苍白，舌淡；阳气虚脱，失于温煦，则肌肤凉、四肢冷；阳气亏虚，阴寒内盛，则口淡不渴或渴喜热饮；阳气外泄，气虚于内，则呼吸微弱；阳气虚衰，神失所养，则精神委靡，甚则神志模糊、昏迷。阳气外脱，无力温运血脉，则脉微欲绝。

亡阴证与亡阳证均出现于疾病的危重阶段，辨证错误，或救治稍迟，就会导致阴阳离决而死亡。由于人体的阴阳是依存互根的，所以亡阴可以导致亡阳，而亡阳也可以致使阴液更加耗竭。在临床上，宜分别亡阴、亡阳之主次，及时救治。

## 2.1.5 Relationship among the eight principal syndromes

In syndrome differentiation of eight principles, complicated diseases are generalized into four pairs of principal syndromes, i. e. external and internal syndromes, cold and heat syndromes, asthenia and sthenia syndromes and yin and yang syndromes. These four pairs of principal syndromes, however, are not solitary, absolute and static. In fact, they are correlated and inseparable. In clinical differentiation of syndromes, trials are not only made to distinguish the principal syndromes, but also their correlation. Only a comprehensive analysis of the eight principal syndromes ensures correct diagnosis.

### 2.1.5.1 Relationship between two principles in a pair

The relationship between two principles in a pair manifests as combination or mixture of the syndromes, transformation of syndromes and false manifestations in certain syndromes.

#### 2.1.5.1.1 Relationship between external and internal syndromes

During the course of disease and under certain conditions, there may appear simultaneous internal and external disorder, transmission of pathogenic factors from the exterior into the interior and from the interior to the exterior.

**Simultaneous external and internal disorder**: At the same stage, there appear both external syndrome and internal syndrome. The causes of such a morbid condition are various. It may be caused by invasion of pathogenic

## 五、八纲证候间的关系

八纲辨证从疾病本质的不同角度,把错综复杂的病证归纳为表证与里证、寒证与热证、虚证与实证、阴证与阳证等四对纲领性证候。然而,这四对纲领性证候并不是孤立、绝对对立和静止不变的,它们之间互相联系,不可分割。临床辨证时,不仅要识别八纲基本证候,更应注意它们之间的相互关系,将八纲联系起来对病情作综合分析,才能作出全面、正确的诊断。

### (一) 同一对纲领间的关系

同一对纲领证候间的关系,主要表现为证候相兼或错杂、证候转化和某些证候可以出现假象等。

**1. 表证和里证的关系**

疾病发展过程中,在一定的条件下,可出现表里同病与表邪入里和里邪出表。

(1) 表里同病:患者在同一时期,既出现表证,又出现里证,称为表里同病。形成表里同病的原因有以下几种:外

factors into both the external and internal phases marked by appearance of both external syndrome and internal syndrome at the early stage, or by transmission of pathogenic factors into the interior when the external syndrome is not cured yet, or by contraction of new disease when old one is not cured yet, such as internal impairment followed by contraction of exogenous disease or contraction of exogenous disease followed by improper diet, etc.

Simultaneous appearance of both external and internal syndromes often appears together with cold and heat as well as asthenia and sthenia, usually manifesting as external heat and internal cold, external cold and internal heat as well as external sthenia and internal asthenia, etc. which will be discussed in the following sections.

**External and internal transmission:** During the course of disease and under certain conditions, external pathogenic factors fail to be relieved and transmit into the interior, bringing about internal syndrome; in some internal syndromes, pathogenic factors transmit from the interior to the exterior and produce some external symptoms.

Transmission of exterior pathogenic factors into the interior: Internal syndrome appears after external syndrome and external syndrome disappears with the appearance of the internal syndrome. Such a morbid condition is caused by hyperactivity of pathogenic factors, or by frequent deficiency of healthy qi, or by improper nursing, or by delayed or erroneous treatment that reduces resistance of the body and leads to transmission of pathogenic factors from the external to the internal. This morbid condition is usually seen in the course of exogenous diseases. For example, external syndrome manifests such symptoms like aversion to cold, fever, headache and body pain, whitish thin fur and floating pulse, etc. Transmission of exterior pathogenic factors into the interior and external syndrome

邪同时侵犯表里,初病即既见表证又见里证;或表证未愈,病邪又传及于里;或旧病未愈,又加新病,如本有内伤,复又外感,或先有外感,又伤饮食等。

表里同病的出现,往往与寒热、虚实互见,常见的有表热里寒、表寒里热、表实里虚等,详见后述。

(2) 表里出入:表里出入,是指疾病发展过程中,在一定条件下,表邪不解,内传入里,出现里证;某些里证,病邪从里透达于外,出现某些肌表的症状。

表邪入里:是指先出现表证,后出现里证,而表证随之消失,称为表邪入里。多因病邪亢盛,或正气素虚,或护理不当,或失治、误治等因素致机体抗邪能力降低,表邪内传所导致。常见于外感病的发展过程中。例如:原病表证,出现恶寒发热、头痛身痛、苔薄白、脉浮等症。若恶寒消失,不恶寒反恶热,并见壮热、口渴引饮、舌红苔黄、脉数等症,即为表邪入里,表证转化为里证。

transforming into internal syndrome can be distinguished by such changes like disappearance of aversion to cold and aversion to heat together with high fever, thirst with desire to drink, reddish tongue with yellowish fur and fast pulse, etc.

Transmission of pathogenic factors from the interior to the exterior: Under certain conditions in some internal syndromes, pathogenic factors transmit from the interior to the exterior, leading to the appearance of some external symptoms and alleviation of the internal syndrome. This is the result of proper treatment and nursing that have strengthened the resistance of the body and driven pathogenic factors out of the body. For example, high fever, restlessness, chest oppression, cough and dyspnea in primary disease followed by disappearance of fever after sweating, or eruption of measles and milliaria alba as well as alleviation of restlessness, chest oppression, cough and dyspnea is the sign of pathogenic factors transmitting from the internal to the external.

Transmission of pathogenic factors from the exterior to the interior is a sign of aggravation of pathological changes, while transmission of pathogenic factors from the interior to the exterior signifies the decline of disease. Cognition of such changes is significant for judging the development and changes of diseases.

### 2.1.5.1.2 Relationship between cold syndrome and heat syndrome

Cold syndrome and heat syndrome, though different in nature, are correlated. They may simultaneously appear in one patient and manifest as mixture of cold and heat. Under certain conditions, they may transform into each other. During the development of diseases, especially at severe stage, there may appear such phenomena like false cold and false heat.

里邪出表：某些里证，在一定的条件下，病邪从里透达于外，出现某些肌表的症状，里证随之减轻，称为里邪出表。这是由于治疗、护理得当，机体抗邪能力增强，祛邪外出的结果。例如：原病壮热烦躁、胸闷、咳嗽喘息，继而汗出热退，或斑疹、白痦外透，烦躁、胸闷、咳嗽、喘息等症随之减轻，这是病邪由里出表的表现。

表邪入里表示病势加重，里邪出表反映邪有去路，病势减轻。掌握表里出入的变化，对于推断疾病的发展转归有重要意义。

### 2. 寒证与热证的关系

寒证和热证虽有本质的不同，但又相互联系，它们既可以在同一病人身上同时出现，表现为寒热错杂的证候；又可以在一定的条件下，互相转化，表现为寒证转化为热证，或热证转化为寒证；在疾病发展过程中，特别是危重阶

**Mixture of cold and heat**: Cold syndrome and heat syndrome appear at the same time in one patient. It may be one stage at the development of a disease or signify two syndromes in one patient, i.e. a cold syndrome and a heat syndrome. The commonly encountered ones are upper heat and lower cold, upper cold and lower heat, external cold and internal heat as well as external heat and internal cold.

Upper heat and lower cold syndrome: For example, there are heat symptoms like feverish sensation in the chest, halitosis and swelling pain of gums in the upper part of the body accompanied by cold symptoms like abdominal pain and preference for warmth and loose stool in the lower part of the body.

Upper cold and lower heat syndrome: For example, there are cold symptoms like cold stomachache, reduced appetite and vomiting clear drool in the upper part of the body accompanied by heat syndromes like scanty brownish urine, frequent micturition and painful urination in the lower energizer due to cold in the stomach and heat in the bladder.

External heat and internal cold syndrome: This syndrome is usually caused by frequent existence of internal cold complicated by invasion of pathogenic heat; or by impairment of yangqi in the spleen and stomach in external heat syndrome due to excessive taking of cold drugs. For example, in patients with asthenia of spleen and kidney yang complicated by invasion of exogenous pathogenic heat, there appear borborygmus, abdominal pain and diar-

段,有时还会出现假寒或假热的现象。

(1)寒热错杂:患者在同一时期,既出现寒证,又出现热证,称为寒热错杂。寒热错杂可以是一种疾病发展过程中的一个阶段,也可能是一位患者同时患有两种病证,其中一种为寒,一种为热,常见的有上热下寒、上寒下热、表寒里热、表热里寒等几种情况。

上热下寒证:患者同时上部表现为热,下部表现为寒的证候,为上热下寒证。例如:患者既见胸中烦热、口臭、牙龈肿痛等上热的表现,又见腹痛喜暖、大便稀溏等下寒的症状,此为上热下寒证。

上寒下热证:患者同时上部表现为寒,下部表现为热的证候,为上寒下热证。例如:患者素患胃脘冷痛、食少、呕吐清涎之寒证,又出现小便短赤、尿频、尿痛等热在下焦的症状,此为胃中有寒、膀胱有热的上寒下热证。

表热里寒证:患者同时出现热在其表,寒在其里的证候。常见于素有里寒,又感风热之邪;或表热证因过服寒凉药物,损伤脾胃阳气而形成。例如:脾肾阳虚患者,复感风热之邪,出现既肠鸣腹痛、下利清谷,又见发热微恶风寒、

rhea with indigested food complicated by fever, slight aversion to wind and cold, headache and swelling sorethroat, etc.

External cold and internal heat syndrome: This syndrome may be caused in two ways. One is frequent existence of internal heat complicated by invasion of wind and cold. For example, manifestations of hyperactivity of liver fire like susceptibility to irritation, flushed complexion, red eyes, dizziness, distending headache, bitter taste and dryness in the mouth are complicated by external cold symptoms like aversion to cold, fever, anhidrosis and cough. The other is cold pathogenic factors transmitting into the internal and transforming into heat prior to the relief of external cold. For example, symptoms of external cold syndrome like severe aversion to cold and slight fever, pain of head and body, anhidrosis and floating pulse followed by internal transmission of pathogenic cold and continuous existence of external cold with the symptoms of internal heat syndrome like aggravation of fever, thirst, restlessness and reddish tongue.

In dealing with simultaneous appearance of cold syndrome and heat syndrome, trials should be made to distinguish the upper and the lower as well as the external and the internal. The differentiation of whether the cold is principal or secondary or whether heat is principal or secondary is also essential for establishing therapeutic principles and deciding treatment.

**Inter-transformation of cold and heat**: Cold syndrome or heat syndrome of diseases signifies the conditions of yin and yang in the body. Under certain conditions, the states of yin and yang in the body vary. The cold or heat nature of the syndrome changes accordingly.

Transformation of cold syndrome into heat syndrome:

头痛、咽喉肿痛等症状,即为表热里寒证。

表寒里热证:患者同时出现寒在其表,热在其里的证候。其形成有两种情况:一是素有内热,又感风寒,如患者本有急躁易怒、面红目赤、头晕胀痛、口苦口干等肝火上炎的表现,又见恶寒发热、无汗、咳嗽等表寒证的表现,即为表寒里热证。二是寒邪入里化热而表寒未解,如初起出现恶寒重发热轻、头身疼痛、无汗、脉浮等表寒证的表现,继则寒邪入里化热而表寒仍在,发热由轻转重,又出现口渴、烦躁、舌红等里热证的表现,为表寒里热证。

寒证与热证同时并见,除了要分清上下、表里之外,还要分清寒热孰多孰少和标本先后主次。这些鉴别十分重要,是治疗立法用药的依据。

(2)寒热转化:疾病表现为寒证或热证,是机体阴阳盛衰的反映。在一定的条件下,机体的阴阳盛衰发生了变化,则证候的寒热属性亦随之转化。

寒证转化为热证:患者先

The patient shows cold syndrome first, and then heat syndrome. The cold syndrome disappears after the appearance of the heat syndrome. For example, the patient is attacked by pathogenic cold and shows symptoms of external cold syndrome, such as aversion to cold, fever, headache and body pain, no sweating, white fur and floating-tense pulse. As the pathological conditions further develop, the cold pathogenic factors transmit into the interior and transform into heat, bringing about symptoms of internal heat syndrome, such as disappearance of aversion to cold, high fever, dysphoria, thirst, yellow fur and fast pulse, etc.

Transformation of heat syndrome into cold syndrome: The patient shows heat syndrome first, and then cold syndrome. When cold syndrome appears, heat syndrome disappears. Such a transformation may be either sudden or gradual. For example, chronic heat dysentery consumes yangqi and gradually transforms into asthenic cold dysentery. This transformation is slow. In patients with high fever, yang leakage with profuse sweating or yang exhaustion with excessive vomiting and diarrhea will lead to symptoms of asthenic cold syndrome (depletion of yang), such as sudden decrease of body temperature, cold limbs, pale complexion and indistinct pulse. This transformation is sudden.

The transformation between cold syndrome and heat syndrome lies in the confliction between pathogenic factors and healthy qi. Transformation of cold syndrome into heat syndrome indicates that the healthy qi is strong, yangqi is exuberant and pathogenic factors transforms into heat with yang. Such a morbid condition, though indicating further development of the pathological conditions, suggests normal strength of the healthy qi that is capable enough of resisting invasion of pathogenic factors.

出现寒证，后出现热证，热证出现后，寒证便随之消失，即为寒证转化为热证。例如：患者感受寒邪，出现恶寒发热、头痛身痛、无汗、苔白、脉浮紧等症，为表寒证，病情进一步发展，寒邪化热入里，恶寒等症消退，壮热、心烦口渴、苔黄、脉数等症相继出现，即为由表寒证转化为里热证。

热证转化为寒证：患者先出现热证，后出现寒证，寒证出现后，热证便随之消失，即为热证转化为寒证。这种转化可缓可急。如热痢日久，阳气日耗，转化为虚寒痢。这是缓慢转化的过程。如高热病人，由于大汗不止，阳随汗泄，或吐泻过度，阳随津脱，出现体温骤降、四肢厥冷、面色苍白、脉微欲绝的虚寒证（亡阳），这是急骤转化的过程。

寒证与热证的转化，关键在于邪正双方力量的对比。寒证转化为热证，是人体正气尚强，阳气旺盛，邪气从阳化热，虽为病进，但提示机体正气未衰，犹能抗邪；热证转化为寒证，是机体正气虚衰，阳气耗伤，无力抗邪的表现，提示邪盛正虚，正不胜邪，病情

Transformation of heat syndrome into cold syndrome indicates decline of the healthy qi, consumption of yangqi and no strength to resist pathogenic factors, suggesting predominance of pathogenic factors and asthenia of healthy qi, failure of the healthy qi to dominate over pathogenic factors and worsening of the pathological conditions.

**False and true manifestations of cold and heat:** In the development of certain diseases, especially at the critical stage of some severe diseases, cold syndrome or heat syndrome may show some manifestations contrary to the nature of the disease, therefore bringing about true cold and false heat syndrome or true heat and false cold syndrome. False manifestations usually cover up the nature of disease. In clinical treatment, cares should be taken to distinguish true manifestations from the false ones to avoid erroneous diagnosis.

True cold and false heat syndrome: Cold syndrome shows false heat symptoms. For example, in some patients with severe yang asthenia and internal cold syndrome, there appear such symptoms like cold limbs, dispiritedness, indigested diarrhea, clear and profuse urine and pale tongue with white fur together with the symptoms like heat syndrome, such as flushed complexion, feverish body, thirst and large pulse. However, flushed complexion only occasionally appears on the cheeks with pale complexion; the body is feverish, but the patient still wants more clothes and quilt; though thirsty, the patient prefers hot water and does not drink much; though large, the pulse is weak when pressed. Such a morbid condition is caused by internal exuberance of cold which drives declining yang outward known as "predominant yin rejecting yang".

True heat and false cold syndrome: Heat syndrome shows false cold manifestations. For example, in some

恶化。

（3）寒热真假：某些疾病的发展过程中，尤其是病情危重阶段，寒证或热证有时会出现与疾病本质相反的一些假象，从而形成真寒假热证或真热假寒证。假象的出现往往会掩盖疾病的本质，临证时应仔细辨别，以免误诊。

真寒假热证：是指疾病的本质是寒证，而外见假热征象的证候。例如某些严重的阳虚内寒证患者，出现四肢厥冷、精神委靡、下利清谷、小便清长、舌淡苔白等症，同时又出现面红、身热、口渴、脉大等类似热证的表现。但是，患者虽面红，却是在面色苍白的基础上仅颧颊部泛红如妆，时隐时现；虽身热，却反欲盖衣被；虽口渴，却喜热饮，且饮水不多；虽脉大却按之无力。这是由于阴寒内盛，将已非常虚衰的阳气格拒于外所致。因此，亦称"阴盛格阳"。

真热假寒证：是指疾病的本质是热证，而外见假寒征象

patients with severe internal heat syndrome, there appear symptoms of fever, thirst with preference for cold drinks, restlessness, scanty brownish urine, retention of dry feces and reddish tongue with yellow fur together with symptoms like cold syndrome, such as cold limbs and sunken pulse, etc. However, the patient feels cold in limbs, but scorching feverish over the chest and abdomen with aversion to heat; though sunken, the pulse is fast and powerful. This is due to internal exuberant heat stagnates yangqi and prevents it to reach the limbs. Such a morbid condition is caused by internal exuberant yang driving yin outward, known as "exuberant yang rejecting yin". Under such a condition, the severer the internal heat, the colder the limbs, which is known as "severer heat and severer cold".

Key points for differentiating false and true cold and heat syndromes:

Firstly, false manifestations usually appear over the complexion, limbs and superficies. However, the changes of viscera, qi, blood and body fluid are essential. So the manifestations of internal syndrome should be taken as the evidence for diagnosis, such as whether there are thirst, preference and aversion and how the tongue conditions and pulse states are.

Secondly, pay attention to the difference between false manifestations and true ones. For example, in false heat syndrome, flushed complexion only appears on the forehead and cheeks, and the colour is light, tender, floating and occasional; while flushed complexion in the true heat syndrome involves the whole face. Take false cold syndrome for example, though the limbs are cold, the patient does not want more clothes and quilt and the chest and abdomen feel scorching feverish; in true cold syndrome, cold limbs appears together with huddled pos-

的证候。例如某些严重的里实热证患者，出现壮热、口渴饮冷、烦躁不宁、小便短赤、大便燥结、舌红苔黄等症，同时又有四肢厥冷、脉沉等类似寒证的表现。但是，患者虽肢冷，却胸腹灼热，且反恶热；脉虽沉，却数而有力。这是由于里热炽盛，致阳气郁闭于内，不能外达于四肢所形成，即阳盛于内，格阴于外。因此，亦称"阳盛格阴"。其里热愈甚，则四肢厥冷愈严重，即所谓"热深厥亦深"。

寒热真假的辨证要点：

首先，假象多出现在面色、四肢、体表等方面，而脏腑、气血、津液等方面的变化是疾病的本质，故应以里证的表现为诊断的依据，如口渴与否、喜恶之情、舌象、脉象等。

其次，注意假象与真象的区别。例如假热证的面红仅表现在额颊上，且颜色浅红而娇嫩，浮在肤表，时隐时现；真热证的面红是满面通红。又如假寒证虽见肢冷但反不欲盖衣被，且胸腹灼热；真寒证肢冷的同时常并见身蜷卧、欲盖衣被等症。

ture in sleep and need more clothes and quilt.

#### 2.1.5.1.3 Relationship between asthenia syndrome and sthenia syndrome

In the development of diseases, asthenia of healthy qi and sthenia of pathogenic factors oppose each other and are also related to each other. Therefore, asthenia syndrome and sthenia syndrome may appear simultaneously or transform into each other and appear in sequence. At the critical stage of diseases, there may appear false sthenia and false asthenia manifestations.

**Mixture of asthenia and sthenia**: Asthenia of healthy qi and sthenia of pathogenic factors exist simultaneously at the same stage in a patient. This morbid conditions is usually caused by pathogenic factors in a sthenia syndrome impairing healthy qi, or by invasion of new pathogenic factors in an asthenia syndrome with deficiency of healthy qi, or by accumulation of pathological substances in the body due to deficiency of healthy qi and dysfunction of viscera in an asthenia syndrome. Mixture of asthenia and sthenia may be a stage in the development of a disease or may appear as two syndromes at the same time in a patient in which one is asthenia and the other sthenia. This morbid condition may be further divided into asthenia syndrome complicated by sthenia, sthenia syndrome complicated by asthenia and equality of asthenia and sthenia according to the levels of asthenia and sthenia.

Sthenia syndrome complicated by asthenia: This syndrome is marked by predominance of pathogenic factors complicated by asthenia of healthy qi. For example, in an internal sthenic heat syndrome with the manifestations of high fever, flushed complexion, dysphoria, sweating, reddish tongue and full and large pulse, there appear at the same time such symptoms like thirst, scanty brownish urine and retention of dry feces. Such a morbid

3. 虚证与实证的关系

在疾病过程中，正气虚与邪气盛，既相互对立，又相互联系，往往还互为因果。因此，虚证与实证既可以相互夹杂而同时出现，又可以由于转化而先后出现。此外，在疾病的危重阶段，有时还会出现假实或假虚的现象。

（1）虚实夹杂：同一患者，同一时期，存在着正虚与邪实两方面的病变，即为虚实夹杂证。多因病为实证，病邪损伤正气，正气已伤而病邪仍在；或病为虚证，正气不足，又感新邪；或病为虚证，因正气不足，脏腑功能失调，致病理产物停积体内而形成。虚实夹杂可以是一种疾病发展过程中的一个阶段，也可能是一位患者同时患有两种病证，其中一种为虚，一种为实。根据虚实之多少，可分为虚证夹实、实证夹虚以及虚实并重等多种情况。

实证夹虚：是指以邪气盛实为主，兼有正气虚弱所表现的一类证候。例如壮热、面赤、烦躁、汗出、舌红、脉洪大的里实热证，同时又出现口渴、小便短赤、大便干结等症，此属热盛伤津所致，以热邪炽盛为主的虚实夹杂证。

condition is due to consumption of body fluid by predominant heat and exuberance of pathogenic heat.

Asthenia syndrome complicated by sthenia: This syndrome is marked by deficiency of healthy qi complicated by retention of sthenic pathogenic factors. For example, at the advanced stage of seasonal febrile disease, there appear such symptoms like low fever, dispiritedness, dry mouth, poor appetite, furless tongue and thin pulse, etc. Such a morbid condition is typical of asthenia syndrome complicated by sthenia marked by deficiency of healthy qi due to impairment of qi and yin by remaining heat.

Equality of asthenia and sthenia: This syndrome is marked by equal degree of the deficiency of healthy qi and sthenia of pathogenic factors. For example, tympanites due to failure of asthenic spleen and kidney yang to transform qi and transport fluid is marked by manifestations of sthenia syndrome like drum-like abdomen and scanty urine as well as by symptoms of asthenia syndrome like aversion to cold, cold limbs, pale complexion, aching weakness of loins and knees and deep-thin pulse, etc. In such a morbid condition, the degree of the deficiency of healthy qi and the degree of the sthenia of pathogenic factors are practically equal.

**Transformation of asthenia and sthenia**: In the development of a disease, the confliction of pathogenic factors and healthy qi is usually signified by transformation of asthenia and sthenia. Such a transformation usually appears as transformation of sthenia into asthenia and development of asthenia into sthenia in clinical practice.

Transformation of sthenia syndrome into asthenia: This transformation is marked by sthenia syndrome followed by asthenia syndrome in the course of a disease. Such a transformation of syndrome is usually due to

虚证夹实：是指以正气亏虚为主，兼有实邪停积所表现的一类证候。例如温病后期阶段，出现低热、神疲、口干、纳少、舌苔光剥、脉细等症，此属余热未尽，气阴两伤所致，以正气亏虚为主的虚实夹杂证。

虚实并重：是指正气虚弱与邪气盛实的程度大致相当所表现的一类证候。例如脾肾阳虚，不能化气行水所致的鼓胀病，既有腹大胀满如鼓、小便短少之实证的表现，又有畏寒肢冷，面色㿠白，腰膝酸冷，脉沉细等虚证的表现，正虚邪实程度大致相当，难分主次，故为虚实并重的虚实夹杂证。

(2) 虚实转化：疾病过程中，邪正斗争往往表现为证候的虚实变化。临床常见的有实证转虚和因虚致实。

实证转虚：疾病过程中先出现实证，后出现虚证，而实证表现随之消失，即为实证转化为虚证。多因病邪亢盛或

hyperactivity of pathogenic factors, or retention of pathogenic factors in the body and impairment of healthy qi due to erroneous treatment and delayed treatment. For example, at the primary stage of exogenous disease, there appear such symptoms like high fever, flushed complexion, restlessness, or even coma and delirium, reddish tongue with yellow fur as well as full and large pulse which are the manifestations of sthenic heat syndrome. At the advanced stage, there appear such symptoms like dispiritedness, emaciation, dry throat and mouth, tremor of hands and feet, reddish and dry tongue, furless tongue as well as thin and fast pulse which signify the transformation of sthenia syndrome into asthenia syndrome due to prolonged retention of pathogenic heat exhausting liver and kidney yin in spite of the fact that pathogenic heat has already been eliminated.

Development of asthenia into sthenia: Such a development is marked by appearance of symptoms of sthenia syndrome in an asthenia syndrome due to deficiency of healthy qi, hypofunction of viscera and retention of such substances like phlegm, food, dampness, fluid and blood stasis in the body. For example, in the aged there usually appear such symptoms like palpitation and shortness of breath (which is worsened after movement and difficult to heal) followed by occasional chest oppression and stabbing pain, purplish tongue and thin and astringent pulse, etc. Such pathological changes are due to gradual asthenia of yangqi in the heart in the aged. The prolonged asthenia of yangqi in the heart is unable to transport blood, leading to slow circulation of blood and obstruction of the heart vessels. Though there appear chest oppression and stabbing pain, purplish coloration of the tongue and retention of blood stasis, asthenia of yangqi in the heart still exists. That is why the nature of the syndrome

久羁体内，及失治、误治等损伤正气而致。例如外感病极期出现壮热、面赤、烦躁，甚或神昏谵语、舌红苔黄、脉洪大等症，属实热证。病至后期，由于邪热久羁，劫灼肝肾之阴，虽热邪已去，却出现精神委靡、形体消瘦、口咽干燥、手足蠕动、舌红而干、舌苔光剥、脉细数等症，即为实证转化为虚证。

因虚致实：病本为虚证，由于正气不足，脏腑功能减退，致痰、食、水湿、瘀血等阻滞体内，而表现出实证的症状，即为因虚致实。例如年高体弱，心之阳气渐虚，常见心悸、气短，动则尤甚，久治不愈，继则又出现心胸憋闷刺痛、时发时止、舌紫暗、脉细涩等。此因心之阳气亏虚日久，无力温运血行，致血行缓滞，痹阻心脉而形成。虽有心胸憋闷刺痛、舌紫暗等瘀血阻滞的表现，但心之阳气亏虚仍然持续存在，故其证候性质应属虚实夹杂。

is mixture of asthenia and sthenia.

**False and true manifestations of asthenia and sthenia:** During the development of a disease, some asthenia syndromes and sthenia syndromes may show some false manifestations contrary to the nature of the disease known as true asthenia and false sthenia syndrome and true sthenia and false asthenia syndrome. In the differentiation of syndromes, trials should be made to distinguish the false from the true in the complicated manifestations so as to differentiate the nature of disease.

True sthenia and false asthenia syndrome: The disease is essentially sthenic with the manifestations of some asthenic symptoms. Such a syndrome is usually caused by retention of sthenic pathogenic factors preventing yangqi or qi and blood from warming and nourishing the body. For example, in the sthenic heat syndrome due to retention of heat in the intestines and stomach, the appearance of cold limbs, loose stool and deep and slow pulse are like the manifestations of asthenic cold syndrome. However, the patient feels cold in limbs but scorching feverish over the chest and abdomen; the stool is loose, but foul in smell and yellow in colour, and the abdomen is painful and unpalpable; the pulse is deep and slow, but appears powerful when pressed. True sthenia and false asthenia syndrome is just what was known as "asthenic manifestations in severe sthenia condition" in the past. Clinically attention should be paid to the differentiation of mixture of asthenia and sthenia syndrome due to consumption of healthy qi by sthenic pathogenic factors.

True asthenia and false sthenia syndrome: The disease is essentially asthenic with the manifestations of sthenia-like symptoms. Such a syndrome is usually caused by deficiency of yangqi due to prolonged disease fails to warm and transport, leading to hypofunction of the viscera.

（3）虚实真假：疾病过程中,某些虚证和实证会出现与疾病本质相反的一些假象,形成真虚假实和真实假虚证候。辨证时应注意从复杂的证候表现中,识别真假,辨清证候本质。

真实假虚证：是指疾病本质为实证,却出现某些类似虚证表现的一类证候。多因实邪阻遏,致使机体阳气或气血失于温运、濡养而形成。如热结肠胃的实热证,出现肢冷、便下稀水、脉沉迟等类似虚寒证的表现。但是,患者虽肢冷,却胸腹灼热;虽便下稀水,却色黄臭秽,且腹胀痛拒按;脉虽沉迟,却按之有力。真实假虚证即前人所谓"大实有羸状"。临床应注意与实邪伤正所致的虚实夹杂证相鉴别。

真虚假实证：是指疾病本质为虚证,却出现某些类似实证表现的一类证候。多因久病阳气亏虚,温运无力,以致脏腑功能减退,但实邪尚未产

However, sthenic pathogenic factors have not been developed yet. For example, insufficiency of gastrosplenic qi and dysfunction of the spleen bring about some sthenia-like symptoms, such as abdominal distension and fullness or pain. Though there is abdominal distension and fullness, it is alleviated occasionally, unlike that of sthenia syndrome which never attenuates; though there is abdominal pain, but it is palpable, unlike that of sthenia syndrome which is unpalpable. True asthenia and false sthenia syndrome was known as "sthenia manifestations in severe asthenia syndrome" in the past. Clinically attention should be paid to the differentiation of mixture of asthenia and sthenia syndrome due to development of asthenia into sthenia syndrome.

Key points for differentiate true and false asthenia and sthenia:

Tongue states: Tough tongue with thin fur is usually of sthenia syndrome; bulgy and tender tongue with thin fur is usually of asthenia syndrome.

Pulse conditions: Powerful pulse with spirit is of sthenia syndrome; weak pulse without spirit is of asthenia syndrome. Attention should be taken to differentiate whether the sunken pulse is weak or strong.

Voice: Sonorous voice is of sthenia syndrome; low and timid voice is of asthenia syndrome.

History of disease: This includes the constitution of the patient, causes of illness, duration of illness and treatment. Generally speaking, patients with strong constitution usually suffer from sthenia syndrome, while patients with weak constitution usually suffer from asthenia syndrome; diseases caused by six exogenous pathogenic factors are of sthenia, while diseases due to overstrain and chronic diseases are often of asthenia; new disease is

生所形成。如中气不足,脾运失健,出现腹部胀满或痛等类似实证的表现。但是,患者虽腹胀满却有时减轻,不似实证的常满不减;虽腹痛,却喜按,按之痛减,不似实证之疼痛拒按。真虚假实证即前人所谓"至虚有盛候"。临床应注意与因虚致实的虚实夹杂证相鉴别。

辨别虚实真假的要点如下:

① 舌象:舌质苍老、舌苔厚者多为实证;舌质胖嫩、舌苔薄者多为虚证。

② 脉象:脉象有力有神者,多为实证;无力无神者,多为虚证。尤其需注意沉候有力与无力。

③ 语声:语声高亢洪亮者,多为实证;低微虚怯者,多为虚证。

④ 病史:包括患者体质的强弱,发病的原因,病程的长短,以及治疗经过等。一般来说,患者体质强壮者多实证,体质虚弱者多虚证;外感六淫多致实证,劳倦内伤、病久不愈多致虚证;新病多实,久病多虚。

usually sthenic, while chronic disease is often asthenic.

### 2.1.5.2 Relationship between different pairs of principles

In the eight principles, external and internal, cold and heat as well as asthenia and sthenia generalize the nature of diseases from the aspects of the location and nature of diseases as well as the conditions of the healthy qi and pathogenic factors. However, different aspects of the nature of diseases are inter-related. For example, cold and heat nature of diseases as well as the predominant and deficient states of healthy qi and pathogenic factors cannot exist independent of the external or internal location of diseases; accordingly, external syndrome or internal syndrome cannot exist independent of cold and heat as well as asthenia and sthenia nature of diseases. The inter-relation between the internal and external, cold and heat as well as asthenia and sthenia may bring about various syndromes. The following is a brief discussion of the major ones.

#### 2.1.5.2.1 External cold syndrome

External cold syndrome refers to the symptoms of exogenous disease at the primary stage caused by pathogenic wind and cold attacking the surface of the body.

Clinical manifestations: Severe aversion to cold, light fever, pain of head and body, stuffy and running nose, no sweating, whitish thin and moist tongue fur, floating and tense pulse.

Analysis of symptoms: Aversion to cold is due to pathogenic cold attacking the superficies and stagnating yang in the superficies; fever is due to healthy qi fighting against pathogenic factors; pain of head and body is due to pathogenic cold stagnating the meridians and preventing meridian qi from free flowing; stuffy and running nose is due to failure of the lung to disperse; no sweating is due

（二）不同对纲领间的关系

八纲中，表里、寒热、虚实，分别从病位、病性、邪正盛衰等不同方面，概括疾病的本质。然而疾病本质的各个方面是互相联系的，寒热病性、邪正盛衰不能离开表里病位而单独存在，也没有可以离开寒热、虚实而独立存在的表证或里证。由于表里、寒热、虚实的互相联系，即可形成多种证候，兹分述如下：

**1. 表寒证**

表寒证，是指风寒之邪侵袭肌表引起的外感病初期阶段所表现的证候。

临床表现：恶寒重，发热轻，头身疼痛，鼻塞流涕，无汗，苔薄白而润，脉浮紧。

证候分析：寒邪袭表，卫阳郁遏，肌表失于温煦则恶寒；正气抗邪则发热；寒邪凝滞经脉，经气不利则头身疼痛；肺气失宣，其窍不利，则鼻塞流涕；寒性收引，腠理闭塞则无汗。苔薄白而润，脉浮

to obstruction of the muscular interstices by cold which tends to contract; whitish thin and moist tongue fur as well as floating and tense pulse are signs of pathogenic cold encumbering the surface of the body.

#### 2.1.5.2.2 External heat syndrome

External heat syndrome refers to symptoms of exogenous febrile disease at the primary stage caused by wind and heat attacking the surface of the body.

Clinical manifestations: Fever, slight aversion to wind and cold, headache, or sweating, slight thirst, swelling sore-throat, red margin and tip of tongue, whitish thin tongue fur or yellowish thin and dry tongue fur, floating and fast pulse.

Analysis of symptoms: Slight aversion to cold and fever are due to wind and heat attacking the surface of the body and the fact that heat is a pathogenic factor of yang nature; headache and swelling sore-throat are due to upper disturbance by pathogenic heat; sweating is due to upper floating of pathogenic heat that loosens the muscular interstices; slight thirst is due to mild impairment of body fluid by pathogenic heat; red margin and tip of tongue as well as floating and fast pulse are signs of wind and heat attacking the surface of the body.

#### 2.1.5.2.3 External sthenic syndrome

External sthenic syndrome refers to symptoms of exogenous disease at the primary stage caused by pathogenic cold attacking the surface of the body. This syndrome is marked by severe aversion to cold, no sweating and floating and tense pulse, also known as external sthenic syndrome of cold attack which is discussed in the section of external cold syndrome.

#### 2.1.5.2.4 External asthenia syndrome

External asthenia syndrome usually refers to two kinds of syndromes. One is the external syndrome caused

紧,是寒邪束表的征象。

**2. 表热证**

表热证,是指风热之邪侵袭肌表引起的外感温热病初期阶段所表现的证候。

临床表现:发热,微恶风寒,头痛,或有汗,口干微渴,咽喉肿痛,舌边尖红,苔薄白或薄黄欠润,脉浮数。

证候分析:风热犯表,热为阳邪,故发热明显而恶寒轻;热邪上扰,故头痛、咽喉肿痛;热性升散,致腠理疏松,故汗出;热邪伤津不甚故口干微渴。舌边尖红,脉浮数均为风热犯表的征象。

**3. 表实证**

表实证,是指寒邪侵袭肌表引起的外感病初期阶段所表现的证候。以恶寒重,无汗,脉浮紧为特征,又称为伤寒表实证。具体内容见表寒证。

**4. 表虚证**

习惯上所说的表虚证有两种,一是指外感风邪而引起

by exogenous wind attack and marked by aversion to wind, spontaneous sweating and floating and moderate pulse. This syndrome is called exogenous external asthenia syndrome as compared with external sthenia syndrome of cold attack marked by severe aversion to cold, no sweating and floating-tense pulse. The other is external asthenia syndrome of internal impairment caused by looseness of weiqi resulting from asthenia of pulmonary and splenic qi.

Clinical manifestations: Light fever, aversion to wind, headache, sweating, whitish thin tongue fur, floating and moderate pulse, or frequent spontaneous sweating, susceptibility to common cold, accompanied by pale complexion, lassitude, shortness of breath, asthma right after movement, poor appetite, loose stool, pale tongue with white fur and thin and weak pulse.

Analysis of symptoms: Fever, sweating and aversion to cold seen in exogenous external asthenia syndrome are due to disharmony between weiqi and yingqi and looseness of muscular interstices resulting from pathogenic invasion of the surface of the body by wind which tends to open and outburst; headache is due to wind attacking the superfices and inhibited flow of meridian qi; whitish thin tongue fur and floating and moderate pulse are signs of pathogenic wind lingering in the surperficies. In external asthenia syndrome of internal impairment, frequent spontaneous sweating and susceptibility to common cold are due to looseness of muscular interstices and weakness of weiqi and yingqi due to qi asthenia in the lung (which governs skin and hair) and the spleen (which governs muscles). The lung governs qi and manages respiration; while the spleen governs transformation and transportation; both of which are the production source of qi and blood. Asthenia of pulmonary and splenic qi and hypofunction of the lung

的表证,以恶风、自汗、脉浮缓为特征,与以恶寒重,无汗,脉浮紧为特征的伤寒表实证相对而言,称为外感表虚证,又称为中风表虚证。二是指由于肺脾气虚,致卫气不能固密所表现的证候,属内伤表虚证。

临床表现:发热轻,恶风,头痛,汗出,苔薄白,脉浮缓;或经常自汗出,容易感冒,兼面色淡白,倦怠乏力,气短,动则气喘,纳少便溏,舌淡苔白,脉细弱等。

证候分析:外感表虚证,由于风邪外袭,风性开泄外越,致营卫不和,腠理疏松,故发热、汗出而恶风;风邪外袭,经气不利,故头痛。苔薄白,脉浮缓,为风邪在表的征象。内伤表虚证,因肺脾气虚,肺主皮毛,脾主肌肉,其气既虚则肌表疏松,卫表不固,故经常自汗出,易被外邪侵袭而感冒。肺主气,司呼吸;脾主运化,为气血生化之源。肺脾气虚,功能减退,故见面色淡白、倦怠乏力、气短、动则气喘、纳少便溏、舌淡苔白、脉细弱等气虚证的表现。

and the spleen lead to such symptoms like pale complexion, lassitude, shortness of breath, asthma right after movement, poor appetite, loose of stool, pale tongue with white fur as well as thin and weak pulse, etc.

#### 2.1.5.2.5 Internal sthenic cold syndrome

Internal sthenic cold syndrome refers to symptoms of internal exuberance of yin cold frequently caused by invasion of pathogenic yin cold into the viscera, or excessive intake of uncooked and cold food which stagnate yangqi.

Clinical manifestations: Clinical manifestations are various due to difference in causes. The usual ones are cold limbs, pale complexion, moist mouth without thirst, or thirst with preference for hot drinks, unpalpable pain of abdomen, clear and profuse urine, loose stool, whitish moist tongue fur as well as deep and slow pulse or deep and tense pulse.

Analysis of symptoms: Cold limbs and pale complexion are due to invasion of pathogenic cold into the viscera which stagnates yangqi and deprives the body of warmth; moist mouth without thirst, or thirst with preference for hot drinks and profuse clear urine are due to internal exuberance of yin cold and non-impairment of body fluid; unpalpable pain of abdomen is due to stagnation of yin cold and inhibited movement of qi; loose stool is due to pathogenic cold stagnating gastrosplenic yang and failure of the spleen to transport and transform; whitish moist tongue fur and deep and slow pulse or deep and tense pulse are signs of internal cold.

#### 2.1.5.2.6 Internal asthenia cold syndrome

Internal asthenia cold syndrome refers to symptoms of deficiency of yangqi which is discussed in the section of yang asthenia syndrome.

#### 2.1.5.2.7 Internal sthenic heat syndrome

Internal sthenic heat syndrome refers to symptoms of

5. 里实寒证

里实寒证,是指阴寒内盛所表现的证候。多由于阴寒之邪内侵脏腑,或过食生冷等,困遏阳气而形成。

临床表现:由于形成原因不同,临床表现各异。常见的有:形寒肢冷,面白,口润不渴,或渴喜热饮,腹痛拒按,小便清长,大便稀溏,舌苔白润,脉沉迟有力,或沉紧。

证候分析:寒邪内侵脏腑,困遏阳气,机体失于温煦,故形寒肢冷,面白;阴寒内盛,津液不伤,故口润不渴,或渴喜热饮,小便清长;阴寒凝滞,气机不畅,故腹痛拒按;寒邪困阻中阳,运化失职,故大便稀溏。舌苔白润,脉沉迟或紧,均为里寒的征象。

6. 里虚寒证

里虚寒证,是指由于阳气亏虚所表现的证候。具体内容见阳虚证。

7. 里实热证

里实热证,是指阳热之邪

internal exuberance of pathogenic yang heat usually caused by internal invasion of pathogenic yang heat, or by pathogenic cold transforming into heat and invading the internal, or by emotional impairment and emotional transformation of fire, or by improper diet which accumulates into heat.

Clinical manifestations: The clinical manifestations are various due to difference in causes. The usual ones are flushed complexion and somatic fever, aversion to heat and preference for cold, thirst with preference for cold drinks, restlessness, or even coma with delirium, yellowish thick sputum and snivel, vomiting blood and epistaxis, unpalpable pain of abdomen, scanty brownish urine, retention of dry feces, reddish and dry tongue, yellowish tongue fur, full pulse, or slippery pulse, or fast and sthenic pulse.

Analysis of symptoms: Flushed complexion and somatic fever as well as aversion to heat and preference for cold are due to exuberant internal heat fumigating the exterior; thirst with preference for cold drinks, dry tongue and yellowish urine are due to heat consuming body fluid; heat disturbing heart spirit may lead to restlessness in mild case and coma with delirium in severe case; yellowish thick sputum and snivel is due to heat scorching body fluid; hematemesis and epistaxis are due to heat impairing blood collaterals and driving blood to extravasate; unpalpable abdominal pain and retention of dry feces are due to retention of heat in the intestines and stagnation of intestinal qi; reddish tongue with yellow fur and full, slippery, fast and sthenic pulse conditions are signs of internal heat.

### 2.1.5.2.8 Internal asthenia heat syndrome

Internal asthenia heat syndrome refers to symptoms of consumption of body fluid which is discussed in the section of yin asthenia syndrome.

内盛所表现的证候。多由于阳热之邪内侵，或寒邪化热入里，或情志所伤，五志化火，或饮食不节，积蓄为热所形成。

临床表现：由于形成原因不同，临床表现各异。现以热邪内侵为例，可见：面红身热，恶热喜冷，口渴喜冷饮，烦躁不宁，甚或神昏谵语，痰涕黄稠，吐血衄血，腹胀满痛拒按，小便短赤，大便干结，舌红而干，苔黄，脉洪，或滑，或数实。

证候分析：里热亢盛，蒸腾于外，故面红身热，恶热喜冷；热伤津液，故口渴喜冷饮，舌干，小便黄赤；热扰心神，轻者烦躁不安，重者神昏谵语；热灼津液，故痰涕黄稠；热伤血络，迫血妄行，故吐血衄血；热结于肠，腑气不通，故腹胀满痛拒按，大便秘结。舌红苔黄，脉洪滑数实，均为里热的征象。

### 8. 里虚热证

里虚热证，是指由于体内阴液亏虚所表现的证候。具体内容见阴虚证。

## 2.2 Syndrome differentiation of qi, blood and body fluid

Syndrome differentiation of qi, blood and body fluid is a method used to analyze the pathological changes of qi, blood and body fluid during the course of a disease and differentiate the symptoms according to the theory of TCM about qi, blood and body fluid.

The pathological changes of qi, blood and body fluid can be generalized into two major aspects. One is the asthenia of qi, blood and body fluid, which pertains to asthenia syndrome in syndrome differentiation of eight principles; the other is the disturbance of the transportation and metabolism of qi, blood and body fluid with the manifestations of stagnation and adverse flow of qi, blood stasis and retention of fluid, which pertains to sthenia syndrome in syndrome differentiation of eight principles.

Qi, blood and body fluid are the material basis for the functional activities of the viscera. The production, transportation and distribution of qi, blood and body fluid are dependent on the functional activities of the viscera. So, visceral disorders may affect the changes of qi, blood and body fluid. On the other hand, the disorders of qi, blood and body fluid also affect the functions of the viscera. Therefore, the disorders of qi, blood and body fluid are closely related to the conditions of the viscera. Clinically, the differentiation of syndromes of qi, blood and body fluid is made in combination with the differentiation of syndromes of the viscera.

### 2.2.1 Syndrome differentiation of qi disorders

The disorders of qi are various and clinically divided

第二节 气血津液辨证

气血津液辨证,是运用中医学有关气血津液的理论,分析疾病过程中人体气、血、津液的病理变化,辨认其所反映的不同证候的辨证方法。

气、血、津液病证的病理变化,一般可归纳为两个方面,一是气、血、津液的亏虚,属于八纲辨证中虚证的范畴;二是气、血、津液的运行、代谢障碍,而表现为气滞、气逆、血瘀、水液停滞等,多属八纲辨证中实证的范畴。

人体的气、血、津液是脏腑功能活动的物质基础,而它们的生成及运行、输布又有赖于脏腑的功能活动。因此,脏腑发生病变,可以影响到气、血、津液的变化;而气、血、津液的病变,也必然影响到脏腑的功能。所以,气、血、津液的病变是与脏腑密切相关的。临床上,气血津液辨证应与脏腑辨证互相结合运用。

一、气病辨证

气的病变颇多,临床常见

into four categories, i.e. qi asthenia, qi sinking, qi stagnation and qi reversion. Qi asthenia and qi sinking syndromes are asthenic in nature, while qi stagnation and qi reversion syndromes are sthenic in nature.

### 2.2.1.1 Qi asthenia syndrome

Qi asthenia syndrome refers to insufficiency of primordial qi and asthenia symptoms of hypofunction of the viscera and tissues. This syndrome is usually caused by excessive consumption of primordial qi due to chronic disease, severe disease or overstrain, or by deficiency of primordial qi due to congenital defects and postnatal improper diet, or by decline of primordial qi due to weakness and hypofunction of the viscera and tissues resulting from senility.

Clinical manifestations: Lack of qi, no desire to speak, low voice, shortness of breath, dispiritedness, lassitude, dizziness, spontaneous sweating, aggravation of all the symptoms after movement, pale and tender tongue, as well as weak pulse.

Analysis of symptoms: Lack of qi, no desire to speak, low voice, shortness of breath, dispiritedness and lassitude are due to insufficiency of primordial qi and hypofunction of the viscera; dizziness is due to failure of asthenic qi to nourish the head; spontaneous sweating is due to failure of weakened weiqi to protect the superficies of the body; all the symptoms are aggravated after movement because "overstrain consumes qi"; pale and tender tongue and weak pulse are signs of qi asthenia and insufficiency of qi and blood.

Key points for syndrome differentiation: The essential symptoms for diagnosis are lack of qi, lassitude, dispiritedness, spontaneous sweating and weak pulse.

### 2.2.1.2 Qi sinking syndrome

Qi sinking syndrome refers to symptoms of asthenia

证候可概括为气虚、气陷、气滞、气逆等四种主要类型。气虚证与气陷证属虚，气滞证与气逆证多属实。

（一）气虚证

气虚证是指元气不足，脏腑组织功能活动减退所表现的虚弱证候。本证多由于久病、重病或劳累过度，使元气耗损过多；或因先天禀赋不足、后天饮食失调，使元气生成匮乏；或因年老体弱，脏腑功能衰退而元气自衰等原因所导致。

临床表现：少气懒言，声音低微，呼吸气短，神疲乏力，头晕目眩，自汗，活动或劳累后诸症加重，舌淡嫩，脉虚弱。

证候分析：元气不足，脏腑功能衰退，则少气懒言，声音低微，呼吸气短，神疲乏力；气虚不能上荣头目，则头晕目眩；卫气虚弱，不能固护肌表，则自汗；"劳则气耗"，故活动劳累后诸症加重。舌淡嫩、脉虚弱，为气虚鼓动无力，气血不充的征象。

辨证要点：本证以少气、乏力、神倦、自汗、脉虚为诊断依据。

（二）气陷证

气陷证是指气虚无力升

marked by prolapse of the viscera due to inability of qi to lift and sinking of lucid yang. Qi sinking syndrome is usually due to splenic asthenia. That is why this syndrome is also called syndrome of sinking of gastrosplenic qi or qi sinking due to splenic asthenia. This syndrome is usually the further development of qi asthenia or caused by overstrain.

Clinical manifestations: Prolapsing distension of epigastrium and abdomen, or prolapse of rectum due to chronic diarrhea, prolapse of uterus, dizziness, lassitude, pale tongue with whitish thin fur and weak pulse, etc.

Analysis of symptoms: Prolapsing distension of epigastrium and abdomen, or prolapse of rectum and uterus are due to inability of asthenic qi to lift and maintain the viscera in the normal position; dizziness, chronic diarrhea and lassitude are due to inability of asthenic qi to lift and lucid yang to rise; pale tongue, whitish thin fur and weak pulse are signs of the decline of the functions of the body due to qi asthenia.

Key points for syndrome differentiation: Prolapse of the viscera, dizziness, lack of qi and lassitude.

### 2.2.1.3 Qi stagnation syndrome

Qi stagnation syndrome refers to symptoms caused by qi stagnation in a certain region or a certain viscera in the human body. The causes of qi stagnation syndrome are various, such as emotional upsets, improper diet, attack by exogenous pathogenic factors, asthenia of yangqi, or trauma, falling, contusion and sprain which all may lead to dysfunction and disturbance of qi and bring about qi stagnation.

Clinical manifestations: Distending oppression, pain (distension is more serious than pain) or migratory pain and attacking pain are felt over the chest, hypochondrium, epigastrium and abdomen. The location of pain and distension is usually unfixed. The distension cannot be felt by palpation but is alleviated after sighing, borborygmus and breaking wind. It may be attenuated or worsened with the changes of emotions.

Analysis of symptoms: Normally qi should be free and smooth in flowing, stagnation will lead to distending oppression in mild case and pain in severe case; qi sometimes gathers up and sometimes disperses, so the location of pain is not fixed, pain is now serious and then light and it cannot be felt by palpation; sighing, borborygmus and breaking wind smooth the flow of qi, that is why distension and pain are alleviated; hyponchondriac distension and pain are due to emotional upsets and stagnation of liver qi which prevent free dispersion and inhibit flow of meridian qi; distending oppression of chest is due to stagnation of pulmonary qi; epigastric and abdominal distending pain is due to stagnation of gastric and intestinal qi; oppression and pain over the chest is due to obstruction of heart qi and inhibited flow of blood in vessels.

Key points for syndrome differentiation: Local distending oppression and pain. The symptoms are usually various due to different causes of qi stagnation and pathological changes of different viscera. So cares should be taken to differentiate the location of distending oppression and pain as well as the accompanied symptoms.

## 2.2.1.4　Qi reversion syndrome

Qi reversion syndrome refers to symptoms of disorder of qi to ascend and descend, or excessive ascent. This syndrome is usually caused by exogenous pathogenic factors, or phlegm, retention of food, retention of cold fluid, or emotional upsets which lead to upward reversion of pulmonary and gastric qi as well as excessive ascent of

痛、攻痛,部位多不固定,按之无形,触之无物,常随嗳气、肠鸣、矢气后而减轻,亦随情绪的变化而减轻或加重。

证候分析:气机以通顺为贵,一旦有所郁滞,轻则胀闷,重则疼痛;气时聚时散,故疼痛部位不定,时轻时重,按之无形,触之无物;嗳气、肠鸣、矢气后气机得以通顺,则胀痛得以减轻。情志不舒,肝气郁滞,疏泄失职,经气不畅,则胁肋胀痛;肺气壅滞,则胸部痞闷而胀;胃肠气滞,则脘腹胀痛;心气郁阻,血脉运行不畅,则心胸部憋闷疼痛。

辨证要点:本证以局部胀闷、疼痛为诊断依据。由于引起气滞的病因不同,病变的脏腑不同,其证候表现尚有各自的特点,故应分辨胀闷、疼痛的部位及兼症以审证求因。

## (四) 气逆证

气逆证是指气机升降失常,当降不降,逆而向上,或升发太过所表现的证候。本证多由感受外邪,或痰浊、食滞、寒饮内停,或情志不遂,致肺、胃之气上逆,肝气升发太过而

liver qi.

Clinical manifestations: Cough and asthmatic breath in upward reversion of pulmonary qi; hiccup, belching, nausea and vomiting in upward reversion of gastric qi; headache, dizziness, even coma and hematemesis in upward reversion of liver qi.

Analysis of symptoms: Cough and asthmatic breath are due to invasion of exogenous pathogenic factors, or accumulation of phlegm which drive the pulmonary qi to flow adversely upwards; hiccup, belching, nausea and vomiting are due to invasion of exogenous pathogenic factors, or retention of food and retention of phlegm and fluid in the stomach which prevents the gastric qi from descending and drives it to flow adversely upwards; headache, dizziness and even coma are due to emotional upsets and impairment of the liver by rage which prevent the liver qi from free dispersing and drives it to ascend excessively, making stagnant qi transform into fire which moves up to disturb the head and eyes along the meridians; hematemesis is due to upward flow of blood with adverse running of qi and impairment of yang collaterals.

Key points for syndrome differentiation: Upward adverse flow of lung, stomach and liver qi.

## 2.2.2 Syndrome differentiation of blood disease

Blood disease is either of asthenia syndrome due to inability of blood asthenia to nourish the body, or of sthenia syndrome due to blood stasis, blood heat and blood cold resulting from disturbance of blood circulation.

### 2.2.2.1 Blood asthenia syndrome

Blood asthenia syndrome refers to asthenia syndrome caused by failure of insufficient blood to nourish viscera,

引起。

临床表现：肺气上逆则表现为咳嗽、喘息；胃气上逆则表现为呃逆、嗳气、恶心、呕吐；肝气上逆则表现为头痛、眩晕，甚至昏厥、呕血。

证候分析：外邪侵袭，或痰浊壅滞，导致肺气不得肃降而上逆，则咳嗽、喘息；感受外邪，或食积、痰饮停积于胃，导致胃气失于和降而上逆，则呃逆、嗳气、恶心、呕吐；情志不遂，郁怒伤肝，致使肝气失于条达，升发太过，气郁化火，气火循经上逆，犯扰头目，则头痛、眩晕，甚至昏厥；血随气逆而上涌，阳络伤则血上溢，故呕血。

辨证要点：本证以肺、胃、肝等脏腑之气上逆不顺的见症为诊断依据。

## 二、血病辨证

血的病变，一方面是血液亏虚，不能濡养机体，属于虚证；另一方面是血液运行障碍，而为血瘀、血热、血寒，多属实证。

### （一）血虚证

血虚证是指血液亏少，不能濡养脏腑、经络、组织所表

meridians and tissues. This syndrome is usually caused by various chronic and acute bleeding, or by excessive contemplation and anxiety which have consumed blood, or by asthenia of the spleen and stomach which affect blood production, etc.

Clinical manifestations: Pale or sallow complexion, pale eyelids, lips and nails, dizziness, palpitation, insomnia, numbness of hands and feet, scanty, pale and delayed menstruation, or even amenorrhea, pale tongue, and thin and weak pulse.

Analysis of symptoms: Pale or sallow complexion as well as pale eyelids, lips and tongue are due to failure of asthenic blood to nourish the face; dizziness is due to asthenic blood to nourish the head; palpitation and insomnia are due to failure of asthenic blood to nourish heart spirit; numbness of hands and feet as well as pale nails are due to failure of asthenic liver blood to nourish tendons; scanty, pale and delayed menstruation or even amenorrhea is due to insufficiency of blood in uterus and thoroughfare and conception vessels; thin and weak pulses are signs of insufficiency of blood in the vessels due to blood asthenia.

Key points for syndrome differentiation: Lack of proper nutrition of the body with the manifestations of pale complexion, eyelids, lips, tongue and nails as well as hypofunction of the organs with the symptoms of dizziness and palpitation, etc.

### 2.2.2.2 Blood stasis syndrome

Blood stasis syndrome refers to syndrome caused by retention of blood stasis in the body. Blood stasis refers to extravasation of blood that is not excreted or dispersed in time and retained in the body; or refers to stagnation of blood in the meridians, vessels or organs and tissues due to inhibited circulation of blood. This syndrome is usually

现的虚弱证候。本证多由各种急慢性出血；或思虑劳心过度，暗耗阴血；或久病、大病，耗伤营血；或脾胃虚弱，生血乏源等所导致。

临床表现：面色淡白无华或萎黄，眼睑、口唇、爪甲色淡白，头晕眼花，心悸，失眠，手足麻木，妇女月经量少、色淡、衍期，甚或经闭，舌质淡，脉细无力。

证候分析：血虚不能上荣于面，则见面色淡白或萎黄，眼睑、唇、舌淡白；血虚头目失于濡养，则头晕眼花；心血亏虚，不能濡养心神，则心悸、失眠；肝血亏虚，筋脉失养，则手足麻木，爪甲色淡；血海空虚，冲任失充，则妇女月经量少、色淡、衍期，甚或经闭。脉细无力，是血虚无以充盈于脉的征象。

辨证要点：本证以面、睑、唇、舌、爪甲淡白无华等血虚形体失于濡养，以及头晕、心悸等功能虚弱的表现为诊断依据。

### （二）血瘀证

血瘀证是指由瘀血内阻而产生的证候。所谓瘀血，是指离经之血，未能及时排出或消散，滞留于体内；或血液运行不畅，壅滞于经脉或器官组织之内的病理变化。本证多

caused by extravasation and stasis of blood due to trauma or qi asthenia; or by qi stagnation inhibiting blood circulation; or by failure of asthenic qi to propel blood to flow; or by stagnancy of blood due to retention of pathogenic cold in the vessels; or by confliction between heat and blood due to invasion of pathogenic heat into blood phase.

Clinical manifestations: Stabbing and cutting pain with fixed location which is unpalpable and worsened at night; local lumps which appear cyanotic in the superficies and hard and unmovable in the abdomen; repeated bleeding with purplish colour or with clot or with asphalt-like stool; amenorrhea or metrorrhagia in women; blackish complexion, cyanotic lips and nails, subcutaneous purplish petechiae, or squamous skin, or visible abdominal veins, or silk-like red stripes on the skin; cyanotic tongue or with cyanotic petechiae and points, thin and astringent pulse.

Analysis of symptoms: Stabbing pain with fixed position is due to obstruction by blood stasis; severe and unpalpable pain is due to aggravation of inhibited qi movement under pressure; severe pain at night is due to the fact that yinqi is active in the night and blood stagnation becomes more serious; purplish lumps on the superficies and hard, unmovable and unpalpable lumps in the abdomen are due to local retention of blood stasis; repeated bleeding with purplish colour, clot, or asphalt-like stool, or metrorrhagia are due to obstruction of vessels resulting from blood stasis and extravasation of blood; cyanotic lips, tongue and nails, or subcutaneous petechiae, or silk-like red stripes, or local visible veins are due to retention of blood stasis and inhibited flow of qi and blood; blackish complexion and squamous skin are due to prolonged

因外伤或气虚，致血溢脉外瘀积不散；或气滞致血行不畅；或气虚推动无力而血行瘀滞；或阴寒之邪客于血脉，血行凝涩；或热邪侵入血分，血热搏结所致。

临床表现：疼痛，痛如针刺刀割，部位固定，拒按，常于夜间痛甚。局部可有肿块，其在体表者，色呈青紫；其在腹内者，质地坚硬而推之不移。出血反复不止，其血色紫暗或夹有血块，或大便色黑如柏油，妇女可见经闭或崩漏。面色黧黑，唇甲青紫，皮下可见紫斑，或肌肤甲错，或腹部青筋显露，或皮肤出现丝状红缕。舌紫暗，或见紫斑紫点，脉象细涩。

证候分析：瘀血阻滞，不通则痛，故疼痛如针刺刀割，痛处固定；按压则气机更窒，故疼痛益甚而拒按；夜间阴气用事，阴血凝滞更甚，所以夜间疼痛更剧。瘀血蓄积局部不得消散，形成肿块，其在体表者常呈青紫色，在腹内者可触及坚硬有形的肿块，按之疼痛，推之不移。瘀血阻塞脉络，血不循经而外溢，可致出血反复不止，血色紫暗，夹有血块，或大便色黑如柏油，或崩漏。瘀血内阻，气血运行不畅，则见唇、舌、爪甲青紫，或

retention of turbid substance and malnutrition of skin and meridians; amenorrhea is due to stagnation of blood stasis and obstruction of thoroughfare and conception vessels; astringent pulse is a sign of retention of blood stasis in the vessels and inhibited flow of blood.

Key points for syndrome differentiation: Stabbing pain with fixed position, lumps, bleeding with purplish colour, cyanotic lips, tongue and nails.

### 2.2.2.3 Blood cold syndrome

Blood cold syndrome refers to syndrome caused by cold retention and qi stagnation in local meridians and vessels. This syndrome is usually caused by retention of pathogenic cold in the vessels and stagnancy of qi; or by inhibited flow of blood due to cold produced by yang asthenia which deprives blood of warmth and proper circulation.

Clinical manifestations: Local cold pain which alleviates with warmth and aggravates with cold, cyanotic and cold skin over the affected part, delayed menstruation, purplish menorrhea with clot, dysmenorrhea, purplish tongue with white fur, and sunken, slow and astringent pulse.

Analysis of symptoms: Local cold, preference for warmth and purplish and cold skin are due to stagnation of qi and blood resulting from pathogenic cold, or due to inhibited blood circulation resulting from failure of asthenic yang to warm vessels and transport blood; delayed menstruation, purplish menorrhea with clot, dysmenorrhea or even amenorrhea are due to retention of cold in the uterus, disorder of thoroughfare and conception vessels and stagnancy of blood in circulation; purplish tongue with white fur, sunken, slow and astringent pulses are signs of

皮下瘀斑,或丝状红缕,或局部青筋显露。浊瘀久停,肌肤脉络失养,则可见面色黧黑,肌肤甲错。瘀血阻滞,冲任不通,则经闭。脉涩,为瘀阻脉络,血行不畅的征象。

辨证要点:本证以刺痛、部位固定,肿块,出血紫暗,唇、舌、爪甲青紫等为诊断依据。

### (三) 血寒证

血寒证是指局部脉络寒凝气滞,血行不畅所表现的证候。本证多由于寒邪客于血脉,凝滞气机;或阳虚生寒,不能温运血脉,导致血行不畅。

临床表现:局部冷痛,得温痛减,遇寒痛剧,患处肤色紫暗而凉,妇女月经衍期、经色紫暗夹有血块,痛经,舌紫暗,苔白,脉沉迟而涩。

证候分析:寒邪凝滞气血,或阳虚不能温运血脉,血行不畅,故见局部冷痛喜温,肤色紫暗而凉;寒凝胞宫,冲任失调,血行瘀滞,则妇女月经衍期、经色紫暗夹有血块,痛经甚或经闭。舌紫暗,苔白,脉沉迟而涩,为阴寒凝滞血脉,气血运行不畅的征象。

retention of pathogenic cold in the vessels and inhibited flow of blood.

Key points for syndrome differentiation: The syndrome is marked by stagnant blood circulation due to excessive interior cold with local cold pain alleviated with warmth and cyanotic skin.

### 2.2.2.4 Blood heat syndrome

Blood heat syndrome refers to syndrome caused by exuberance of fire and heat in the viscera that invades blood phase. This syndrome is usually caused by extreme emotional disorder which transforms into fire; or by excessive drinking of alcohol which transforms into heat and invades blood phase. Blood heat syndrome can be seen in miscellaneous disease due to internal impairment and exogenous febrile disease which are discussed in the section of syndrome differentiation of wei, qi, ying and blood.

Clinical manifestations: Hemoptysis, or hematemesis, bleeding, hematuria, hematochezia, advanced profuse menstruation, even metrorrhagia, dysphoria, thirst, deep reddish tongue and fast pulse.

Analysis of symptoms: Internal exuberance of fire and heat impairs collaterals and causes various bleeding marked by sudden onset, profuse quantity and deep red colour; fire and heat may lead to different blood syndromes when they have impaired different viscera: impairment of lung collateral causes hemoptysis, impairment of stomach collaterals causes hematemesis, impairment of the kidney or bladder causes hematuria, impairment of the large intestine causes hematochezia and impairment of the thoroughfare and conception vessels causes advanced and profuse menstruation or even metrorrhagia; internal exuberance of fire and heat consumes fluid and causes thirst; heat disturbs heart spirit and causes dysphoria; exuberant heat promotes blood flow and drives blood to the vessels of

辨证要点：本证以局部冷痛、得温痛减，肤色紫暗等阴寒内盛，血行凝滞不畅的表现为诊断依据。

### （四）血热证

血热证是指脏腑火热炽盛，热迫血分所表现的证候。本证多因情志过极，郁而化火；或嗜酒过度，蓄积为热，火热内炽，侵犯血分而形成。血热证既可见于内伤杂病，又可见于外感温热病。此处所述属内伤杂病，外感病血分邪热炽盛，见卫气营血辨证。

临床表现：咳血，或吐血、衄血、尿血、便血，妇女月经先期、量多，甚至崩漏，心烦，口渴，舌红绛，脉数。

证候分析：火热内炽迫血妄行，络伤血溢而致多种出血，且具有来势较急、出血量较多、血色深红的特点。火热伤及不同的脏腑，可出现不同的出血证候：热伤肺络，则见咳血；热伤胃络，则见吐血；热伤肾脏或膀胱，则见尿血；热伤大肠，则为便血；热扰冲任，则见月经先期、量多，甚至崩漏。火热炽灼于内，伤津耗液，则见口渴；热扰心神，则见心烦；热盛血涌，舌之脉络充盈，则见舌红绛；热迫血行加

tongue and makes the tongue appear deep red; heat propels blood and leads to fast pulse.

Key points for syndrome differentiation: This syndrome is marked by various bleeding accompanied by symptoms of internal exuberant fire and heat, such as dysphoria, thirst, deep red tongue and fast pulse, etc.

## 2.2.3 Syndrome differentiation of simultaneous disorder of qi and blood

Qi and blood depend on each other to exist and promote each other to develop. Pathologically, qi and blood affect each other, blood disorder may involve qi and vice versa. If qi disorder and blood disorder appear at the same time, it is known as simultaneous disorder of qi and blood. Clinically, simultaneous disorder of qi and blood is divided into two major categories: asthenia of both qi and blood, loss of blood due to qi asthenia, qi depletion with blood in asthenia syndrome; qi stagnation and blood stasis in sthenia syndrome, and qi asthenia and blood stasis in syndrome of principal asthenia and secondary sthenia.

### 2.2.3.1 Asthenia of both qi and blood

Asthenia of both qi and blood refers to syndrome caused by simultaneous existence of qi asthenia and blood asthenia. This syndrome is usually caused by asthenia of qi and blood in chronic disease; or by asthenia of the spleen and stomach that affects the production of qi and blood; or by qi loss of blood followed by depletion of qi; or by qi asthenia followed by blood asthenia.

Clinical manifestations: Lack of qi, no desire to speak, dispiritedness, fatigue, or spontaneous sweating, dizziness, palpitation, pale or sallow complexion, pale lips and nails, pale and tender tongue, thin and weak pulse.

速,故脉数。

辨证要点:本证以火热迫血妄行所致的各种出血,以及心烦口渴、舌红绛、脉数等火热内炽的表现为诊断依据。

## 三、气血同病辨证

气与血相互依存,相互资生,相互为用。因而在病理变化过程中,气与血相互影响,血病可以及气,气病又可及血。如既见气病,又见血病,即为气血同病。临床常见的气血同病证候,虚证有气血两虚、气虚失血、气随血脱等,实证有气滞血瘀,本虚标实证有气虚血瘀。

### (一)气血两虚证

气血两虚证是指气虚与血虚同时存在所表现的证候。本证多因久病不愈,气血两亏;或脾胃亏虚,气血生化不足;或先有失血,气随血耗;或先因气虚,无以生化而继见血虚所形成。

临床表现:少气懒言,神疲乏力,或有自汗,头晕目眩,心悸失眠,面色淡白或萎黄,唇、爪甲淡白,舌质淡嫩,脉细无力。

Analysis of symptoms: Lack of qi, no desire to speak, dispiritedness, fatigue or spontaneous sweating are due to hypofunction of viscera due to qi asthenia; pale or sallow complexion as well as pale lips and nails are due to inability of qi and blood asthenia to nourish the body; dizziness, palpitation and insomnia are due to the inability of qi and blood asthenia to nourish the head and heart spirit; pale and tender tongue as well as thin and weak pulse are signs of qi and blood asthenia.

Key points for syndrome differentiation: Hypofunction of the viscera due to qi asthenia and inability to nourish viscera and body due to blood asthenia.

### 2.2.3.2 Qi asthenia and hemorrhagia syndrome

Qi asthenia and hemorrhagia syndrome refers to syndrome caused by failure of asthenic qi to control blood. This syndrome is mainly caused by spleen asthenia due to chronic disease, or by inability of asthenic qi to control blood resulting from overstrain.

Clinical manifestations: Hematemesis, hematochezia, or muscular bleeding, or epistaxis, or profuse menstruation, metrorrhagia, accompanied by lack of qi, no desire to speak, lassitude, pale complexion, pale tongue and weak pulse.

Analysis of symptoms: Failure of asthenic qi to control blood and extravasation of blood lead to hematemesis, hematochezia, bleeding and metrorrhagia; lack of qi, no desire to speak and lassitude appearing at the same time or in advance of bleeding are due to hypofunction of the viscera resulting from qi asthenia; pale complexion and tongue as well as weak pulse are signs of asthenia of both qi and blood due to bleeding.

Key points for syndrome differentiation: Hypofunction

证候分析：气虚脏腑功能活动减退，则少气懒言，神疲乏力，或有自汗；血虚不能濡润充养形体，则见面色淡白或萎黄，唇甲淡白；气血亏虚，不能上荣头目、濡养心神，则头晕目眩，心悸失眠。舌质淡嫩，脉细无力，是气血两虚的征象。

辨证要点：本证以气虚而脏腑功能活动减退和血虚不能濡养脏腑形体的表现共见为诊断依据。

### (二) 气虚失血证

气虚失血证是指由于气虚不能统摄血液，而以出血为主要表现的证候。本证多由久病脾虚，或劳累过度等导致气虚，统血无权而形成。

临床表现：呕血、便血，或肌衄，或齿衄，或鼻衄，或妇女月经过多、崩漏，兼见少气懒言，倦怠乏力，面色淡白，舌质淡白，脉弱。

证候分析：气虚无力统摄血液，血溢脉外而形成呕血、便血、衄血、崩漏等多种出血证候。气虚脏腑功能活动减退，故在出血的同时，或在其先出现少气懒言、倦怠乏力等症。失血更使气血双亏，则面色淡白，舌淡，脉弱。

辨证要点：本证以气虚脏

of the viscera and bleeding.

### 2.2.3.3 Depletion of qi with bleeding syndrome

Depletion of qi with bleeding refers to syndrome in which qi depletes due to massive bleeding. This syndrome is usually caused by trauma, or by damage of the viscera, or by massive bleeding from uterus or in delivery of child.

Clinical manifestations: Massive bleeding accompanied by pale complexion, profuse sweating, cold limbs, weak breath, extreme dispiritedness, even coma, pale tongue, indistinct pulse, or hollow pulse, or scattered pulse.

Analysis of symptoms: Blood is the mother of qi, so loss of blood will lead to loss of qi at the same time; pale complexion and cold limbs are due to loss of qi and yang to warm the body; profuse sweating is due to sudden loss of yangqi which weakens the superficies and gives rise to leakage of fluid; weak breath, extreme dispiritedness and even coma are due to loss of proper nutrition of the spirit resulting from depletion of qi and blood; indistinct pulse or hollow pulse or scattered pulse are due to loss of qi and blood that disperses primordial qi and fails to enrich the vessels; pale tongue is the sign of consumption of qi and blood which fail to nourish the head.

Key points for syndrome differentiation: Massive bleeding and simultaneous loss of qi and blood.

### 2.2.3.4 Qi asthenia and blood stasis syndrome

Qi asthenia and blood stasis syndrome refers to syndrome caused by blood stagnation resulting from qi asthenia to transport blood. This syndrome is usually caused by

腑功能活动减退和出血症状共见为诊断依据。

### (三) 气随血脱证

气随血脱证是指由大量出血而引起阳气随之暴脱所表现的证候。常由外伤,或内脏破损,或妇女崩中、分娩等突然大量出血而引起。

临床表现:在突然大量出血的同时,伴见面色苍白,大汗淋漓,四肢厥冷,气息微弱,精神极度委靡,甚则昏厥,舌质淡白,脉微欲绝,或脉芤,或脉散。

证候分析:血为气之母,血脱则气无所附,阳气随之亡脱。气脱阳亡,不能温煦形体,故见面色苍白,四肢厥冷;阳气暴脱,不能固摄肌表,津液外泄,则见冷汗淋漓;血失气脱,神失所养,则气息微弱,精神极度委靡,甚则昏厥;血失气脱,元气涣散,脉失充盈鼓动,故脉微欲绝、或芤、或散。舌质淡白为气血耗散,不能上荣的征象。

辨证要点:本证以大量出血,同时出现气脱阳亡的表现为诊断依据。

### (四) 气虚血瘀证

气虚血瘀证是指气虚运血无力,导致血行瘀滞所表现的证候。常由久病气虚运血

qi asthenia to propel blood in chronic disease and gradual formation of blood stasis due to inhibited flow of blood.

Clinical manifestations: Dispiritedness, lack of qi, no desire to speak, or spontaneous sweating, fixed, unpalpable and stabbing pain over the chest, hypochondrium and other local regions, pale complexion, light purplish tongue or with petechiae, sunken, astringent and weak pulse.

Analysis of symptoms: Dispiritedness, lack of qi, no desire to speak, spontaneous sweating and pale complexion are due to hypofunction of the viscera and tissues; fixed, unpalpable and stabbing pain is due to inhibited flow of blood; light purplish tongue or with petechiae, sunken, astringent and weak pulse conditions are signs of qi asthenia and blood stasis.

Key points for syndrome differentiation: The syndrome is marked by the manifestations of both qi deficiency and stagnant blood circulation.

### 2.2.3.5 Qi stagnation and blood stasis syndrome

Qi stagnation and blood stasis syndrome refers to syndrome caused by stagnation of qi and stasis of blood. This syndrome is usually caused by emotional upsets, or by invasion of pathogenic cold and stagnation of qi and blood. Qi can promote blood circulation and blood can carry qi. Since qi and blood circulate continuously inside the body, qi stagnation and blood stasis frequently affect each other and often appear at the same time.

Clinical manifestations: Depression or restlessness, distending pain or migratory pain over chest and hypochondrium, or accompanied by mass formation, unpalpable stabbing pain, purplish tongue or with purplish petechiae, taut and astringent pulse, distending pain of breast before or after menstruation, dysmenorrhea, purplish menstruation with blood clot, or amenorrhea, etc.

无力,渐致血行不畅而瘀滞所形成。

临床表现:神倦乏力,少气懒言,或有自汗,胸胁或其他局部刺痛,部位固定,拒按,面色淡白,舌质淡紫或有紫斑,脉沉涩无力。

证候分析:气虚脏腑组织功能活动减退,故神倦乏力,少气懒言,自汗,面色淡白;血行瘀滞不畅,故局部刺痛,部位固定,拒按;舌质淡紫或有紫斑,脉沉涩无力,为气虚鼓动无力,血行瘀滞的征象。

辨证要点:本证以气虚功能活动减退和血行瘀滞不畅的表现共见为诊断依据。

### (五)气滞血瘀证

气滞血瘀证是指气机郁滞,血行瘀阻所表现的证候。多由情志不遂,或寒邪侵袭,使气血瘀滞而形成。气能行血,血能载气,气血于人体内环流不息,故气滞与血瘀往往又互为因果,相兼为病。

临床表现:性情抑郁或急躁,胸胁胀满疼痛或窜痛,或兼胁下痞块,刺痛拒按,舌质紫暗,或有紫斑,脉弦涩。妇女可见经前或经期乳房胀痛,痛经,经色紫暗、有血块,或经闭等。

Analysis of symptoms: The symptoms in this syndrome vary due to the location of qi stagnation and blood stasis in different viscera and meridians. Clinically the common manifestations are qi stagnation and blood stasis due to stagnancy of qi activity and failure of liver to disperse and convey because the liver governs dispersion and conveyance and stores blood. Depression or restlessness, distending fullness of the chest and hypochondrium, migratory pain and distending pain of the breast are due to stagnation of liver qi and failure of the liver to disperse and convey; hypochondriac lumps and unpalpable stabbing pain are due to internal retention of blood stasis resulting from prolonged stagnation of qi and inhibited flow of blood; dysmenorrhea, purplish menorrhea with blood clot and even amenorrhea are due to qi stagnation and blood stasis; purplish tongue or with purplish petechiae as well as taut and astringent pulse are signs of qi stagnation and blood stasis.

Key points for syndrome differentiation: Stagnancy of qi activity, inhibited blood circulation and blood stasis.

## 2.2.4 Syndrome differentiation of fluid disorder

The disorders of body fluid mainly include deficiency of body fluid as well as retention of phlegm and fluid and edema. The former is caused by insufficiency of the production of body fluid or excessive loss of body fluid, the latter is caused by dysfunction of the viscera and disturbance of the distribution and excretion of body fluid which leads to the retention and accumulation of fluid.

### 2.2.4.1 Insufficiency of body fluid

Insufficiency of body fluid refers to syndrome due to deficiency of body fluid which fails to nourish and moisten viscera, tissues and organs. This syndrome is mainly

证候分析：气滞血瘀证因病变所在的脏腑、经络部位不同，其临床表现亦各有差异。由于肝主疏泄，又主藏血，故临床一般以肝失疏泄，气机郁结所导致的气滞血瘀者居多。肝气郁结，疏泄失职，故见性情抑郁或急躁，胸胁胀满，走窜疼痛，乳房胀痛；气滞日久，血行不畅，终致瘀血内停，渐成胁下痞块，刺痛拒按；气血瘀滞，妇女则痛经，经色紫暗、有血块，甚则经闭。舌质紫暗或有紫斑，脉弦涩为气滞血瘀的征象。

辨证要点：本证以气机郁滞和血行瘀阻不畅的表现共见为诊断依据。

## 四、津液病辨证

津液的病变，一方面是津液的生成不足或丧失过多，出现津液亏虚的证候；另一方面是脏腑功能失调，津液的输布、排泄障碍，导致水液停聚，而产生痰、饮、水肿等病理变化。

### （一）津液不足证

津液不足证是指由于津液亏虚，脏腑组织器官失其滋润所表现的证候。本证主要

caused by excessive consumption of body fluid due to high fever, profuse sweating, excessive vomiting, excessive diarrhea and profuse urine or consumption of fluid by dryness and heat; or by insufficiency of body fluid due to scanty drinking of water and decline of visceral qi.

Clinical manifestations: Dry mouth and throat, dry or fissured lips, sunken orbit, dry skin, thirst with desire for water, scanty urine, retention of dry feces, dry tongue with scanty saliva and thin and astringent pulse.

Analysis of symptoms: Dry mouth, lips, tongue, throat and skin as well as sunken orbit and thirst with desire for water are due to failure of deficient body fluid to nourish and moisten the viscera and body; scanty urine is due to deficiency of body fluid to transform urine; retention of dry feces is due to scanty body fluid to lubricate the large intestine; scanty saliva is due to deficiency of body fluid to moisten the tongue; thin and fast pulse is due to insufficiency of qi and blood.

Key points for syndrome differentiation: Dry mouth, lips, tongue, throat and skin as well as scanty urine and dry stool.

### 2.2.4.2 Phlegm syndrome

Phlegm syndrome refers to syndrome due to local retention of phlegm or migration of phlegm. Phlegm is produced by such factors like six exogenous pathogenic factors, emotional impairment, improper food, overstrain and lack of necessary physical activities which affect the transforming functions of the lung, spleen and kidney, leading to stoppage of fluid distribution and production of phlegm. The retention of phlegm in viscera, meridians and tissues results in phlegm syndrome.

Clinical manifestations: Cough with sticky sputum,

因高热、大汗、大吐、大泻、多尿或燥热伤津等，使津液耗损过多；亦可因饮水过少、脏气虚衰，津液生化不足所致。

临床表现：口燥咽干，唇焦或裂，眼眶凹陷，皮肤干燥甚或枯瘪，渴欲饮水，小便短少，大便干结，舌干少津，脉细涩。

证候分析：津液亏虚，不能濡养滋润脏腑形体，则口、唇、舌、咽及肌肤干燥失润，目眶凹陷，渴欲饮水；津液亏虚，尿无化源，则小便短少；津亏液少，大肠失于滋润，则大便干结；津液亏虚，舌失滋润，则舌干少津；脉失充盈，则脉细数。

辨证要点：本证以口、唇、舌、咽、肌肤干燥及尿少便干为诊断依据。

### （二）痰证

痰证是指由于痰阻于局部或流窜全身所表现的病证。痰的形成，多由于外感六淫、内伤七情、饮食不当、过劳体虚、过逸少动等诸种因素，影响肺、脾、肾的气化功能，以致水液失于输布而停聚成痰。痰之已成，留于体内，停于脏腑、经络、组织之间则形成本证。

临床表现：咳嗽，咯痰质

chest oppression, or dizziness, or epigastric mass, anorexia, nausea, vomiting, or coma with sputum rale, or mental derangement with mania, dementia and epilepsy, or numbness of limbs, hemiplegia, or scrofula, goiter, breast nodules, phlegm nodules, greasy fur and slippery pulse.

Analysis of symptoms: Phlegm is marked by variability in causing disease. So there is a saying that "all diseases are caused by phlegm". Chest oppression and cough with sticky sputum are due to retention of phlegm in the lung which affects the lung to disperse and descend; dizziness is due to phlegm invading the head and preventing lucid yang from rising; epigastric mass, anorexia, vomiting and nausea are due to retention of phlegm in the middle energizer that prevents the spleen from transforming and the stomach from descending; coma with sputum rale or mental derangement with mania, dementia and epilepsy are due to phlegm confusing the mind; numbness of limbs, or hemiplegia is due to retention of phlegm in the meridians and inhibited flow of qi and blood; scrofula, goiter, breast nodules and phlegm nodules are due to retention of phlegm in the skin and muscles; greasy fur and slippery pulse are signs of internal exuberance of phlegmatic dampness.

Key points for syndrome differentiation: This syndrome is marked by vomiting of sputum or dizziness, vomiting, or coma with sputum rale, or numbness of limbs, or phlegm nodules, greasy fur and slippery pulse. Phlegm syndrome may be divided into cold phlegm, heat syndrome, damp phlegm, dry phlegm and stagnant phlegm according to the nature of phlegm and the complication which should be carefully differentiated.

粘,胸闷,或头目晕眩,或脘痞纳呆、恶心呕吐,或神昏而喉中痰鸣,或神乱而为癫、狂、痴、痫,或肢体麻木、半身不遂,或为瘰疬、瘿瘤、乳癖、痰核等。舌苔腻,脉滑。

证候分析:痰之为病,病变多端,故有"百病多由痰作祟"之说。痰阻于肺,肺失宣降,则胸闷咳嗽,咯痰质粘;痰浊上蒙,清阳不升,则头晕目眩;痰湿中阻,脾失健运,胃失和降,则脘痞纳呆,呕恶;痰迷心窍,则神昏而喉中痰鸣,或神乱而为癫、狂、痴、痫;痰阻经络,气血不畅,则肢体麻木,或半身不遂;痰气交阻,停滞于皮下、肌肉之间,则为瘰疬、瘿瘤、乳癖、痰核等。苔腻,脉滑,为痰湿内盛的征象。

辨证要点:本证以咯痰或眩晕,呕吐,或神昏而喉中痰鸣,或肢体麻木,或见痰核,苔腻,脉滑等为诊断依据。由于痰的性状及其兼见证候的不同,痰证又有寒痰、热痰、湿痰、燥痰及风痰、瘀痰等不同,故应根据其不同的表现特点及兼症进行鉴别。

### 2.2.4.3 Fluid-retention syndrome

Fluid-retention syndrome refers to syndrome caused by retention of fluid in the viscera and tissues, usually caused by stoppage of fluid and retention of fluid resulting from six exogenous pathogenic factors, or overstrain and weakness.

Clinical manifestations: Epigastric and abdominal fullness and distension, borborygmus, vomiting of clear fluid; or cough and asthma, profuse thin sputum, chest oppression and palpitation, even inability to lie flat on bed; or thoracic and hypochondriac fullness, distending pain, aggravation of pain after cough, spitting or rotating the body; or dizziness, dysuria, dropsy and aching heaviness of the limbs; whitish slippery fur and taut pulse.

Analysis of symptoms: The symptoms are various due to different location of fluid-retention. In his Synopsis of Golden Chamber, Zhang Zhongjing divided fluid-retention syndrome into phlegmatic fluid-retention (in a narrow sense), suspended fluid-retention, sustained fluid-retention and extravasating fluid-retention. Phlegmatic fluid-retention is marked by epigastric and abdominal distension, borborygmus and vomiting of clear fluid due to retention of fluid in the stomach and intestines, inactivation of gastrosplenic yang and dysfunction of transportation and transformation; suspended fluid-retention is marked by chest and hypochondrium fullness, distending pain, aggravation of pain after cough, spitting or rotating the body due to retention of fluid in the chest and hypochondrium; sustained fluid-retention is marked by cough and asthma, profuse thin sputum, chest oppression and palpitation, even inability to lie flat on bed due to retention of fluid in the lung and fluid-retention invading the heart; extravasating fluid-retention is marked by dizziness, dysuria, dropsy and aching heaviness of the limbs due to retention of

### （三）饮证

饮证是指因饮邪停滞于脏腑、组织所表现的病证。多由外感六淫，或劳倦体虚等，以致水液失布，停聚为饮而形成。

临床表现：脘腹痞胀，水声辘辘，泛吐清水；或咳嗽气喘，痰多而稀，胸闷心悸，甚至倚息不能平卧；或胸胁饱满，支撑胀痛，咳唾或转侧牵引痛甚；或头晕目眩，小便不利，肢体浮肿而沉重酸痛。苔白滑，脉弦。

证候分析：饮停部位的不同，可见不同的症状。张仲景之《金匮要略》根据饮邪停聚于机体的不同表现，将饮证分为痰饮（狭义）、悬饮、支饮、溢饮四种。饮停于胃肠，中阳不振，运化失职，则见脘腹痞胀，水声辘辘，泛吐清水，谓之痰饮（狭义）；饮停胸胁，则胸胁饱满、支撑胀痛，咳唾或转侧牵引痛甚，谓之悬饮；饮停于肺，则咳嗽气喘，痰多而稀，胸闷，甚或倚息不能平卧，水饮凌心，则心悸，谓之支饮；水饮留溢于四肢肌肤，则肢体浮肿沉重，小便不利，谓之溢饮。饮邪阻遏清阳，故头晕目眩。苔白滑，脉弦，为水饮停滞的征象。

fluid in the muscles of the four limbs; whitish slippery tongue and taut pulse are signs of fluid-retention.

Key points for syndrome differentiation: Phlegmatic fluid-retention is marked by epigastric and abdominal fullness and distension as well as borborygmus; suspended fluid-retention is marked by thoracic and hypochondriac fullness, distending pain, aggravation of pain due to spitting, cough or rotation of the body; sustained fluid-retention is marked by cough and asthma, profuse and thin sputum, chest oppression and palpitation; extravasating fluid-retention is marked by dropsy of limbs and dysuria.

### 2.2.4.4 Edema

Edema refers to dropsy of eyelid, face, four limbs, chest and abdomen or even the whole body due to accumulation of fluid in the muscles resulting from disturbance of the lung, spleen and kidney in distributing and excreting fluid. Clinically, edema is divided into yang edema and yin edema.

#### 2.2.4.4.1 Yang edema

Yang edema, of sthenia in nature, is marked by swelling above the waist and short duration due to exogenous pathogenic wind or spreading of fluid and dampness.

Clinical manifestations: Dropsy of face and eyelids, eventually involving the whole body with rapid development, smooth and bright skin, scanty urine, accompanied by fever, aversion to wind and cold, aching pain of limbs, sore-throat, thin fur and floating pulse; or dropsy of the whole body with slow development, depression under pressure, heaviness of the limbs, epigastric and abdominal fullness and oppression, poor appetite, nausea and regurgitation, whitish greasy tongue fur as well as soft and slow pulse.

辨证要点：痰饮（狭义）以脘腹痞胀，水声辘辘为诊断依据。悬饮以胸胁饱满、胀痛，咳唾或转侧牵引痛甚为诊断依据。支饮以咳嗽气喘，痰多而稀，胸闷心悸为诊断依据。溢饮以肢体浮肿，小便不利为诊断依据。

### （四）水肿

水肿是指由于肺、脾、肾的输布、排泄水液功能失常，以致水液停聚体内，泛溢肌肤，引起眼睑、头面、四肢、胸腹甚至全身浮肿的病证。临床上可分为阳水、阴水两大类。

#### 1. 阳水

阳水是指由外邪侵袭所引起，腰以上肿甚，病程较短，属于实证的水肿。多由外感风邪，或水湿浸淫等因素所致。

临床表现：头面、眼睑浮肿，继则遍及全身，来势迅速，皮肤薄而光亮，小便短少，伴发热恶风寒，肢体酸痛，咽痛，苔薄，脉浮等症。或全身浮肿，来势较缓，按之没指，肢体困重，脘腹痞闷，纳呆，泛恶欲吐，舌苔白腻，脉濡缓。

Analysis of symptoms: Dysuria and sudden dropsy are due to disorder of fluid distribution and spreading of fluid in the muscles resulting from dysfunction of the lung to disperse and regulate caused by wind attack; dropsy of head and eyelids with the involvement of the whole body due to the fact that wind tends to float upwards and change and that wind comes into combination with fluid; fever, aversion to wind and cold, aching pain of limbs, sore-throat, thin fur and floating pulse are due to pathogenic wind invading the lung and failure of the lung to disperse; general edema and heaviness of limbs are due to encumbrance of the spleen by fluid and dampness which leads to failure of yangqi to rise, dysfunction of transformation and extravasation of fluid; dysuria or scanty urine is due to internal accumulation of fluid and dampness, dysfunction of the triple energizer to control fluid and disturbance of the bladder to transform qi; epigastric and abdominal fullness and oppression, poor appetite, regurgitation and nausea are due to encumbrance of the spleen and stomach by dampness which affects ascent and descent.

Key points for syndrome differentiation: This syndrome is marked by rapid onset and development of edema primarily involving the eyelids, face and head as well as severe edema of the upper part of the body.

#### 2.2.4.4.2　Yin edema

Yin edema is marked by asthenia of spleen and kidney qi, severe edema of the part below the waist and long duration, usually caused by asthenia of the healthy qi due to prolonged illness, internal impairment due to overstrain and consumption of spleen and kidney yang.

Clinical manifestations: Repeated relapse of edema, severity below the waist, depression under pressure, epigastric and abdominal distension and oppression, poor

证候分析：风邪外袭，肺卫受病，宣降失常，通调失职，水津失布，泛溢肌肤，故小便不利而浮肿骤起；风性轻扬，善行数变，风水相搏，故水肿多始于头面，眼睑尤为明显，迅即遍及全身；风邪束表犯肺，肺卫失宣，则出现发热恶风寒，肢体酸痛，咽痛，苔薄，脉浮等卫表症状。若水湿浸淫，脾土受困，阳气不得舒展，健运失职，水泛肌肤，则全身水肿，肢体困重；水湿内聚，三焦决渎失司，膀胱气化失常，则小便不利或短少；湿困脾胃，升降失常，则脘腹痞闷，纳呆，泛恶欲吐。苔白腻，脉濡缓，为脾失健运，水湿困阻的征象。

辨证要点：本证以水肿发病急，来势猛，先见于眼睑、头面，上半身肿甚为诊断依据。

#### 2. 阴水

阴水是指脾肾阳气虚弱，腰以下肿甚，病程较长的水肿。多因病久正虚，劳倦内伤，耗损脾肾阳气而引起。

临床表现：水肿反复发作，腰以下为甚，按之凹陷不起，脘腹胀闷，纳呆便溏，神倦

appetite and loose stool, dispiritedness, fatigue of limbs, cold body and limbs, preference for warmth, or aching cold sensation of loins and knees, scanty urine, dull or pale complexion, pale and bulgy tongue with white and slippery fur as well as sunken, slow and weak pulse.

Analysis of symptoms: Edema and scanty urine are due to spreading of fluid and dampness resulting from failure of the asthenic spleen yang to warm and transport and failure of asthenic kidney yang to transform qi; repeated relapse of edema, severity below the waist and depression under pressure are due to asthenia of spleen and kidney yang, accumulation of fluid and dampness, downward migration of dampness as well as heavy and sticky nature of dampness; cold body and limbs, aching cold sensation of loins and knees, dull or pale complexion, dispiritedness and fatigue of limbs are due to asthenia of spleen and kidney yang and decline of mingmen fire to warm and nourish the body; epigastric and abdominal distension and oppression, poor appetite and loose stool are due to asthenia of spleen yang and inability to transport and transform; pale and bulgy tongue, white and slippery fur as well as sunken, slow and weak pulse are signs of yang asthenia and internal exuberance of dampness.

Key points for syndrome differentiation: Repeated relapse of edema, long duration, severity below the waist, accompanied by asthenia of spleen and kidney yang.

## 2.3 Syndrome differentiation of viscera

Syndrome differentiation of viscera means to differentiate syndromes according to the physiological functions and pathological changes of the viscera.

肢困,形寒肢冷喜温,或腰膝酸冷,小便短少,面色晦滞或㿠白,舌淡胖,苔白滑,脉沉迟无力。

证候分析:脾阳虚温运无权,肾阳虚无以气化,开合不利,水湿泛溢,则水肿,小便短少;脾肾阳虚,水湿停聚,湿性趋下,重浊粘滞,故见水肿反复发作,尤以腰以下肿甚,按之凹陷不起;脾肾阳虚,命门火衰,不能温养形体,故见形寒肢冷,腰膝酸冷,面色晦滞或㿠白,神倦肢困;脾阳虚衰,运化无权,水停气滞,则脘腹胀闷,纳呆便溏。舌质淡胖,苔白滑,脉沉迟无力,是阳虚水湿内盛的征象。

辨证要点:本证以水肿反复发作,病程长,尤以腰以下肿甚,兼见脾肾阳虚的表现为诊断依据。

## 第三节 脏腑辨证

脏腑辨证是根据脏腑的生理功能、病理表现,对疾病进行辨证。

Syndrome differentiation of viscera is the base for syndrome differentiation in the clinical specialties of TCM and is an important part in the syndrome differentiation system in TCM. Syndrome differentiation of viscera, a further progress of syndrome differentiation of eight principles as well as qi, blood and body fluid, is helpful for differentiation of the location, cause and nature of disease, the conditions of healthy qi and pathogenic factors as well as the pathological states of the viscera, making it more specific for treatment.

## 2.3.1 Syndrome differentiation of heart disease

Pathological changes of the heart refer to the dysfunction of the heart and its functions to govern the mind and blood vessels, clinically marked by palpitation, heart pain, dysphoria, insomnia, dreaminess, amnesia, derangement, knotted pulse, slow regular intermittent pulse or rapid irregular intermittent pulse. Since the heart opens to the tongue, so some of the tongue disorders, such as tongue pain and tongue sore, are also related to the heart.

The heart disease is either asthenic or sthenic. Asthenic heart disease is usually due to excessive anxiety, congenital defects, asthenia of visceral qi in senility or impairment of the heart by prolonged illness which leads to asthenia of heart qi, asthenia of heart blood, asthenia of heart yin and sudden loss of heart yang. Sthenic heart disease is due to phlegm retention, fire disturbance, cold coagulation, qi stagnation and blood stasis which lead to obstruction of heart vessels, hyperactivity of heart fire, confusion of heart by phlegm and phlegmatic fire disturbing the heart, etc.

### 2.3.1.1 Asthenia of heart qi

Asthenia of heart qi refers to asthenia symptoms of

脏腑辨证是临床各科辨证的基础,是中医辨证体系中的重要组成部分。脏腑辨证是八纲辨证和气血津液辨证的深化,能具体地辨认病证所在的脏腑部位及病因、病性、邪正盛衰和脏腑病理,从而使治疗有更强的针对性。

## 一、心病辨证

心的病变主要反映在心脏本身及其主神明、主血脉的功能失常方面,临床以心悸、怔忡、心痛、心烦、失眠、多梦、健忘、神昏、神识错乱、脉结代或促等为常见症状。此外,由于心开窍于舌,所以某些舌体病变,如舌痛、舌疮等症,亦常归属于心。

心病的证候有虚实之分。虚证多由思虑劳神太过,或先天不足,或年高脏气虚弱,或久病伤心,导致心气虚、心阳虚、心血虚、心阴虚及心阳暴脱;实证多由痰阻、火扰、寒凝、气郁、血瘀等原因,导致心脉痹阻、心火亢盛、痰迷心窍及痰火扰心等。

### (一) 心气虚证

心气虚证是指由于心气

palpitation and shortness of breath resulting from insufficiency of heart qi and failure of heart qi to propel. This syndrome is due to frequent weakness, or malnutrition with prolonged disease, or deficiency of visceral qi caused by senility, which leads to asthenia of heart qi, weakness in propelling and malnutrition of the heart.

Clinical manifestations: Palpitation, shortness of breath, spiritual lassitude, aggravation after movement, pale complexion, or spontaneous sweating, pale tongue and weak pulse, seen in cardiac insufficiency (compensatory period) due to coronary atherosclerotic cardiopathy, viral myocarditis, chronic rheumatic heart disease, hypotension, primary myocardiopathy, chronic pulmonary heart disease, and mitral valve prolapse syndrome as well as patients with cardiac neurosis.

Analysis of symptoms: Insufficiency of heart qi, lack of proper moisture and nourishment of the heart and irregular beating of the heart lead to palpitation; shortness of breath and spiritual lassitude are due to functional decline resulting from qi asthenia; spontaneous sweating is due to qi asthenia and weakness of weiqi to protect the superficies; aggravation after movement is due to consumption of qi after movement; pale complexion, pale tongue and weak pulse are due to failure of asthenic qi to propel and insufficiency of qi and blood.

Key points for syndrome differentiation: Palpitation, shortness of breath, spiritual lassitude, aggravation after movement and decline of functional activities due to qi asthenia.

### 2.3.1.2 Heart yang asthenia syndrome

Heart yang asthenia syndrome refers to asthenia cold syndrome marked by palpitation, aversion to cold and cold limbs due to asthenia of heart yang to warm and propel.

不足,鼓动无力,而表现以心悸、气短为主症的虚弱证候。本证多由于素体虚弱,或久病失养,或年高脏气虚衰等因素,导致心气虚弱,鼓动无力,心失濡养。

临床表现:心悸,气短,精神疲惫,活动后加重,面色淡白,或自汗,舌淡,脉虚。可见于冠状动脉粥样硬化性心脏病、病毒性心肌炎、慢性风湿性心脏病、低血压、原发性心肌病、慢性肺源性心脏病、二尖瓣脱垂综合征等所致的心功能不全(代偿期),以及临床常见的心脏神经官能症患者。

证候分析:心气不足,心失濡养,心动失常,则心悸不安;气虚功能活动衰退,故气短、神疲;气虚卫外不固则自汗;动则气耗,故活动后诸症加重;气虚鼓动无力,气血不充,则面色淡白,舌淡,脉虚。

辨证要点:本证以心悸与气短、精神疲惫、活动后加重等气虚功能活动衰退的表现并见为诊断依据。

### (二)心阳虚证

心阳虚证是指由于心阳虚衰,温养鼓动无力,而表现以心悸怔忡、畏寒肢冷为主症

This syndrome is the further development of heart qi asthenia in which asthenia of qi impairs yang and leads to asthenia of heart yang and lack of proper warming and nourishment of the heart as well as inhibited circulation of blood.

Clinical manifestations: Palpitation, chest oppression or pain, shortness of breath, spontaneous sweating, aversion to cold and cold limbs, pale complexion or cyanotic complexion and lips, pale and bulgy tongue or purplish tongue, whitish slippery tongue fur, weak pulse, or knotted pulse, or slow regular intermittent pulse. This syndrome is usually seen in coronary atherosclerotic cardiopathy, infectious endocarditis, viral myocarditis, chronic rheumatic heart disease, hypotension, primary myocardiopathy, chronic pulmonary heart disease, mitral valve prolapse syndrome and cardiac insufficiency (compensatory period) due to cardiac neurosis.

Analysis of symptoms: Palpitation is due to asthenia of heart yang, weakness to propel and irregular heart beating; chest oppression or pain and shortness of breath are due to inactivation of thoracic yang; aversion to cold and cold limbs are due to yang asthenia and lack of proper warming; spontaneous sweating is due to weakness of weiqi to protect the superficies; pale complexion or cyanotic complexion and lips as well as knotted pulse, slow regular intermittent pulse or weak pulse are due to asthenia of heart yang to warm and propel and inhibited circulation of blood; pale and bulgy tongue or purplish tongue as well as white and slippery fur are signs of yang asthenia and exuberant cold.

Key points for syndrome differentiation: Palpitation, chest oppression or pain, weak pulse or knotted pulse and slow regular intermittent pulse as well as aversion to cold and cold limbs.

的虚寒证候。本证常由心气虚进一步发展，气损及阳，导致心阳虚衰，心失温养，心血运行不畅所形成。

临床表现：心悸怔忡，心胸憋闷或痛，气短，自汗，畏寒肢冷，面色㿠白，或面唇青紫，舌淡胖或青紫，苔白滑，脉弱或结代。可见于冠状动脉粥样硬化性心脏病、感染性心内膜炎、低血压、原发性心肌病、慢性肺源性心脏病、二尖瓣脱垂综合征等所致的心功能不全（失代偿期）。

证候分析：心阳虚弱，鼓动无力，心动失常，故心悸怔忡；胸阳不展，则心胸憋闷或痛，气短；阳虚温煦失职，故见畏寒肢冷；卫外不固则自汗；心阳虚温运无力，血行不畅，故见面色㿠白或面唇青紫，脉结代或弱。舌质淡胖或青紫，苔白滑，均为阳虚寒盛的表现。

辨证要点：本证以心悸怔忡、胸闷或痛、脉弱或结代，及畏寒肢冷等虚寒表现并见为诊断依据。

## 2.3.1.3 Sudden loss of heart yang syndrome

Sudden loss of heart yang is a critical condition due to extreme exhaustion of heart yang and sudden loss of yangqi. This syndrome is the further development of heart yang asthenia. It may be caused by severe impairment of heart yang by pathogenic cold or obstruction of the heart by phlegm.

Clinical manifestations: Apart from the symptoms of heart yang asthenia, there appear some other symptoms, such as sudden profuse cold sweating, cold limbs, weak breath, pale complexion, or sharp heart pain, cyanotic lips, indistinct pulse, even or unconsciousness and coma, usually seen in cardiogenic shock due to various diseases.

Analysis of symptoms: Profuse cold sweating is due to leakage of body fluid with sudden loss of yangqi; cold limbs is due to decline of yangqi to warm the limbs; weak breath is due to asthenia of yangqi and leakage of thoracic qi to help the lung perform respiration; pale complexion is due to sudden loss of yangqi, weakness in warming the body, inhibited circulation of blood and vacuity of the vessels; sharp heart pain and cyanotic lips are due to inhibited circulation of blood and stagnation of blood in the heart vessels; unconsciousness or coma are due to declination of yangqi, lack of necessary warmth and nourishment of the heart and dispersion of the spirit; indistinct pulse is a sign of the declination of yangqi.

Key points for syndrome differentiation: Asthenia of yangqi, sudden profuse cold sweating, cold limbs, weak breath, pale complexion, cyanotic lips and indistinct pulse.

## （三）心阳暴脱证

心阳暴脱证是指心阳衰极，阳气暴脱所表现的危重证候。本证常是心阳虚证进一步发展的结果，亦有因寒邪暴伤心阳或痰瘀阻塞心窍所致者。

临床表现：在心阳虚证表现的基础上，更见突然冷汗淋漓，四肢厥冷，呼吸微弱，面色苍白，或心痛剧烈，口唇青紫，脉微欲绝，甚或神志模糊，昏迷不醒。可见于各种疾病所导致的心源性休克。

证候分析：阳气暴脱，津液随之外泄，则冷汗淋漓；阳气衰亡，不能温煦肢体，故四肢厥冷；心阳衰，宗气泄，不能助肺以行呼吸，故呼吸微弱；阳气亡脱，温运无力，血行迟涩，脉络失充，故面色苍白；血行不畅，瘀阻心脉，则心痛剧烈，口唇青紫。阳气衰微，心失温养，神散不收，导致神志模糊，或昏迷不醒。脉微欲绝，为阳气衰微的征象。

辨证要点：本证以心阳虚和突然冷汗淋漓，四肢厥冷，呼吸微弱，面色苍白，口唇青紫，脉微欲绝等亡阳的临床表现同时出现为诊断依据。

### 2.3.1.4 Heart blood asthenia syndrome

Heart blood asthenia syndrome is caused by asthenia of heart blood and lack of proper moisture and nourishment of the heart. This syndrome is caused by weakness of the spleen in producing blood, or by excessive loss of blood, or by lack of proper nursing in chronic disease, or by consumption of heart blood.

Clinical manifestations: Palpitation, dizziness, insomnia, dreaminess, amnesia, pale complexion or sallow complexion, pale lips and tongue as well as thin and weak pulse, seen in various hemorrhagia, disturbance of blood production and anemia due to various chronic and consumptive diseases.

Analysis of symptoms: Palpitation is due to insufficiency of heart blood, lack of proper nourishment of the heart, and irregular heart beating; insomnia and dreaminess are due to failure of blood to nourish the heart and anxiety; dizziness, amnesia, pale or sallow complexion as well as light whitish lips and tongue are due to failure of asthenic blood to nourish the head and face; thin and weak pulse is due to insufficiency of blood in the vessels.

Key points for syndrome differentiation: The syndrome is marked by palpitation, insomnia, dizziness, pale or sallow complexion, light whitish lips and tongue due to failure of deficient blood to nourish the body.

### 2.3.1.5 Heart yin asthenia syndrome

Heart yin asthenia syndrome refers to the syndrome caused by depletion of heart yin and internal disturbance of asthenic heat. This syndrome is usually caused by excessive contemplation which consumes heart yin; or by consumption of yin fluid at the advanced stage of febrile disease; or by deficiency of liver and kidney yin involving the heart.

### （四）心血虚证

心血虚证是指由于心血亏虚，不能濡养心脏所表现的证候。本证多因脾虚生血之源亏乏，或失血过多，或久病失养，或劳心耗血所致。

临床表现：心悸，头晕，失眠多梦，健忘，面色淡白或萎黄，唇、舌色淡，脉细弱。可见于各种出血，造血功能障碍，以及由慢性消耗性疾病引起的贫血症。

证候分析：心血不足，心失所养，心动失常，故见心悸；血不养心，心神不安，则失眠多梦；血虚不能上荣于头面，故见头晕，健忘，面色淡白或萎黄，唇舌淡白；血少脉道失充，故脉细无力。

辨证要点：本证以心悸，失眠，以及头晕，面色淡白或萎黄，唇舌淡白等血虚机体失于荣养的表现共见为诊断依据。

### （五）心阴虚证

心阴虚证是指由于心阴亏损，虚热内扰所表现的证候。本证多因思虑劳神太过，暗耗心阴；或因热病后期，耗伤阴液；或肝肾等脏阴亏累及于心所致。

Clinical manifestations: Dysphoria, palpitation, insomnia, dreaminess, afternoon tidal fever, feverish sensation over five centers (palms, soles and chest), flushed cheeks, night sweating, reddish tongue with scanty saliva, thin and fast pulse, usually seen in viral myocarditis, chronic rheumatic heart disease, mitral valve prolapse syndrome, pericarditis, arrhythmia, cardiac neurosis and rehabilitative stage of various infectious diseases.

Analysis of symptoms: Palpitation is due to insufficiency of heart yin, lack of proper nutrition of the heart and irregular heart beating; dysphoria, insomnia and dreaminess are due to lack of proper nutrition of the heart, asthenic heat disturbing the heart and anxiety; feverish sensation over the five centers, afternoon tidal fever, flushed cheeks and night sweating are due to failure of yin to control yang and internal generation of asthenic heat; reddish tongue with scanty saliva and thin and fast pulse are signs of yin asthenia and internal heat.

Key points for syndrome differentiation: Palpitation, dysphoria, insomnia, dreaminess, feverish sensation over the five centers, afternoon tidal fever and flushed cheeks.

## 2.3.1.6 Heart vessels obstruction syndrome

Heart vessels obstruction syndrome refers to symptoms of palpitation, chest oppression and heart pain due to obstruction of the heart vessels by blood stasis, phlegm, yin cold and qi stagnation. This syndrome is caused by primary asthenia of healthy qi, inactivation of heart yang and obstruction of the heart vessels by substantial pathogenic factors. According to different causes, this syndrome may be divided into different types, such as obstruction of heart vessels by stagnation, obstruction of

临床表现：心烦心悸，失眠多梦，午后潮热，五心烦热，颧红盗汗，舌红少津，脉细数。可见于慢性风湿性心脏病、病毒性心肌炎、感染性心内膜炎、心包炎、二尖瓣脱垂综合征、心律失常、心脏神经官能症，以及多种感染性疾病的恢复阶段。

证候分析：心阴亏少，心失所养，心动失常，故见心悸；心失濡养，且虚热扰心，心神不安，则心烦，失眠，多梦；阴不制阳，虚热内生，故五心烦热，午后潮热，颧红，盗汗。舌红少津，脉细数，为阴虚内热的表现。

辨证要点：本证以心悸心烦不宁，失眠多梦及五心烦热、午后潮热、颧红等阴虚内热的表现共见为诊断依据。

## （六）心脉痹阻证

心脉痹阻证是指由于瘀血、痰浊、阴寒、气滞等因素阻痹心脉，而出现以心悸怔忡、胸闷心痛为主症的一类证候。本证多因正气先虚，心阳不振，有形之邪阻滞心脉所致。根据其成因之不同，又有瘀阻心脉、痰阻心脉、寒凝心脉、气滞心脉等不同的证型。

heart vessels by phlegm, obstruction of heart vessels by cold coagulation and stagnation of qi in heart vessels, etc.

Clinical manifestations: Palpitation, chest oppression and pain, pain involving the shoulder, back and inner part of arm and occasional occurrence; or stabbing chest pain, dull tongue or tongue with purplish petechiae, thin and astringent pulse or knotted pulse and slow regular intermittent pulse; or chest oppression and pain, obesity and profuse sputum, heaviness of body and lassitude, whitish greasy tongue fur, sunken and slippery pulse or sunken and astringent pulse; or aggravation of pain with cold, alleviation with warmth, cold body and limbs, pale tongue with white fur, sunken and slow pulse or sunken and tense pulse; or pain and distension, hypochondriac distension, sighing, light reddish tongue and taut pulse. Such symptoms are usually seen in coronary atherosclerotic cardiopathy, angina pectoris, myocardiac infarction and primary cardiac myopathy, etc.

Analysis of symptoms: Palpitation is due to inactivation of heart yang, lack of warmth and irregular heart beating; chest oppression and pain are due to failure of yangqi to disperse, weak flow of blood and obstruction of heart vessels; pain involving the shoulder, back and inner side of the arm is due to the fact that the heart meridian distributes directly to the lung, comes out from the armpit and moves along the inner side of the arm. Stasis in the heart vessels is marked by dull pain, usually accompanied by dull or purplish tongue with petechiae, thin and astringent pulse or knotted pulse and slow regular intermittent pulse; obstruction of heart vessels by phlegm is marked by dull pain, usually accompanied by obesity, profuse phlegm, heaviness and lassitude of the body, whitish greasy fur, sunken and slippery pulse or sunken and astringent pulse that indicate internal exuberance of

临床表现：心悸怔忡，心胸憋闷作痛，痛引肩背内臂，时作时止。或胸痛如针刺，舌暗或有青紫斑点，脉细涩或结代；或为心胸闷痛，体胖痰多，身重困倦，舌苔白腻，脉沉滑或沉涩；或遇寒痛剧，得温痛减，形寒肢冷，舌淡苔白，脉沉迟或沉紧；或疼痛而胀，胁胀，喜太息，舌淡红，脉弦。可见于冠状动脉粥样硬化性心脏病、心绞痛、心肌梗死、原发性心肌病等。

证候分析：心阳不振，失于温养，心动失常，故见心悸怔忡；阳气不宣，血行无力，心脉痹阻，故心胸憋闷疼痛；手少阴心经之脉直行上肺出腋下，循内臂，故痛引肩背内臂。瘀阻心脉以刺痛为特点，伴见舌暗或有青紫色瘀斑瘀点，脉细涩或结代等瘀血内阻的症状；痰阻心脉以闷痛为特点，多见体胖痰多，身重困倦，苔白腻，脉沉滑或沉涩等痰浊内盛的症状；寒凝心脉以痛势剧烈，突然发作，得温痛减为特点，伴见畏寒喜温，肢冷，舌淡苔白，脉沉迟或沉紧等寒邪内

phlegm; obstruction of heart vessels by cold coagulation is marked by sharp pain, sudden onset, alleviation with warmth, accompanied by aversion to cold and preference for warmth, cold limbs, pale tongue with white fur, sunken and slow pulse or sunken and tense pulse that indicate internal exuberance of cold; obstruction of heart vessels by qi stagnation is marked by distending pain and close relation of occurrence with psychological factors, often accompanied by hypochondriac distension, susceptibility to sighing and taut pulse that indicate stagnation of qi.

Key points for syndrome differentiation: The key points are palpitation, chest oppression and pain. Since obstruction of heart vessels is caused by various factors, such as blood stasis, phlegmatic turbidity, cold coagulation and qi stagnation, so trials must be made in differentiating pain and complications to specify the causes of disease.

### 2.3.1.7 Exuberance of heart fire syndrome

Exuberance of heart fire syndrome refers to sthenic heat syndrome due to internal exuberance of heart fire. This syndrome is caused by mental depression, transformation of fire from qi stagnation, or internal invasion of pathogenic heat and fire, or excessive intake of acrid, hot and tonic food, transformation of fire from prolonged accumulation in the heart.

Clinical manifestations: Dysphoria, insomnia, flushed complexion, thirst, fever, constipation, yellow urine, deep reddish tongue tip, yellow fur and fast pulse; or ulceration and pain of tongue, or hematemesis, hemorrhagia, or even mania, delirium and unconsciousness, usually seen in hypertension, thyroidism, endocarditis, periodontitis, infection of urinary system and craniocerebral infection, etc.

Analysis of symptoms: Dysphoria and insomnia are

due to internal exuberance of fire heat and disturbance of heart spirit; thirst, constipation and yellow urine are due to consumption of fluid by pathogenic fire; flushed complexion and deep reddish tip of tongue are due to up-flaming of fire and heat; fast pulse is due to exuberant heat promoting blood circulation; sores, ulceration and pain of mouth and tongue are due to heart fire affecting the tongue through meridians; hematemesis and hemorrhagia are due to heart fire driving blood to extravasate; fever, mania, delirium and unconsciousness are due to exuberance of pathogenic heat that disturbs heart spirit.

Key points for syndrome differentiation: Dysphoria and insomnia as well as manifestations of exuberant fire and heat on the tongue and pulse.

### 2.3.1.8 Mind confusion by phlegm

Mind confusion by phlegm refers to symptoms of unconsciousness due to phlegm confusing heart spirit. This syndrome is usually caused by damp turbid substance that hinders qi movement; or by emotional upsets, stagnation of qi, failure of qi to promote fluid flow and accumulation of fluid into phlegm; or by internal disturbance of phlegmatic turbid substance combined with liver wind, leading to confusion of heart spirit by phlegmatic turbid substance.

Clinical manifestations: Mental confusion, even unconsciousness, or mental depression, dull facial expressions, dementia, murmuring, abnormal behaviour; or sudden coma, unconsciousness, drooling, sputum rale in the throat; dull complexion, chest oppression, nausea, whitish greasy fur, slippery pulse. Such symptoms are usually seen in craniocerebral infection and depressive schizophrenia, etc.

Analysis of symptoms: Mental confusion and coma are due to phlegmatic turbid substance confusing mind and disorder of spirit; dementia, mental depression, dull facial expressions, murmuring and abnormal behaviour are due to qi stagnation and phlegm coagulation, mixture of phlegm and qi and confusion of spirit; sudden syncope, unconsciousness, drooling and sputum rale in the throat are due to mixture of phlegm with liver wind to hinder heart spirit; dull complexion is due to internal retention of phlegmatic turbid substance, failure of lucid yang to rise and upper movement of turbid qi; chest oppression and vomiting are due to failure of the stomach to descend and adverse flow of gastric qi; whitish greasy tongue fur and slippery pulse are signs of internal exuberance of phlegmatic turbid substance.

Key points for syndrome differentiation: Mental confusion or dementia, sputum rale in the throat and whitish greasy tongue fur that indicate internal exuberance of phlegmatic turbid substance.

### 2.3.1.9 Disturbance of the heart by phlegmatic fire

Disturbance of the heart by phlegmatic fire refers to the syndrome of mental derangement due to fire, heat and phlegmatic turbid substance disturbing the heart spirit. This syndrome is usually caused by emotional stimulation, transformation of fire from qi stagnation scorching fluid into phlegm; or by exogenous damp heat that accumulates into fire; or by exogenous pathogenic heat that scorches fluid into phlegm and leads to internal disturbance of phlegmatic fire.

Clinical manifestations: Fever, restlessness, or coma with delirium, flushed complexion, thirst, hoarse breath, constipation, yellow urine, or sputum rale in the throat, chest oppression, dysphoria, insomnia, or even mania, fighting against people, breaking objects, ravings, emotional disorder, reddish tongue, yellow and greasy fur as

甚则昏不知人。气郁痰凝，痰气搏结，阻蔽神明，则神识痴呆，精神抑郁，表情淡漠，喃喃独语，举止失常。若痰浊挟肝风闭阻心神，则突然昏仆，不省人事，口吐涎沫，喉中痰鸣。痰浊内阻，清阳不升，浊气上泛，故面色晦暗；胃失和降，胃气上逆，则胸闷作呕。舌苔白腻，脉滑，均为痰浊内盛的征象。

辨证要点：本证是以神志昏蒙不清或神识痴呆，喉有痰声，舌苔白腻等痰浊内盛见症为诊断依据。

### （九）痰火扰心证

痰火扰心证是指由于火热痰浊侵扰心神，表现以神志狂乱为主症的证候。本证多因情志刺激，气机郁滞化火，煎熬津液为痰；或外感湿热之邪，蕴成痰火；或外感热邪，灼津为痰，致痰火内扰而引起。

临床表现：发热烦躁，或神昏谵语，面赤口渴，气粗，便秘尿黄，或喉间痰鸣，胸闷，心烦不寐，甚则狂越妄动，打人毁物，胡言乱语，哭笑无常，舌质红，苔黄腻，脉滑数。可见

well as slippery and fast pulse, usually seen in craniocerebral infection and manic schizophrenia, etc.

Analysis of symptoms: Disturbance of the heart by phlegmatic fire is due to either exogenous pathogenic factors or internal impairment. Fever, restlessness, or even coma with delirium and mania are due to phlegmatic fire disturbing heart spirit in exogenous febrile disease; flushed complexion, red eyes and hoarse breath are due to fumigation of internal heat; yellow urine and constipation are due to heat scorching fluid; yellowish thick sputum, or sputum rale in the throat and chest oppression are due to internal exuberance of phlegmatic fire and stagnation of qi; in miscellaneous diseases due to internal impairment, internal exuberance of phlegmatic fire and disturbance of heart spirit lead to dysphoria and insomnia in mild case and mania, ravings, emotional disorder, fighting against people and breaking objects in severe case. Reddish tongue, yellowish greasy fur and slippery and fast pulse are signs of internal exuberance of phlegmatic fire.

Key points for syndrome differentiation: High fever, restlessness or coma with delirium and sputum rale in the throat in exogenous febrile diseases; mania and internal exuberance of phlegmatic fire in miscellaneous diseases with internal impairment.

## 2.3.2 Syndrome differentiation of lung disease

Lung disease mainly reflects dysfunctions of the lung and its functions in governing qi and breath as well as in regulating water passage. The usual clinical symptoms include cough, asthmatic breath, expectoration, stuffy nose, nasal discharge and edema.

Lung disease is either asthenic or sthenic. Asthenic

lung disease is usually caused by prolonged disease with cough, or insufficiency of qi and yin production, or consumption of qi and yin in febrile disease that leads to asthenia of pulmonary qi and asthenia of pulmonary yin. Sthenic lung disease is usually due to invasion of pathogenic wind, cold, dryness and heat, or internal exuberance of phlegmatic dampness that leads to failure of pulmonary qi to disperse and descend, resulting in such syndromes like invasion of the lung by wind cold, invasion of the lung by dryness, invasion of the lung by wind heat, exuberance of pulmonary heat, accumulation of phlegmatic heat in the lung, retention of phlegm and fluid in the lung and mixture of wind and fluid.

### 2.3.2.1 Pulmonary qi asthenia syndrome

Pulmonary qi asthenia syndrome refers to asthenia syndrome due to insufficiency of pulmonary qi and hypofunction of the lung in governing qi and weakness of weiqi to protect the superficies. This syndrome is caused by chronic disease with cough and consumption of pulmonary qi; or by insufficiency of essence and tonification of the lung due to spleen asthenia that fails to transform food.

Clinical manifestations: Weak cough, shortness of breath with aggravation after movement, cough with thin sputum, low and timid voice, spiritual lassitude, pale complexion, spontaneous sweating, aversion to wind, susceptibility to invasion of exogenous pathogenic factors and weak pulse. These symptoms are usually seen in chronic bronchitis, chronic obstructive pulmonary emphysema, insufficiency of lung (compensatory stage) due to chronic and pulmogenic heart disease, remission stage of bronchial asthma, rehabilitative stage of pneumonia and influenza and various diseases due to hypofunction of immunity.

虚证多由久病咳喘,或气阴生化不足,或热病耗伤气阴,导致肺气虚、肺阴虚;实证多由风、寒、燥、热等邪气侵袭,或痰湿内盛,导致肺气失于宣降,而形成风寒犯肺、风热犯肺、燥邪犯肺、肺热炽盛、痰热壅肺、痰饮停肺、风水相搏等证。

### (一) 肺气虚证

肺气虚证是指由于肺气不足,其主气、卫外功能减弱所表现的虚弱证候。本证多由久病咳喘,耗伤肺气;或因脾虚水谷精气化生不足,肺失充养所致。

临床表现:咳喘无力,少气息短,动则益甚,咳痰清稀,语声低怯,神倦乏力,面色淡白,自汗畏风,易感外邪,舌淡苔白,脉弱。可见于慢性支气管炎、慢性阻塞性肺气肿、慢性肺源性心脏病等所导致肺功能不全(代偿期),支气管哮喘缓解期,肺炎及流行性感冒的恢复期,以及多种免疫功能低下疾病。

Analysis of symptoms: Weak cough and asthma are due to asthenia of pulmonary qi, upper adverse flow of qi and failure of dispersion and descent; aggravation of cough and asthma after movement is due to consumption of qi; expectoration of thin and clear sputum is due to failure of the lung to distribute fluid due to asthenia and accumulate fluid into phlegm which is brought upwards with the adverse flow of qi; shortness of breath, low and timid voice are due to insufficiency of thoracic qi due to lung asthenia; spontaneous sweating, aversion to wind and susceptibility to invasion of exogenous pathogenic factors are due to asthenia of pulmonary qi and weakness of weiqi to protect the superficies; dispiritedness and lassitude, pale complexion, light-colored tongue with whitish fur and weak pulse are signs of functional decline due to qi asthenia.

Key points for syndrome differentiation: Weak cough, expectoration with thin and clear sputum and functional decline due to qi asthenia.

#### 2.3.2.2　Lung yin asthenia syndrome

Lung yin asthenia syndrome refers to syndrome of asthenic internal heat due to insufficiency of lung yin and failure of depuration. If internal disturbance of asthenic heat is not evident, it is called fluid consumption and lung dryness syndrome. This syndrome is mainly caused by consumption of lung yin due to dry heat impairing the lung or consumptive disease damaging the lung; or by consumption of fluid due to sweating; or by asthenia of lung yin due to chronic cough impairing lung yin.

Clinical manifestations: Dry cough with scanty sputum, or scanty and sticky sputum difficult to expectorate, or sputum mixed with blood, hoarseness, dry mouth and throat, emaciation, feverish sensation over five centers (palms, soles and chest), afternoon tidal fever, flushed cheeks and night sweating, reddish tongue with scanty fluid as well as thin and fast pulse. These symptoms are seen in the rehabilitative stage of various infective diseases (such as pneumonia, bronchitis and whooping cough) as well as pulmonary tuberculosis, endobronchial tuberculosis, bronchiectasis and lung cancer, etc.

Analysis of symptoms: Dry cough with scanty sputum or with scanty and sticky sputum difficult to expectorate is due to insufficiency of lung yin and internal generation of asthenic heat which deprive the lung of moisture and lead to adverse flow of qi; sputum mingled with blood is due to bleeding resulting from asthenic fire scorching the lung collaterals; hoarseness is due to insufficiency of lung yin, loss of proper moisture of the throat and fumigation of asthenic fire; dry mouth and throat and emaciation are due to insufficiency of lung yin and lack of nutrition; afternoon tidal fever, feverish sensation over the five centers, flushed cheeks, night sweating, reddish tongue with scanty saliva and thin and fast pulse are signs of internal heat due to yin asthenia.

Key points for syndrome differentiation: Dry cough, scanty and sticky sputum and internal heat with yin asthenia.

## 2.3.2.3 Syndrome of wind cold encumbering lung

Syndrome of wind cold encumbering lung refers to the syndrome of failure of pulmonary qi to disperse due to wind cold attacking the lung. This syndrome is usually caused by failure of pulmonary qi to disperse due to exogenous wind cold.

Clinical manifestations: Cough, thin expectoration, stuffy nose with clear snivel and throat itching, accompanied by aversion to cold and fever, or body pain without sweating, whitish thin tongue fur as well as floating and tense pulse, usually seen at the primary stage of upper

等多种感染性疾病的恢复阶段,以及肺结核、支气管内膜结核、支气管扩张、肺癌等。

证候分析:肺阴不足,虚热内生,肺失清润而气逆,故干咳无痰,或痰少而粘,难以咯出;虚火灼伤肺络,络伤血溢,则痰中带血;肺阴不足,咽喉失润,且为虚火所蒸,以致声音嘶哑;阴液不足,失于滋养,则口燥咽干,形体消瘦。午后潮热,五心烦热,颧红,盗汗,舌红少津,脉细数,为阴虚内热的表现。

辨证要点:本证以干咳,痰少而粘和阴虚内热见症为诊断依据。

## (三)风寒束肺证

风寒束肺证是指由于风寒之邪侵袭肺卫,肺卫失宣所表现的证候。本证多由外感风寒之邪,致使肺卫失宣而形成。

临床表现:咳嗽,咳痰清稀,鼻塞,流清涕,喉痒,兼有恶寒发热,或见身痛无汗,舌苔薄白,脉浮紧。可见于上呼吸道感染及肺炎、气管炎等多

respiratory tract infection, bronchitis, pneumonia and various infectious diseases.

Analysis of symptoms: Cough with clear and thin sputum, stuffy nose with clear snivel and throat itching are due to failure of pulmonary qi to disperse resulting from wind cold encumbering the lung; aversion to cold, fever, body pain, no sweating, whitish thin tongue fur and floating and tense pulse are due to wind cold attacking the superficies, stagnation of weiqi, lack of warmth of the surface of the body and obstruction of the muscular interstices.

Key points for syndrome differentiation: Cough, thin and clear sputum, aversion to cold, fever, pain of head and body as well as no sweating.

### 2.3.2.4 Wind heat invading lung syndrome

Wind heat invading lung syndrome refers to the syndrome of the lung failing to disperse resulting from wind heat attacking the lung. This syndrome pertains to weifen syndrome in syndrome differentiation of wei, qi, ying and blood. It is often caused by invasion of wind heat into the lung.

Clinical manifestations: Cough, yellowish thick sputum, stuffy nose with turbid snivel, fever, slight aversion to wind and cold, slight thirst, or sore-throat, reddish tongue tip, thin and yellowish tongue fur, floating and fast pulse, usually seen at the primary stage of various infectious diseases, such as upper respiratory tract infection, pneumonia, bronchitis, lung abscess, mumps, epidemic hemorrhagic fever, scarlet fever and measles, etc.

Analysis of symptoms: Cough, yellowish thick sputum and stuffy nose with turbid snivel are due to wind heat attacking the lung, loss of depuration of the lung and adverse flow of pulmonary qi; sore-throat is due to wind heat disturbing the upper; slight aversion to wind and cold, slight thirst, reddish tongue tip, yellowish thin tongue fur and floating and fast pulse are due to wind heat attacking the superficies, stagnation of weiqi and consumption of body fluid by heat.

Key points for syndrome differentiation: Cough, yellowish thick sputum, fever, slight aversion to wind and cold, slight thirst and reddish tongue tip.

### 2.3.2.5 Syndrome of dryness attacking lung

Syndrome of dryness attacking the lung refers to the syndrome of consumption of fluid in the lung system due to invasion of pathogenic dryness into the lung. This syndrome is divided into febrile dryness syndrome and cool dryness syndrome according to its heat or cold nature. This syndrome is caused by dryness in autumn consuming pulmonary fluid and disturbing weiqi; or by dryness transforming from pathogenic wind and febrile factors consuming body fluid. Dryness in early autumn is febrile and the disease caused is febrile dryness; while dryness in late autumn is cold and the disease caused is cool dryness.

Clinical manifestations: Dry cough with scanty sputum, or sticky sputum difficult to expectorate, even chest pain, sputum mingled with blood, or epistaxis, hematemesis, dryness of mouth, lips, nose and throat, dry feces with scanty urine, thin and dry tongue with scanty saliva, or accompanied by fever, slight aversion to wind cold, no sweating or scanty sweating, floating and fast pulse or floating and tense pulse. These manifestations are usually seen at the primary stage of various infectious diseases, such as upper respiratory tract infection, pneumonia, bronchitis and pharyngitis.

Analysis of symptoms: Dry cough without sputum or

不利,故咽喉疼痛;风热袭表,卫气郁遏,热伤津液,则发热微恶风寒,口微渴,舌尖红,苔薄黄,脉浮数。

辨证要点:本证以咳嗽,痰稠色黄和发热微恶风寒、口微渴、舌尖红等风热表证并见为诊断依据。

### (五)燥邪犯肺证

燥邪犯肺证是指燥邪侵犯肺卫,肺系津液耗伤所表现的证候,又称肺燥(外燥)证。据其偏热、偏寒之不同,又有温燥、凉燥之分。本证多因秋令之季感受燥邪,耗伤肺津,肺卫失和,或因风温之邪化燥伤津所致。初秋感燥,燥偏热,多病温燥;深秋感燥,燥偏寒,多病凉燥。

临床表现:干咳少痰,或痰粘难咯,甚则胸痛,痰中带血,或见鼻衄、咯血,口、唇、鼻、咽干燥,便干尿少,苔薄而干燥少津,或伴发热,微恶风寒,无汗或少汗,脉浮数或浮紧。可见于上呼吸道感染、肺炎、气管炎、咽炎等多种感染性疾病的早期阶段。

证候分析:燥邪犯肺,易

with scanty and sticky sputum difficult to expectorate is due to pathogenic dryness invading the lung, consuming pulmonary fluid and depriving the lung of moisture and depuration; chest pain, sputum mingled with blood, or epistaxis and hematemesis are due to impairment of the pulmonary collaterals due to dryness; dryness of mouth, lips, nose, throat and feces as well as scanty urine and thin tongue fur with scanty saliva are due to pathogenic dryness consuming body fluid; fever and slight aversion to wind cold are due to disorder of weiqi resulting from pathogenic dryness invading the superficies; no sweating and floating and tense pulse are due to mixture of pathogenic dryness with cold which blocks the muscular interstices; scanty sweating and floating and fast pulse are due to mixture of dryness with heat which opens the muscular interstices.

Key points for syndrome differentiation: Dry cough, scanty and sticky sputum difficult to expectorate, dryness of mouth, lips, nose and throat with scanty saliva.

### 2.3.2.6 Syndrome of accumulation of pathogenic heat in lung

Syndrome of accumulation of pathogenic heat in lung refers to the syndrome due to loss of depuration of the lung resulting from exuberant pathogenic heat in the lung. This syndrome pertains to qifen syndrome in syndrome differentiation of wei, qi, ying and blood. This syndrome is usually caused by internal development of exogenous wind heat or accumulation of heat in the lung transforming from internal development of pathogenic wind cold.

Clinical manifestations: Fever, cough, asthmatic breath, even flapping nose with hot breath, red swelling and pain of throat, chest pain, yellowish sticky sputum, or rusty sputum, or foul sputum mingled with blood, thirst, scanty urine, constipation, red tongue with yellow

伤肺津,肺失滋润,清肃失职,故干咳无痰,或痰少而粘,难以咯出;甚则燥伤肺络,而见胸痛,痰中带血,或鼻衄、咯血。"燥胜则干",燥邪伤津,失于滋润,则口、唇、鼻、咽干燥,大便干结,小便短少,苔薄而干燥少津。燥邪袭表,卫气失和,故见发热微恶风寒;若燥与寒并为凉燥,腠理闭塞,故见无汗,脉浮紧;若燥与热合为温燥,腠理开泄,则少汗,脉浮数。

辨证要点:本证以干咳、痰少而粘,难咯及口、唇、鼻、咽干燥少津为诊断依据。

### (六)热邪蕴肺证

热邪蕴肺证是指由邪热内盛于肺,肺失清肃而出现的肺经实热证候,简称肺热证或肺火证。本证在卫气营血辨证中属气分证。多因外感风热入里,或风寒之邪入里化热,蕴结于肺所致。

临床表现:发热,咳嗽,喘息,甚则鼻煽气灼,咽喉红肿疼痛,胸痛,痰黄而粘稠,或咯吐铁锈色痰,或为脓血腥臭痰,口渴,小便短赤,大便秘

fur and fast pulse. These manifestations are usually seen in various respiratory tract infectious diseases (such as pneumonia, infectious common cold, acute bronchitis, lung abscess and bronchial asthma, etc.) as well as measles and scarlet fever, etc.

Analysis of symptoms: Fever is due to fumigation of internal heat; cough and asthma are due to invasion of pathogenic heat in the lung, loss of depuration of the lung and upper adverse flow of qi; flapping nose with hot breath is due to pathogenic heat invading the lung and stagnation of pulmonary qi; red swelling and pain throat is due to fumigation of pulmonary heat and stagnation of qi and blood; chest pain is due to pathogenic heat scorching the pulmonary collaterals; yellow and sticky sputum is due to pathogenic heat scorching fluid into sputum which mixes up with heat and moves adversely upward with pulmonary qi; rusty sputum is due to pathogenic heat impairing the pulmonary collaterals; foul sputum mingled with blood is due to phlegmatic heat accumulation in the lung, qi stagnation and blood coagulation as well as putrid muscles and blood; thirst, constipation and scanty urine are due to exuberant heat consuming fluid; reddish tongue with yellow fur and fast pulse are signs of exuberance of internal heat.

Key points for syndrome differentiation: Fever, cough, asthmatic breath, chest pain and yellowish sticky sputum.

## 2.3.2.7 Syndrome of phlegmatic dampness retention in lung

Syndrome of phlegmatic dampness retention in lung refers to the syndrome due to failure of the lung to disperse and descend resulting from retention of phlegmatic dampness in the lung. This syndrome is caused by retention of phlegm coagulating from fluid in the lung due to

结,舌红苔黄,脉数。可见于肺炎、流行性感冒、急性气管炎、肺脓疡、支气管哮喘等多种呼吸道感染性疾病以及麻疹、猩红热等。

证候分析：里热蒸腾则发热；热邪犯肺,肺失清肃,气逆于上,故咳嗽,气喘；邪热迫肺,肺气郁闭,故鼻煽气灼；肺热上薰咽喉,气血壅滞,故咽喉红肿疼痛；热灼肺络,则胸痛；邪热灼津为痰,痰热互结,随肺气上逆,故咯痰黄而粘稠；热伤肺络,则咯吐铁锈色痰；痰热壅滞于肺,气滞血壅,肉腐血败,则咳吐脓血腥臭痰；热盛伤津,则口渴,便秘,小便短赤。舌红苔黄,脉数,为邪热内盛的征象。

辨证要点：本证以发热,咳嗽,喘息,胸痛,痰黄粘稠为诊断依据。

## （七）痰湿阻肺证

痰湿阻肺证是指由痰湿停滞于肺,肺失宣降所表现的证候。本证常由脾气亏虚,运化无权,水液凝聚为痰,上渍于肺；或久咳伤肺,输布水液

asthenia of splenic qi and failure of transformation and transportation; or by prolonged cough impairing the lung, weakened function of the lung to transport fluid which leads to accumulation of dampness into phlegm and retention of phlegm in the lung system; or by invasion of exogenous cold and dampness into the lung which prevents the lung from dispersing and descending, leading to failure of the lung to transport fluid, accumulation of fluid into phlegm and retention of phlegm in the lung.

Clinical manifestations: Cough with profuse whitish sputum easy to expectorate or with clear, thin and frothy sputum, even asthmatic breath with sputum rale, pale tongue with whitish greasy fur and slippery pulse, usually seen in chronic bronchitis, bronchial asthma, chronic obstructive pulmonary emphysema, chronic pulmonogenic heart disease and lung cancer, etc.

Analysis of symptoms: Cough and profuse sputum are due to retention of phlegmatic dampness in the lung and upper adverse flow of pulmonary qi (whitish, sticky and easy to expectorate sputum is due to retention of phlegmatic dampness in the lung; while clear, thin and frothy sputum is due to retention of fluid in the lung); chest oppression, even asthmatic breath with sputum rale are due to retention of phlegm and fluid in the respiratory tract and inhibited flow of pulmonary qi; pale tongue with whitish greasy or whitish slippery fur, slippery pulse or soft and slow pulse are signs of exuberance of internal phlegmatic dampness.

Key points for syndrome differentiation: Cough, asthmatic breath, profuse whitish sputum which is either sticky and slippery or thin and clear.

### 2.3.2.8 Syndrome of confliction of wind and fluid in lung

Syndrome of confliction of wind and fluid in lung

功能减弱,聚湿酿痰,阻滞肺系;或感受寒湿外邪侵袭肺脏,使肺气宣降失常,肺不布津,水液停聚而为痰湿,停滞于肺。

临床表现:咳嗽,痰多色白,粘滑易咯,或痰液清稀、泡沫多,胸闷,甚则气喘痰鸣,舌淡苔白腻,脉滑。可见于慢性支气管炎、支气管哮喘、慢性阻塞性肺气肿、慢性肺源性心脏病、肺癌等。

证候分析:痰湿停滞于肺,肺气上逆,故咳嗽,痰多。若痰液色白、粘滑易咯者为痰湿阻肺;痰液清稀、泡沫多者为饮停于肺;痰饮阻滞气道,肺气不利,则胸闷,甚则气喘痰鸣。舌淡苔白腻或白滑,脉滑或濡缓,是痰湿内盛的征象。

辨证要点:本证以咳嗽气喘,痰多色白,质粘滑或清稀为诊断依据。

### (八)风水搏肺证

风水搏肺证是指风邪侵

refers to the syndrome due to invasion of pathogenic wind which prevents the lung from dispersing, descending and regulating water passage as well as causes extravasation of fluid and dampness in the skin. This syndrome pertains to yang edema, usually caused by exogenous pathogenic wind attacking the lung and failure of the lung to disperse, descend and regulate water passage which give rise to stagnation of wind, retention of fluid, confliction between wind and fluid as well as extravasation of fluid in the skin.

Clinical manifestations: Primary dropsy of the eyelids and face, eventual edema of the whole body with rapid development, thin and bright skin, scanty urine, accompanied by aversion to cold, fever, no sweating, whitish thin tongue fur, floating and tense pulse; or accompanied by swelling and pain of throat, reddish tongue as well as floating and fast pulse. These manifestations are usually seen in acute nephritis, pyelonephritis and acute onset of chronic nephritis, etc.

Analysis of symptoms: Primary dropsy of eyelids and face, eventual edema of the whole body with rapid development as well as thin and bright skin are due to invasion of pathogenic wind into the lung which prevents the lung from dispersing, descending and regulating water passage as well as causes confliction between wind and fluid and extravasation of fluid; scanty urine is due to failure of the upper energizer to disperse and loss of qi transformation. If accompanied by aversion to cold, fever, no sweating, whitish thin fur as well as floating and tense pulse, it is the syndrome marked by confliction between wind and fluid with superficial cold; if accompanied by swelling and pain of throat, reddish tongue and floating and fast pulse, it is the syndrome marked by confliction between wind and fluid with superficial heat.

Key points for syndrome differentiation: Sudden

袭,肺失宣降,不能通调水道,水湿泛溢肌肤所表现的证候。本证属于阳水范畴,多由外感风邪,侵袭肺卫,宣降失常,通调失职,以致风遏水阻,风水相搏,泛溢肌肤而成。

临床表现:眼睑头面先肿,继而遍及全身,来势迅猛,皮肤薄而光亮,小便短少,兼见恶寒发热,无汗,舌苔薄白,脉浮紧;或兼见咽喉肿痛,舌红,脉浮数。可见于急性肾炎、肾盂肾炎、慢性肾炎急性发作等。

证候分析:风邪袭肺,肺失宣降,不能通调水道,风水相搏,水湿泛溢,故水肿先起于眼睑头面,继而遍及全身,来势迅猛,皮肤薄而光亮;上焦不宣,气化失司,则小便短少。若伴见恶寒发热,无汗,苔薄白,脉浮紧,为风水夹表寒之证;若兼有咽喉肿痛,舌红,脉浮数,为风水夹表热之证。

辨证要点:本证以水肿骤

onset of edema of the eyelids and face first with quick involvement of the whole body, scanty urine, accompanied by aversion to cold and fever, etc.

### 2.3.3 Syndrome differentiation of spleen disease

Spleen disease is mainly marked by dysfunction of the lung to transport, transform and govern blood. The clinical symptoms are usually poor appetite, abdominal distension or pain, loose stool, dropsy, heaviness of limbs, prolapse of the viscera and bleeding, etc.

Spleen disease is either asthenic or sthenic. Asthenic spleen disease is mainly caused by improper diet, irregular daily life, excessive vomiting and diarrhea as well as other acute or chronic diseases which impair the spleen and lead to such problems like asthenia of splenic qi, asthenia of splenic yang, sinking of qi due to splenic asthenia and failure of the spleen to govern blood; sthenic spleen disease is caused by improper diet or intake of contaminated food or exogenous cold dampness or internal invasion of damp heat which leads to cold dampness encumbering the spleen and accumulation of damp heat in the spleen, etc.

#### 2.3.3.1 Syndrome of asthenia of splenic qi

Syndrome of asthenia of splenic qi refers to the syndrome due to asthenia of splenic qi and failure of transportation and transformation, usually caused by improper diet, overstrain and impairment of splenic qi by chronic and acute diseases.

Clinical manifestations: Poor appetite, abdominal distension, especially after meal, loose stool, or dry feces followed by loose stool, lack of qi, no desire to speak, lassitude of limbs, sallow complexion, emaciation, or dropsy, pale tongue with whitish fur, slow and weak pulse, usually seen in chronic gastritis, digestive ulceration,

起,眼睑头面先肿,迅速遍及全身,小便短少,并兼恶寒发热等表证症状为诊断依据。

### 三、脾病辨证

脾的病变主要反映在脾主运化、主统血的功能失常方面,临床以纳少、腹胀或痛、便溏、浮肿、肢体困重、内脏下垂、出血等为常见症状。

脾病的证候有虚实之分,虚证多由饮食失调,劳逸失常,吐泻过度,以及其他急、慢性疾患损伤于脾,导致脾气虚、脾阳虚、脾虚气陷、脾不统血;实证多由饮食失节,或误食不洁食物,或外感寒湿,或湿热之邪内侵,从而形成寒湿困脾、湿热蕴脾等证。

#### (一)脾气虚证

脾气虚证是指脾气虚弱,运化失健所表现的证候。多因饮食失调,劳累过度,以及其他急、慢性疾患耗伤脾气所致。

临床表现:纳少,腹胀,食后尤甚,大便稀溏或先干后溏,少气懒言,肢体倦怠,面色萎黄,形体消瘦,或浮肿,舌淡苔白,脉缓弱。可见于慢性胃炎、消化性溃疡、慢性肠炎、吸

chronic enteritis and malabsorption syndrome, etc.

Analysis of symptoms: Poor appetite and abdominal distension are due to asthenia of splenic qi, failure of transportation and transformation, weakness to digest, absorb and transport cereal nutrient; aggravation of abdominal distension after meal is due to aggravation of stagnancy of splenic qi after meal; loose stool or dry feces followed by loose stool are due to downward migration of dampness into the large intestine resulting from failure of the spleen to transform dampness; lack of qi and no desire to speak are due to failure of transportation and transformation resulting from asthenia as well as insufficiency of gastrosplenic qi; lassitude, sallow complexion and gradual emaciation are due to insufficiency of splenic qi, insufficient production of qi and blood which fail to nourish the body and skin; dropsy of limbs is due to failure of asthenic spleen to transport, internal generation of dampness and extravasation of fluid in the muscles.

Key points for syndrome differentiation: Poor appetite, abdominal distension, loose stool, lack of qi, no desire to speak and lassitude of limbs.

### 2.3.3.2 Syndrome of asthenia of splenic yang

Syndrome of asthenia of splenic yang refers to the syndrome due to asthenia of splenic yang and internal exuberance of yin cold. This syndrome is caused by further development of the asthenia of splenic qi; or by excessive intake of uncooked or cold food; or by asthenia of splenic yang and failure of fire (heart) to generate (promote) earth (spleen).

Clinical manifestations: Poor appetite, abdominal distension, lingering abdominal cold pain, preference for warmth and palpation, aversion to cold, cold sensation of

收不良综合征等。

证候分析：脾气虚弱，运化失健，消化、吸收、输布精微乏力，故纳少，腹胀；食后脾气益困，则腹胀愈甚；脾虚水湿不化，下趋大肠，则大便稀溏或先干后溏；脾虚运化失健，中气生成不足，则少气懒言；脾主四肢肌肉，脾气不足，气血生化乏源，不能充养形体肌肤，可见倦怠乏力，面色萎黄，形体逐渐消瘦；脾虚不运，水湿内生，泛溢肌表，则肢体浮肿；舌淡苔白，脉缓弱，是脾气虚弱的征象。

辨证要点：本证以纳少，腹胀，大便溏薄和少气懒言、肢体倦怠等气虚功能减退的表现共见为诊断依据。

### （二）脾阳虚证

脾阳虚证是指脾阳虚衰，阴寒内盛所表现的证候。本证多由脾气虚进一步发展而成；或过食生冷，损伤脾阳；或肾阳虚，火不生土所致。

临床表现：纳少，腹胀，腹部冷痛，绵绵不休，喜温喜按，畏寒，四肢不温，面色㿠白，口

four limbs, light whitish complexion, bland taste in the mouth without thirst, loose stool, or stool with indigested food, heaviness of limbs, or dropsy of limbs, dysuria, profuse and thin leukorrhagia, pale, bulgy and tender tongue, or tongue with tooth prints, whitish slippery fur, sunken, slow and weak pulse. Such manifestations are usually seen in chronic gastritis, digestive ulceration, chronic enteritis, malabsorption syndrome, Crohn's disease, irritable intestinal syndrome and chronic nephritis and IgA nephropathy.

Analysis of symptoms: Poor appetite and abdominal distension are due to asthenia of splenic yang and failure of transportation and transformation; lingering abdominal cold pain, preference for warmth and palpation are due to asthenia of yang and exuberance of yin, internal generation of cold as well as cold coagulation and qi stagnation; bland taste in the mouth without thirst and loose stool, or even stool with indigested food are due to failure of splenic yang to warm and transport food because of asthenia; aversion to cold, cold sensation of limbs and light whitish complexion are due to failure of yang to warm because of asthenia; heaviness of limbs, even general edema and dysuria are due to inactivation of gastrosplenic yang, internal retention of dampness and extravasation of dampness; profuse and thin leukorrhagia is due to asthenia of splenic yang, weakness of belt vessel and downward migration of dampness; pale, bulgy and tender tongue, or tongue with tooth prints, whitish slippery pulse, as well as sunken, slow and weak pulse are signs of yang asthenia and internal exuberance of yin cold.

Key points for syndrome differentiation: Poor appetite, abdominal distension, lingering abdominal cold pain and loose stool.

淡不渴,大便溏薄清稀,或完谷不化,肢体困重,或肢体浮肿,小便不利,妇女可见带下量多清稀,舌质淡白胖嫩或有齿痕,苔白滑,脉沉迟无力。可见于慢性胃炎、消化性溃疡、慢性肠炎、吸收不良综合征、克罗恩病、肠易激综合征,以及慢性肾炎、IgA肾病等。

证候分析:脾阳虚弱,运化无权,则纳少腹胀;阳虚阴盛,寒从中生,寒凝气滞,故腹部冷痛,绵绵不休,喜温喜按;脾阳虚不能温运水谷,故口淡不渴,大便溏薄清稀,甚则完谷不化;阳虚温煦失职,故畏寒,四肢不温,面色㿠白;中阳不振,水湿内停,流溢肌肤,则肢体困重,甚则全身浮肿,小便不利;脾阳虚弱,带脉不固,水湿下渗,可见妇女白带清稀量多。舌质淡白胖嫩或有齿痕,苔白滑,脉沉迟无力,皆为阳虚阴寒内盛的征象。

辨证要点:本证以纳少,腹胀,腹部冷痛绵绵,大便溏薄清稀等脾失温运及阳虚阴寒内盛的表现共见为诊断依据。

## 2.3.3.3 Syndrome of sinking of splenic qi

Syndrome of sinking of splenic qi refers to the syndrome due to asthenia of splenic qi and failure of splenic qi to rise. This syndrome is mainly caused by further development of asthenia of splenic qi; or by chronic diarrhea or dysentery, or overstrain; or by multiple delivery and improper nursing after labor which over consume splenic qi.

Clinical manifestations: Prolapsing sensation and distension of epigastrium and abdomen, especially after meal, frequent desire for defecation, prolapsing sensation of anus, or chronic diarrhea, or even prolapse of rectum, or prolapse of uterus, or turbid urine, accompanied by lack of qi, fatigue, lassitude of limbs, low voice or no desire to speak, dizziness, pale tongue with whitish fur and weak pulse. Such manifestations are usually seen in chronic gastritis, digestive ulceration, chronic enteritis, malabsorption syndrome, Crohn's disease, irritable intestinal syndrome, gastroptosis, hepatoptosis, nephroptosis and hysteroptosis, etc.

Analysis of symptoms: Prolapsing sensation and distension of epigastrium and abdomen, especially after meal, frequent desire to defecate, prolapsing sensation of anus and chronic diarrhea are due to insufficiency of splenic qi, failure of transformation and transportation, sinking of splenic qi resulting from weakness to rise; gastroptosis, prolapse of rectum and hysteroptosis are due to insufficiency of splenic qi and failure of the viscera to remain in the normal position; turbid urine is due to failure of the sinking splenic qi to transport cereal nutrient, separate the lucidity from turbidity and transmit it to the bladder; lack of qi, fatigue, lassitude of limbs, low voice, no desire to speak, dizziness, pale tongue with white fur and weak pulse are signs of insufficiency of gastrosplenic qi,

## （三）脾气下陷证

脾气下陷证是指脾气亏虚，升举无力而反下陷所表现的证候。本证多由脾气虚进一步发展；或久泄久痢，或劳累过度，或妇女孕产过多，产后失于调护等原因，导致脾气耗损太过而形成。

临床表现：脘腹重坠作胀，食后更甚，或便意频数，肛门重坠，或久泻不止，甚或脱肛，或子宫下垂，或小便混浊如米泔，伴见少气乏力，肢体倦怠，声低懒言，头晕目眩，舌淡苔白，脉弱。可见于慢性胃炎、消化性溃疡、慢性肠炎、吸收不良综合征、克罗恩病、肠易激综合征，以及胃下垂、肝下垂、肾下垂、子宫下垂等。

证候分析：脾气不足，运化失健，升举无力而反下陷，则脘腹重坠作胀，食后更甚，便意频数，肛门重坠，久泻不止；脾气亏虚，脏器失于升举固摄而下垂，则见胃下垂、脱肛、子宫下垂等；脾虚气陷，精微不能正常输布，清浊不分，反注膀胱，则小便混浊如米泔；中气不足，清阳不升，脏腑组织功能活动减退，则少气乏力，肢体倦怠，声低懒言，头晕目眩，舌淡苔白，脉弱。

failure of lucid yang to rise and hypofunction of viscera and tissues.

Key points for syndrome differentiation: Prolapsing sensation and distension of epigastrium and abdomen, chronic diarrhea, prolapse of anus and dizziness, etc.

### 2.3.3.4 Syndrome of failure of the spleen to govern blood

Syndrome of failure of the spleen to govern blood refers to the syndrome of bleeding due to failure of the spleen to control blood caused by asthenia of the spleen. This syndrome is usually caused by spleen asthenia due to chronic disease, or by overstrain and impairment of the spleen which lead to asthenia of the splenic qi.

Clinical manifestations: Hematemesis, or hematochezia, or hematuria, or hematohidrosis, or epistaxis, or hypermenorrhea and profuse uterine bleeding, accompanied by poor appetite, abdominal distension, loose stool, sallow complexion or lusterless complexion, dispiritedness, lassitude, lack of qi, no desire to speak, pale tongue, thin and weak pulse. Such symptoms are usually seen in various hemorrhagic diseases, such as upper digestive tract bleeding, hematuria, purpura, hematopathy and dysfunctional uterine bleeding.

Analysis of symptoms: Asthenia of splenic qi, failure of the spleen to govern blood and extravasation of blood lead to various bleeding; extravasation of blood in the stomach and intestines leads to hematemesis and hematochezia; extravasation of blood in the bladder leads to hematuria; extravasation of blood in the muscles leads to hematohidrosis; extravasation of blood in the nose leads to epistaxis; weakness of the thoroughfare and conception vessels leads to hypermenorrhea and profuse uterine bleeding; asthenia of splenic qi and failure of the spleen to

辨证要点：本证以脘腹重坠作胀，久泻，脱肛，头晕目眩等脾虚气陷、脏器下垂的表现为诊断依据。

（四）脾不统血证

脾不统血证是指由于脾气虚弱，不能统摄血液，而致以出血为主要表现的证候。本证多由久病脾虚，或劳倦过度，损伤脾气，以致气虚统血失职而形成。

临床表现：呕血，或便血，或尿血，或肌衄，或鼻衄，或妇女月经过多、崩漏等各种出血，并伴见食少，腹胀，便溏，面色萎黄或无华，神疲乏力，少气懒言，舌淡，脉细无力。可见于消化道出血、血尿、紫癜、血液病、功能失调性子宫出血等各种出血性疾病。

证候分析：脾气亏虚，统血无权，血溢脉外，则见各种出血：血溢胃肠则呕血、便血，血溢膀胱则尿血，血溢肌肤则肌衄，血溢鼻窍则鼻衄，冲任不固则妇女月经过多、崩漏等。脾气虚弱，运化失健，则食少，腹胀，便溏；脾虚气血生化乏源，则面色萎黄或无华，神疲乏力，少气懒言。舌淡，

transport and transform lead to poor appetite, abdominal distension and loose stool; asthenia of splenic qi and insufficient production of qi and blood lead to sallow or lusterless complexion, lack of qi and no desire to speak; pale tongue, thin and weak pulse are signs of asthenia of both qi and blood.

Key points for syndrome differentiation: Various bleeding, poor appetite, abdominal distension and loose stool.

### 2.3.3.5 Syndrome of cold and dampness encumbering the spleen

Syndrome of cold and dampness encumbering the spleen refers to the syndrome due to internal exuberance of cold and dampness and stagnancy of gastrosplenic yang. This syndrome is usually caused by improper diet, excessive intake of cold and uncooked food, walking in rain or in water, prolonged living in damp area and frequent internal exuberance of dampness.

Clinical manifestations: Abdominal fullness and oppression, poor appetite, nausea and vomiting, abdominal pain and loose stool, bland taste in the mouth and no thirst, heavy sensation of the head and body, or dropsy of the limbs, scanty urine, or yellow and dull coloration of the body and eyes, or leukorrhagia, bulgy tongue, whitish greasy or whitish slippery fur, slow and weak or sunken and thin pulse. Such symptoms are usually seen in acute gastritis, chronic gastritis, digestive ulceration, chronic enteritis, disturbance of gastrointestinal functions, chronic hepatitis, cirrhosis of liver, stomach cancer and liver cancer, etc.

Analysis of the symptoms: Abdominal fullness and oppression, poor appetite, nausea and vomiting, abdominal pain and loose stool are caused by exuberance of internal cold and dampness which leads to encumbrance of

脉细无力，为脾虚气血双亏的征象。

辨证要点：本证以各种出血与食少，腹胀，便溏等脾气虚弱的表现共见为诊断依据。

（五）寒湿困脾证

寒湿困脾证是指由于寒湿内盛，中阳受困所表现的证候。本证多由饮食不节，过食生冷，淋雨涉水，久居湿处，以及内湿素盛等因素所引起。

临床表现：脘腹痞闷，纳少，恶心呕吐，腹痛便溏，口淡不渴，头身困重，或肢体浮肿、小便短少，或身目发黄、其色晦暗，或妇女白带量多，舌胖，苔白腻或白滑，脉缓弱或沉细。可见于急性胃炎、慢性胃炎、消化性溃疡、慢性肠炎、胃肠功能紊乱，以及慢性肝炎、肝硬化、胃癌、肝癌等。

证候分析：寒湿内盛，中阳被困，脾胃运纳失司，升降失常，则脘腹痞闷，纳少，恶心呕吐，腹痛便溏；寒湿内盛，津

gastrosplenic yang, dysfunction of the spleen and stomach as well as disturbance of descent and ascent; bland taste in the mouth and no thirst are due to internal exuberance of cold and dampness and non-consumption of body fluid; heavy sensation of the head and body, or dropsy of the limbs and scanty urine are due to stagnation of qi and lucid yang by dampness which spreads in the skin and muscles; yellow and dull coloration of the body and eyes is due to extravasation of the bile caused by encumbrance of dampness and cold which affects the functions of the liver; leukorrhagia is caused by downward migration of cold and dampness which impairs the belt vessel; bulgy tongue, whitish greasy or whitish slippery fur, slow and weak or sunken and thin pulse are the signs of internal exuberance of cold and dampness.

Key points for syndrome differentiation: Symptoms due to dysfunction of the stomach and spleen, such as abdominal fullness and oppression, poor appetite, nausea and vomiting, abdominal pain and loose stool; symptoms of internal exuberant cold and dampness, such as heavy sensation of the head and body, or dropsy of the limbs, yellow and dull coloration of the body and eyes, etc.

### 2.3.3.6 Syndrome of damp heat encumbering the spleen

Syndrome of damp heat encumbering the spleen refers to the syndrome caused by dysfunction of the spleen and stomach due to retention of damp heat in the middle energizer. This syndrome usually results from attack of damp heat or endogenous production of heat due to excessive intake of pungent and greasy food as well as alcohol and cheese.

Clinical manifestations: Fullness and oppression in the epigastrium and abdomen, anorexia, vomiting, nausea, thirst with oligodipsia, loose stool, unsmooth defecation,

液未伤，则口淡不渴；水湿困遏气机，阻遏清阳，泛溢肌肤，则头身困重，肢体浮肿，小便短少；寒湿困阻，肝胆疏泄失职，胆汁外溢，则面目肌肤黄而晦暗；寒湿下注，带脉失约，则妇女白带量多。舌胖，苔白滑或白腻，脉缓弱或沉细，为寒湿内盛的表现。

辨证要点：本证以脘腹痞闷，纳呆，恶心呕吐，便溏等胃脾受纳运化功能障碍与头身困重，或肢体浮肿，或身目发黄，其色晦暗等寒湿内盛的表现并见为诊断依据。

### （六）湿热蕴脾证

湿热蕴脾证是指由于湿热内蕴中焦，脾胃运纳功能失职所表现的证候。本证多由于感受湿热之邪，或过食辛辣、肥甘、酒酪，酿湿生热所致。

临床表现：脘腹痞闷，纳呆呕恶，渴不多饮，大便溏泄不爽，小便短黄，肢体困重，身

scanty and yellow urine, heaviness of limbs, dull fever, failure to relieve fever after sweating, or yellow coloration of the skin and eyes, or pruritus of the skin, reddish tongue, yellowish and greasy tongue coating as well as soft pulse. Such manifestations are usually seen in acute gastritis, chronic gastritis, acute enteritis, chronic enteritis, indigestive ulceration, viral hepatitis, chronic hepatitis, cirrhosis of liver, gastrocarcinoma and liver cancer as well as some infectious diseases, such as typhoid fever and paratyphoid fever.

Analysis of the symptoms: Fullness and oppression in the epigastrium and abdomen, anorexia, vomiting, nausea, loose stool and unsmooth defecation are caused by dysfunction of the spleen and stomach as well as abnormal changes in ascending and descending due to retention of damp heat in the middle energizer; heaviness of the limbs is caused by stagnancy of qi activity due to encumbrance of dampness; dull fever, failure to relieve fever after sweating, thirst with oligodipsia and scanty-yellowish urine are caused by internal retention of dampness; yellow coloration of the skin and eyes are caused by extravasation of bile due to retention of damp heat in the spleen and stomach that steams the liver and gallbladder; reddish tongue, yellowish greasy tongue fur and soft pulse are the signs of internal retention of damp heat.

Key points for syndrome differentiation: The diagnostic evidences for this syndrome are fullness and oppression in the epigastrium and abdomen, anorexia, vomiting, nausea, loose stool, unsmooth defecation, dull fever, failure to relieve fever after sweating or yellow coloration of the skin and eyes.

## 2.3.4 Syndrome Differentiation of liver disease

Liver disease mainly manifests in the liver proper and

热不扬,汗出热不解,或见身目鲜黄,或皮肤发痒,舌质红,苔黄腻,脉濡数。可见于急性胃炎、慢性胃炎、急性肠炎、慢性肠炎、消化性溃疡、病毒性肝炎、慢性肝炎、肝硬化、胃癌、肝癌等消化系统疾病,以及伤寒、副伤寒等传染病。

证候分析:湿热蕴结中焦,脾胃运纳失司,升降失常,则脘腹痞闷,纳呆呕恶,大便溏泄不爽;湿困气机,则肢体困重;湿遏热伏,郁蒸于内,则身热不扬、汗出热不解,口渴不多饮,小便短黄;湿热蕴结脾胃,薰蒸肝胆,疏泄失职,胆汁外溢,则见身目鲜黄,或皮肤发痒。舌质红,苔黄腻,脉濡数,为湿热内蕴的征象。

辨证要点:本证以脘腹痞闷、纳呆、呕恶、大便溏泄不爽等脾胃运化受纳失职,以及身热不扬、汗出热不解,或身目鲜黄等湿热内蕴表现并见为诊断依据。

## 四、肝病辨证

肝的病变主要反映在肝

its abnormal changes in dispersing as well as in storing blood. The clinical manifestations are depression, or irritability, susceptibility to rage, distending pain in chest, hypochondrium and lower abdomen, dizziness, tremor of limbs, spasm of hands and feet, bitter taste in the mouth and jaundice. Besides, eye disorders and irregular menstruation are usually believed to be caused by disorder of the liver because the liver opens into the eyes and the liver is the essential organ in woman.

The liver disease is either asthenia or sthenia. The asthenia syndrome of liver is often caused by insufficiency of liver yin and liver blood due to malnutrition after prolonged duration of disease, or involvement in the disorder of other organs, or bleeding; sthenia syndrome of liver is usually caused by liver depression and qi stagnation, exuberance of liver fire, hyperactivity of liver yang, damp heat in the liver and gallbladder and retention of cold in the liver vessel due to emotional impairment, transformation of fire from qi stagnation, upward adverse flow of qi and fire, or internal invasion of pathogenic cold, fire and damp heat. If pathogenic fire scorches liver yin and yin asthenia fails to control yang, yang will become hyperactive and transform into wind, therefore leading to endogenous of liver wind.

### 2.3.4.1　Asthenia syndrome of liver blood

Asthenia syndrome of liver blood is the syndrome caused by malnutrition of the liver and the related tissues and organs due to insufficiency of liver blood. This syndrome is usually caused by insufficiency of blood production due to asthenia of the spleen and stomach, or by consumption of blood due to hemorrhage and chronic disease.

Clinical manifestations: Vertigo, dizziness, pale complexion, dry and irritating sensation in the eyes, blurred vision or night blindness, dry and lusterless nails,

脏本身及其主疏泄、主藏血的功能失常方面，临床以精神抑郁或急躁易怒、胸胁少腹胀痛、眩晕、肢体震颤、手足抽搐、口苦、黄疸等为肝病的常见症状。此外，由于肝开窍于目，女子以肝为本，所以目疾、月经不调等病证，亦常归属于肝。

肝的病证有虚实之分。虚证多因久病失养，或它脏病变所累，或失血，致使肝阴、肝血不足；实证多由情志所伤，气郁化火，气火上逆，或寒邪、火邪、湿热之邪内犯，导致肝郁气滞、肝火炽盛、肝阳上亢、肝胆湿热、寒凝肝脉等证。若火灼肝阴，阴虚不能制阳，阳亢失制化风，则致肝风内动。

### （一）肝血虚证

肝血虚证是指由于肝血不足，肝脏与所系组织器官失养所表现的证候。本证多因脾胃虚弱，生血不足，或因失血、久病，耗伤营血所致。

临床表现：头晕目眩，面白无华，两目干涩，视物模糊或夜盲，爪甲干枯不荣，或见

or numbness of limbs, inflexibility of joints, tremor of hands and feet, or scanty and light-coloured menstruation, or even amenorrhea, whitish tongue and thin pulse. Such symptoms are seen in anemia caused by various hemorrhage, dysfunction of blood production and chronic consumptive disease.

Analysis of the symptoms: Dizziness, pale complexion and whitish tongue are caused by insufficiency of blood to nourish the head and face; vertigo, dry and irritating sensation in the eyes, blurred vision or night blindness are caused by insufficiency of liver blood to nourish the eyes; dry and lusterless nails, numbness of limbs, inflexibility of joints and tremor of hands and feet are caused by malnutrition of the nails and tendons and vessels due to blood asthenia; scanty and light-coloured menstruation or even amenorrhea are caused by deficiency of thoroughfare vessel and insufficiency of blood source due to insufficiency of liver blood.

Key points for syndrome differentiation: Malnutrition of head, eyes, nails, tendons and vessels as well as general malnutrition due to blood asthenia.

### 2.3.4.2 Syndrome of liver yin asthenia

Syndrome of liver yin asthenia is the syndrome resulting from failure of yin to control yang due to consumption of liver yin. This syndrome is usually caused by emotional upsets, transformation of fire from qi stagnation and fire scorching liver yin; or by consumption of liver yin in the late stage of febrile disease; or by insufficiency of liver yin due to insufficiency of kidney yin and failure of water to strengthen wood.

Clinical manifestations: Dull scorching pain in the hypochondria, dizziness, dry and irritating sensation in the eyes, hypopsia, feverish sensation over the cheeks, tidal fever and night sweating, feverish sensation over the five centers (palms, soles and chest), reddish cheeks in the afternoon, dry mouth and throat, or tremor of the hands and feet, reddish tongue with scanty fluid as well as taut, thin and rapid pulse. Such symptoms are usually seen in chronic hepatitis, cirrhosis of liver, liver cancer, gallbladder cancer and pancreas cancer as well as various infectious diseases at the late stage.

Analysis of the symptoms: Dull pain in the hypochondria is caused by malnutrition of the liver due to consumption of liver yin; dizziness, dry and irritating sensation in the eyes and hypopsia are caused by failure of insufficiency of liver yin to nourish the head and eyes; feverish sensation of the cheeks and tidal fever in the afternoon, reddish cheeks, night sweating, feverish sensation over the five centers (palms, soles and chest) as well as dry mouth and throat are caused by asthenic fire disturbing inside due to yin asthenia and yang hyperactivity; tremor of hands and feet is caused by malnutrition of tendons and vessels due to asthenia of liver yin; reddish tongue with scanty fluid and taut, thin and rapid pulse are the signs of endogenous heat due to yin asthenia.

Key points for syndrome differentiation: The diagnostic evidences for this syndrome are dull scorching pain in the hypochondria, dizziness, dry and irritating sensation in the eyes, hypopsia, feverish sensation of the cheeks, tidal fever, night sweating, feverish sensation over the five centers (palms, soles and chest) and dry mouth and throat.

### 2.3.4.3 Syndrome of liver qi stagnation

Syndrome of liver qi stagnation refers to the syndrome due to failure of the liver to disperse and stagnation of qi. This syndrome is usually caused by emotional upsets, impairment of the liver due to depression and rage; or by failure of liver qi to act freely and to disperse normally due to retention of pathogenic factors in the liver vessels.

Clinical manifestations: Emotional depression, migratory pain in the chest, hypochondria or lower abdomen, chest oppression, frequent sigh, thin and white tongue fur as well as taut pulse; or sensation of foreign body in the throat, or goiter and scrofula, or lump in the hypochondria; distending pain of breast, dysmenorrhea, irregular menstruation and even amenorrhea in woman. Such symptoms are usually seen in neurasthenia, depression, throat-esophagus neurosis, hyperthyroidism, simple thyroid enlargement, chronic hepatitis and climacteric syndrome, etc.

Analysis of the symptoms: Depression and frequent sigh are due to stagnation of liver qi and dysfunction of liver dispersion; migratory distending pain in the chest, hypochondria, breast and lower abdomen is caused by liver depression, qi stagnation and inhibited flow of meridian qi; sensation of foreign body in the throat, or goiter, scrofula and hypochondriac lump are caused by retention of phlegm transformed from qi stagnation in the throat, neck and hypochondria; irregular menstruation, dysmenorrhea, or even amenorrhea are caused by liver depression, qi stagnation and inhibited circulation of blood because the liver is fundamental in woman; thin and whitish tongue fur and taut pulse are the signs of the liver that fails to act freely and disperse normally.

Key points for syndrome differentiation: Emotional depression, migratory distending pain in the chest, hypochondria, breast and lower abdomen as well as irregular menstruation.

### 2.3.4.4 Syndrome of liver fire hyperactivity

Syndrome of liver fire hyperactivity refers to the syndrome due to exuberant fire in the liver meridian and 常而形成。

临床表现：情志抑郁,胸胁或少腹胀满窜痛,胸闷,善太息,舌苔薄白,脉弦。或见咽部异物感,或见瘿瘤瘰疬,或见胁下肿块；妇女可见乳房胀痛,痛经,月经不调,甚则经闭。可见于神经衰弱、抑郁症、咽喉—食管神经官能症、甲状腺功能亢进症、单纯性甲状腺肿、慢性肝炎、更年期综合征等。

证候分析：肝气郁结,疏泄失常,则情志抑郁,胸闷善太息；肝郁气滞,经气不利,故胸胁、乳房、少腹胀满窜痛；气郁生痰,痰气搏结于咽喉、颈项、胁下,故咽部有异物感,或见瘿瘤、瘰疬、胁下肿块；女子以肝为本,肝郁气滞,血行不畅,冲任失调,则月经不调、痛经,甚则闭经。舌苔薄白,脉弦,为肝失条达,疏泄失职的征象。

辨证要点：本证以情志抑郁,胸胁、乳房、少腹胀满窜痛,妇女月经不调等肝失疏泄的表现为诊断依据。

### （四）肝火上炎证

肝火上炎证是指由于肝经火盛,气火上逆,而表现以

upward adverse rising of fire. This syndrome is mainly caused by emotional upsets and transformation of fire from liver depression; or by exogenous pathogenic heat and fire; or by exuberant fire in the other organs that involves the liver.

Clinical manifestations: Dizziness, distending headache, flushed face and red eyes, bitter taste and dryness of mouth, irritability and susceptibility to rage, tinnitus and deafness, insomnia or nightmare, or scorching pain in the hypochondria, or hematemesis and epistaxis, constipation, scanty and yellow urine, red tongue, yellow fur and taut and rapid pulse. These symptoms are usually seen in hypertension, hyperthyroidism, neurasthenia, manic depression, migraine, cerebral arteriosclerosis and climacteric syndrome.

Analysis of the symptoms: Dizziness, distending headache, flushed face and red eyes, bitter taste and dryness of mouth are caused by pathogenic heat and fire disturbing the upper part of the body along the liver meridian; insomnia or nightmare is caused by mental distraction due to internal disturbance of heat and fire; irritability and susceptibility to rage are caused by liver depression; scorching pain in the hypochondria is caused by stagnation of qi and fire in the liver meridian; hematemesis and epistaxis with fresh blood are caused by extravasation of blood due to upward adverse rise of qi and fire; constipation, scanty yellowish urine, reddish tongue with yellowish fur and taut and rapid pulse are caused by fire scorching body fluid.

Key points for syndrome differentiation: The diagnostic evidences of this syndrome are irritability and susceptibility to rage, insomnia or nightmare, dizziness, distending headache, flushed cheeks and red eyes, bitter taste and dryness of the mouth and scorching pain in the

火热炽盛于上为特征的证候。本证多由于情志不遂，肝郁化火；或外感火热之邪，或它脏火热炽盛，累及于肝所致。

临床表现：头晕胀痛，面红目赤，口苦口干，急躁易怒，耳鸣耳聋，不寐或恶梦纷纭，或胁肋灼痛，或吐血、衄血，大便秘结，小便短黄，舌质红，苔黄，脉弦数。可见于高血压病、甲状腺功能亢进症、神经衰弱、躁狂抑郁症、偏头痛、脑动脉硬化症、更年期综合征等。

证候分析：火热循肝经上扰，则头晕胀痛，耳鸣耳聋，面红目赤，口苦口干；火热内扰，神魂不安，则致不寐或恶梦纷纭；肝郁不达而失其条达柔顺之性，则急躁易怒；气火壅滞肝脉，则胁肋灼痛；气火上逆，迫血妄行，则吐血衄血，血色鲜红；火灼津伤，则大便秘结，小便短黄，舌质红，苔黄，脉弦数。

辨证要点：本证以急躁易怒，不寐或恶梦纷纭，以及头晕胀痛，面红目赤，口苦口干，胁肋灼痛等头、目、耳、胁等肝经循行部位表现的实火炽盛

hypochondria and sides.

### 2.3.4.5 Syndrome of liver yang hyperactivity

Syndrome of liver yang hyperactivity refers to the syndrome marked by upper sthenia and lower asthenia due to consumption of liver and kidney yin, failure of yin to control yang and hyperactivity of liver yang. This syndrome is usually caused by impairment due to excessive rage, transformation of fire from qi stagnation and consumption of liver and kidney yin by fire and heat; or by excessive sexual intercourse that exhausts kidney yin; or by consumption of kidney yin due to senility and failure of water to nourish wood which lead to failure of yin to control yang and hyperactivity of liver yang.

Clinical manifestations: Distending headache, dizziness, tinnitus, flushed cheeks and red eyes, irritability and susceptibility to rage, insomnia and dreaminess, aching pain and weakness of loins and knees, top-heaviness, reddish tongue with scanty fluid, taut pulse or taut and thin pulse. Such symptoms are usually seen in hypertension, cerebral arteriosclerosis, Parkinson's disease, hyperthyroidism, neurasthenia, manic depression, migraine and climacteric syndrome, etc.

Analysis of the symptoms: Distending headache, dizziness, tinnitus, flushed cheeks and red eyes, irritability and susceptibility to rage, insomnia and dreaminess are caused by failure of liver and kidney yin to control liver yang and hyperactivity of liver yang due to consumption of liver and kidney yin; aching and weakness of loins and knees are caused by malnutrition of tendons and bones due to asthenia of liver and kidney yin; top-heaviness is caused by hyperactivity of liver yang and consumption of liver and kidney yin; reddish tongue with scanty fluid, taut pulse or taut and thin pulse are the signs of asthenia of liver and kidney yin and hyperactivity of liver yang.

症状为诊断依据。

### （五）肝阳上亢证

肝阳上亢证是指由于肝肾阴亏，阴不制阳，肝阳亢扰于上所表现的上实下虚的证候。本证多由于恼怒所伤，气郁化火，火热耗伤肝肾之阴；或房劳所伤，耗劫肾阴；或年老肾阴亏虚，水不涵木，乃致阴不制阳，肝阳上亢而形成。

临床表现：头目胀痛，眩晕耳鸣，面红目赤，急躁易怒，失眠多梦，腰膝酸软，头重脚轻，舌红少津，脉弦或弦细数。可见于高血压病、脑动脉硬化症、帕金森病、甲状腺功能亢进症、神经衰弱症、躁狂症、偏头痛、更年期综合征等。

证候分析：肝肾阴亏，不能制约肝阳，肝阳亢逆升腾于上，故头目胀痛，眩晕耳鸣，面红目赤，急躁易怒，失眠多梦；肝肾阴虚，筋骨失养，故腰膝酸软；肝阳亢于上，肝肾之阴亏于下，故头重脚轻。舌红少津，脉弦或弦细数，为肝肾阴虚阳亢的征象。

Key points for syndrome differentiation: Dizziness, distending headache, tinnitus, flushed cheeks and red eyes as well as top-heaviness and aching and weakness of loins and knees.

#### 2.3.4.6 Syndrome of endogenous liver wind

Syndrome of endogenous liver wind is the syndrome marked by dizziness, convulsion and tremor. According to the causes, this syndrome is clinically further divided into syndrome of liver yang transforming into wind, syndrome of extreme heat generating wind, syndrome of yin asthenia disturbing wind and syndrome of blood asthenia generating wind.

##### 2.3.4.6.1 Syndrome of liver yang transforming into wind

Syndrome of liver yang transforming into wind refers to wind syndrome due to consumption of liver and kidney yin and hyperactivity of liver yang. This syndrome is usually caused by emotional upsets and qi stagnation transforming into fire and consuming yin; or by constant asthenia of liver and kidney yin, failure of yin to control yang and hyperactivity of liver yang which transforms into wind, therefore leading to the wind syndrome marked by root asthenia and branch sthenia as well as exuberance in the upper and deficiency in the lower.

Clinical manifestations: Dizziness, shaking head, headache, neck stiffness, tremor of limbs, stuttering, numbness of hands and feet, abnormal gait, red tongue with white or greasy fur, powerful pulse, even sudden coma, facial distortion, hemiplegia, aphasia and sputum rale in the throat. Such symptoms are usually seen in hypertension, cerebral arteriosclerosis, cerebral infarction, cerebral hemorrhage, cerebrovascular accident sequela, Parkinson's disease, epilepsy and injury of spinal cord,

辨证要点：本证以头目胀痛、眩晕耳鸣、面红目赤等肝阳亢于上，与头重脚轻、腰膝酸软等肝肾之阴亏于下的表现共见为诊断依据。

（六）肝风内动证

肝风内动证泛指患者出现眩晕欲仆、抽搐、震颤等具有"动摇"特点为主症的一类证候。根据病因病性的不同，临床常见有肝阳化风、热极生风、阴虚动风和血虚生风等不同证候。

1. 肝阳化风证

肝阳化风证是指由于肝肾阴亏，肝阳亢逆无制所导致的动风证候。本证多由于情志不遂，气郁化火伤阴；或素体肝肾阴亏，阴不制阳，肝阳上亢，阳亢无制而化风，从而形成本虚标实、上盛下虚的动风之证。

临床表现：眩晕欲仆，头摇，头痛，项强，肢体震颤，语言謇涩，手足麻木，步履不正，舌红，苔白或腻，脉弦有力。甚或突然昏倒，不省人事，口眼歪斜，半身不遂，舌强不语，喉中痰鸣。可见于高血压病、脑动脉硬化症、脑梗死、脑出血、脑血管意外后遗症、帕金

Analysis of the symptoms: Dizziness, shaking head and headache are caused by hyperactive liver yang transforming into wind and disturbing the upper part of the body; neck stiffness and tremor of limbs are caused by endogenous liver wind and spasm of tendons and vessels; stuttering is caused by wind and yang rising up to disturb the tongue collaterals; numbness of hands and feet is caused by malnutrition of the tendons and vessels due to consumption of liver and kidney yin; abnormal gait is caused by hyperactivity of liver yang and consumption of liver and kidney yin; red tongue with white or greasy fur and powerful pulse are the signs of consumption of yin and hyperactivity of yang; sudden coma, and sputum rale in the throat are caused by abrupt rise of liver wind and yang, disturbance of qi and blood as well as blockage of the upper orifices by liver wind mingled with phlegm; facial distortion, hemiplegia, stiff tongue and aphasia are caused by wandering of liver wind and phlegm in the meridians.

Key points for syndrome differentiation: This syndrome is marked by frequent dizziness and hyperactivity of liver yang as well as sudden severe vertigo, headache, stiff neck, tremor of limbs, stuttering, numbness of hands and feet, even sudden coma and hemiplegia.

### 2.3.4.6.2 Syndrome of extreme heat generating wind

Syndrome of extreme heat generating wind refers to the syndrome due to exuberant pathogenic heat scorching tendons and vessels. This syndrome is usually seen in exogenous febrile disease in which exuberant pathogenic heat scorching the heart and liver meridians, leading to spasm of tendons and vessels and resulting in endogenous

森病、癫痫、脊髓损伤等。

证候分析：肝阳亢逆无制而化风，风阳上扰，则眩晕欲仆，头摇，头痛；肝风内动，筋脉挛急，则项强，肢体震颤；风阳窜扰舌络，则语言謇涩；肝肾阴亏，筋脉失养，故手足麻木；风阳亢于上，阴亏于下，上盛下虚，故步履不正，行走飘浮。舌红，脉弦有力，为阴亏阳亢的征象。若风阳暴升，气血逆乱，肝风挟痰蒙蔽清窍，则突然昏倒，不省人事，喉中痰鸣；风痰流窜经络，则见口眼歪斜，半身不遂，舌强不语。

辨证要点：本证以平素即有头晕目眩等肝阳上亢的症状，突见眩晕欲仆、头痛、项强、肢体震颤、语言謇涩、手足麻木等动风的表现，甚或卒然昏倒、半身不遂为诊断依据。

### 2. 热极生风证

热极生风证是指由于邪热炽盛，燔灼筋脉所表现的动风证候。本证多见于外感温热病，因邪热亢盛，燔灼心肝二经，筋脉挛急，而致肝风内动。

liver wind.

Clinical manifestations: Continuous high fever, restlessness, spasm of hands and feet, stiff necks, upward staring of eyes, even episthotonos, lackjaw, unconsciousness, deep reddish tongue, yellowish dry fur and taut and rapid pulse. Such symptoms are usually seen in epidemic encephalitis B, epidemic cerebrospinal meningitis, brain abscess, tuberculous encephalitis, epidemic hemorrhagic fever, scarlet fever and puerperal infection.

Analysis of the symptoms: Stiff necks, upward staring of eyes or even episthotonos are caused by exuberant pathogenic heat scorching tendons and vessels and causing liver wind; high fever, restlessness and unconsciousness are caused by invasion of heat into the pericardium and disturbance of the brain; deep reddish tongue, yellowish dry fur and taut and rapid pulse are the signs of exuberant heat consuming body fluid.

Key points for syndrome differentiation: This syndrome is marked by high fever and restlessness accompanied by spasm of the limbs, stiff neck and episthotonos which signify internal stirring of liver wind.

### 2.3.4.6.3 Syndrome of endogenous wind due to yin asthenia

Syndrome of endogenous wind due to yin asthenia refers to the syndrome due to consumption of yin fluid and malnutrition of tendons and vessels. This syndrome is usually caused by consumption of yin fluid at the advanced stage of exogenous febrile disease; or by consumption of yin fluid due to internal impairment and chronic disease which lead to malnutrition of tendons and vessels and endogenous asthenia wind.

Clinical manifestations: Tremor or flaccidity of hands and feet, dizziness and tinnitus, tidal fever in the afternoon

临床表现：高热不退，烦躁不安，手足抽搐，颈项强直，两目上视，甚则角弓反张，牙关紧闭，神志昏迷，舌红绛，苔黄燥，脉弦数。可见于流行性乙型脑炎、流行性脑脊髓膜炎、脑脓疡、结核性脑膜炎、流行性出血热、猩红热、产褥感染等感染性疾病。

证候分析：邪热亢盛，燔灼筋脉，引动肝风，故见手足抽搐，颈项强直，两目上视，甚则角弓反张，牙关紧闭；热陷心包，神明被扰，则高热烦躁，甚则神志昏迷。舌红绛，苔黄燥，脉弦数，为热炽伤津的征象。

辨证要点：本证以高热，烦躁不安，兼见四肢抽搐、颈项强直、角弓反张等肝风内动症状为诊断依据。

### 3. 阴虚动风证

阴虚动风证是指由于阴液亏虚，筋脉失养所表现的动风证候。本证多由于外感热病后期，阴液耗损；或内伤久病，阴液亏虚，致使筋脉失养，虚风内动。

临床表现：手足蠕动，或瘈疭，眩晕耳鸣，午后或入夜

or in the evening, feverish sensation over the five centers (palms, soles and chest) or bone-steaming fever, flushed cheeks, emaciation, dry mouth and throat, red tongue with scanty fluid and thin and rapid pulse. Such symptoms are usually seen at the advanced stage of some infectious diseases, such as epidemic encephalitis B, epidemic cerebrospinal meningitis and scarlet fever as well as at the advanced stage of some chronic and consumptive diseases, such as hematopathy and malignant tumor.

Analysis of the symptoms: Tremor or flaccidity of hands and feet is caused by malnutrition of tendons and vessels and endogenous asthenia wind due to consumption of liver and kidney yin fluid; dizziness and tinnitus are caused by malnutrition of ears and eyes due to asthenia of liver and kidney yin; emaciation, dry mouth and throat are caused by failure of asthenic yin fluid to nourish the body; tidal fever in the afternoon or in the evening, feverish sensation over the five centers (palms, soles and chest) or bone-steaming fever, flushed cheeks, red tongue with scanty fluid and thin and rapid pulse are caused by yin asthenia, yang hyperactivity and upward flaming of asthenic fire.

Key points for syndrome differentiation: This syndrome is marked by tremor of hands and feet accompanied by tidal fever in the afternoon or in the evening, feverish sensation over the five centers or bone-steaming fever.

### 2.3.4.6.4 Syndrome of blood asthenia generating wind

Syndrome of blood asthenia generating wind refers to the syndrome due to consumption of blood and malnutrition of tendons and vessels. This syndrome is usually caused by blood asthenia due to chronic disease, acute or chronic hemorrhage which leads to asthenia of blood, mal-

潮热,五心烦热或骨蒸劳热,颧红,形体消瘦,口燥咽干,舌红少津,脉细数。可见于流行性乙型脑炎、流行性脑脊髓膜炎、猩红热等感染性疾病的后期,以及血液病、恶性肿瘤等慢性消耗性疾病的后期。

证候分析:肝肾阴液亏虚,筋脉失养,虚风内动,则见手足蠕动,或瘛疭;肝肾阴虚,耳目失养,故眩晕耳鸣;阴液亏虚,不能滋养濡润形体,则形体消瘦,口燥咽干;阴虚阳亢,虚火上炎,则午后或入夜潮热,五心烦热或骨蒸劳热,颧红,舌红少津,脉细数。

辨证要点:本证以手足蠕动等虚风内动,兼有午后或入夜潮热、五心烦热或骨蒸劳热等阴虚内热的表现为诊断依据。

### 4. 血虚生风证

血虚生风证是指由于血液亏虚,筋脉失养所表现的动风证候。本证多由于久病血虚,或急、慢性失血,致使营血亏虚,筋脉失养,虚风内动。

nutrition of tendons and vessels as well as endogenous wind.

Clinical manifestations: Tremor of hands and feet, fascicular twitching, numbness of limbs, dizziness, tinnitus, pale complexion, light coloured nails, whitish tongue and thin and weak pulse.

Analysis of the symptoms: Tremor of hands and feet, fascicular twitching and numbness of limbs are caused by consumption of blood, malnutrition of tendons and vessels and endogenous asthenia wind; dizziness and tinnitus are caused by failure of blood asthenia to nourish the head; pale complexion, light coloured nails, whitish tongue and thin and weak pulse are caused by failure of blood asthenia to nourish the body.

Key points for syndrome differentiation: This syndrome is marked by tremor of hands and feet, fascicular twitching, numbness of limbs and accompanied manifestations of blood asthenia.

### 2.3.4.7 Syndrome of cold stagnation in the liver meridian

Syndrome of cold stagnation in the liver meridian refers to the syndrome due to cold pain in the distributing region of liver meridian caused by stagnation of pathogenic cold in the liver vessels. This syndrome is usually caused by pathogenic cold attack, stagnation of qi and blood in the liver meridian, inhibited circulation of qi and blood as well as spasm of meridians and vessels.

Clinical manifestations: Lower abdominal cold pain, sagging distension and pain of the pudendum, or contraction and pain of scrotum, aggravation with cold and alleviation with warmth, or cold pain in the vertex, cold limbs and body, light coloured tongue with whitish and moist fur, sinking and tense pulse or taut and tense pulse. Such symptoms are usually seen in hernia, orchitis, varicocele

临床表现：手足震颤，肌肉瞤动，肢体麻木，眩晕耳鸣，面白无华，爪甲淡白，舌质淡白，脉细弱。

证候分析：营血亏虚，筋脉失养，虚风内动，则手足震颤，肌肉瞤动，肢体麻木；血虚不能上荣头目，则眩晕耳鸣，营血亏虚，不能滋养荣润形体，故见面白无华，爪甲淡白，舌质淡白，脉细弱。

辨证要点：本证以手足震颤，肌肉瞤动，肢体麻木，兼有血虚不荣的表现为诊断依据。

### （七）寒凝肝脉证

寒凝肝脉证是指由于寒邪侵袭，凝滞肝脉，表现以肝经循行部位冷痛为主症的证候。本证多由于寒邪侵袭，肝经气血凝滞，运行不畅，经脉挛急所致。

临床表现：少腹冷痛，阴部坠胀作痛，或阴囊收缩引痛，遇寒加甚，得温则减，或见巅顶冷痛，形寒肢冷，舌淡苔白润，脉象沉紧或弦紧。可见于疝气、睾丸炎、精索静脉曲张、偏头痛等。

and migraine, etc.

Analysis of the symptoms: Lower abdominal cold pain, sagging distension and pain of the pudendum, or cold pain in the vertex, or contraction and pain of scrotum, aggravation with cold and alleviation with warmth are caused by contraction and stagnancy of cold, cold attack on the liver meridian, spasm of meridians and vessels as well as stagnation of qi and blood; cold limbs and body is caused by pathogenic cold attack on the body and stagnation of yangqi from developing outwards; light coloured tongue with whitish and moist fur, sinking and tense pulse or taut and tense pulse are the signs of internal exuberance of yin cold.

Key points for syndrome differentiation: This syndrome is marked by cold pain in the lower abdomen, pudendum and vertex as well as cold limbs and body.

### 2.3.5 Syndrome differentiation of kidney disease

Kidney disease mainly reflects morbid changes in the physiological functions of the kidney proper and its functions, such as storing essence, management of growth and reproduction, governing water and bones, producing marrow and blood, controlling the reception of qi as well as nourishing and warming viscera. Clinically kidney disease is marked by aching and weakness or pain in the loins and knees, tinnitus and deafness, loss of hair and shaking of teeth, impotence and seminal emission, oligospermia and sterility, oligomenorrhea in woman, clear and profuse urine, enuresis, incontinence of urine or oliguria and edema, early morning diarrhea, dyspnea and more exhalation and less inhalation.

Kidney disease is usually of asthenia nature and frequently caused by constitutional asthenia, or insufficiency of essence during childhood, or consumption of essence in

主证分析：寒性收引凝滞，寒袭肝脉，致使经脉挛急，气血凝滞，故见少腹冷痛，阴部坠胀作痛，或阴囊收缩引痛，或见巅顶冷痛，遇寒加甚，得温则减；寒邪外袭，阳气被遏不能外达，故形寒肢冷。舌淡苔白润，脉象沉紧或弦紧，为阴寒内盛的征象。

辨证要点：本证以少腹、阴部、巅顶冷痛，形寒肢冷等为诊断依据。

### 五、肾病辨证

肾的病变，主要反映在肾脏本身和肾藏精、主生殖生长发育、主水、主骨生髓化血、主纳气、濡养温煦脏腑等生理功能失常方面，临床以腰膝酸软或痛、耳鸣耳聋、发脱齿摇、阳痿、遗精、精少不育、女子经少、经闭不孕、小便清长、遗尿、尿失禁，或尿少身肿，五更泄泻，喘息、呼多吸少等为常见症状。

肾病多虚证。多因禀赋不足，或幼年精气未充，或老年精气亏损，或房事不节，或

the aged, or intemperance of sexual life, or involvement of the kidney in the disorders of other viscera, which lead to asthenia or deficiency of yin, yang, essence and qi.

### 2.3.5.1 Syndrome of kidney yang asthenia

Syndrome of kidney yang asthenia refers to the asthenia cold symptoms due to failure of qi to transform resulting from decline of kidney yang and its failure in nourishing the body. This syndrome is usually caused by constitutional asthenia of yang, or decline of Mingmen fire in the aged, or impairment of kidney yang due to chronic disease, or involvement of the kidney in the disorders of the other visceral yang, or intemperance of sexual life and consumption of kidney yang.

Clinical manifestations: Aching and cold sensation in the loins and knees, cold limbs and body, dispiritedness and lassitude, impotence, immature ejaculation, cold sperm, infertility due to cold in the uterus, sexual hypoesthesia, or loose stool, early morning diarrhea, or frequent micturition, clear and profuse urine, profuse noctural urine, bright whitish or blackish complexion and light coloured tongue with white fur as well as sinking, deep and weak (especially over chi region) pulse. These symptoms are usually seen in hypothyroidism, hypoadrenocorticism, hypogonadism and chronic nephritis, etc.

Analysis of the symptoms: Aching and cold sensation in the loins and knees, cold limbs and body, dispiritedness and lassitude are caused by asthenia of kidney yang and its failure in nourishing the body; bright whitish or blackish complexion is caused by asthenia and weakness of the kidney to warm and transport qi and blood, leading to internal exuberance of yin cold; impotence, immature ejaculation, cold sperm, infertility due to cold in the uterus, sexual hypoesthesia are caused by asthenia of kidney yang and Mingmen fire as well as decline in reproduction;

其他脏腑虚损累及于肾，导致肾的阴、阳、精、气亏损。

### （一）肾阳虚证

肾阳虚证是指由于肾阳虚衰，温煦失职，气化失权所表现的虚寒证候。本证多由于素体阳虚，或年高命门火衰，或久病损伤肾阳，或它脏阳虚累及于肾，或房事太过，耗损肾阳所致。

临床表现：腰膝酸冷，形寒肢冷，神疲乏力，男子阳痿、早泄、精冷，女子宫寒不孕，性欲减退，或见大便稀溏，五更泄泻，或小便频数，清长，夜尿多，面色㿠白或黧黑，舌淡苔白，脉沉细无力，尺部尤甚。可见于甲状腺功能减退症、肾上腺皮质功能减退症、性腺功能低下症、慢性肾炎等。

证候分析：肾阳虚，温煦失职，形体失于温养，则膝腰酸冷，形寒肢冷，神疲乏力；阳虚愈，无力温运气血，阴寒内盛，则面色㿠白或黧黑；肾阳虚命门火衰，生殖功能衰退，则男子阳痿、早泄、精冷、女子宫寒不孕；肾阳不足，温运气化无权，则小便频数清长，夜尿多；命门火衰，火不暖

frequent micturition, clear and profuse urine and profuse noctural urine are caused by insufficiency of kidney yang and its failure in warming and transporting qi; loose stool and early morning diarrhea are caused by decline of Mingmen fire and failure of fire to warm earth; light coloured tongue with white fur as well as sinking, deep and weak (especially over chi region) pulse are the signs of insufficiency of kidney yang.

Key points for syndrome differentiation: This syndrome is marked by decline in reproduction accompanied by cold limbs and body as well as aching and cold in the loins and knees.

### 2.3.5.2 Syndrome of edema due to kidney asthenia

Syndrome of edema due to kidney asthenia refers to the symptoms of edema due to kidney yang asthenia and its failure in transforming qi. This syndrome is usually caused by dysfunction due to chronic disease and consumption of kidney yang, or by constitutional asthenia and decline of kidney yang which lead to retention of fluid and cutaneous edema.

Clinical manifestations: Anasarca (especially the region below the waist) rebounding after pressure with fingers, oliguria, aching cold in the loins and knees, aversion to cold and cold limbs, abdominal distension and fullness, or palpitation and shortness of breath, or cough, dyspnea and sputum rale, light-coloured and bulgy tongue, whitish slippery tongue fur, sinking, slow and weak pulse. Such symptoms are seen in chronic nephritis, IgA nephropathy, diabetic nephropathy and lupus nephritis as well as various acute and chronic failure of kidney.

Analysis of the symptoms: Anasarca (especially the region below the waist) rebounding after pressure with fingers and oliguria are caused by insufficiency of kidney

土,则大便稀溏,或五更泄泻。舌淡苔白,脉沉细无力,尺脉尤甚,为肾阳不足的征象。

辨证要点:本证以生殖功能减退,并见形寒肢冷、腰膝酸冷等全身虚寒的表现为诊断依据。

(二) 肾虚水泛证

肾虚水泛证是指由于肾阳亏虚,气化失权,水湿泛滥所表现的证候。本证多由于久病失调,耗损肾阳;或素体虚弱,肾阳虚衰,致使水湿停聚,泛溢肌肤而形成。

临床表现:身体浮肿,腰以下尤甚,按之没指,小便短少,腰膝酸冷,畏寒肢冷,腹部胀满,或见心悸气短,或咳喘痰鸣,舌质淡胖,苔白滑,脉沉迟无力。可见于慢性肾炎、IgA肾病、糖尿病肾病、狼疮性肾炎等,以及各种疾病引起的急、慢性肾功能衰竭。

证候分析:肾主水,肾阳不足,气化失权,水湿内停,泛溢肌肤,则小便短少,身体浮

yang and its failure in transforming qi which lead to retention of fluid and edema; abdominal distension and fullness are caused by retention of fluid due to yang asthenia and inhibited activity; palpitation and shortness of breath are caused by fluid attacking the heart and stagnating heart yang; dyspnea and sputum rale are caused by retention of fluid attacking the lung and failure of the pulmonary qi to disperse and descend; aching cold in the loins and knees, aversion to cold and cold limbs are caused by asthenia of kidney yang and its failure in warming the body as well as internal exuberance of yin cold; light-coloured and bulgy tongue, whitish slippery tongue fur, sinking, slow and weak pulse are the signs of consumption of kidney yang and internal retention of fluid.

Key points for syndrome differentiation: This syndrome is marked by edema (especially over the region below the waist), oliguria, aching and cold sensation in the loins and knees as well as cold limbs and body.

### 2.3.5.3　Syndrome of kidney yin asthenia

Syndrome of kidney yin asthenia refers to the symptoms of endogenous asthenic heat due to consumption of kidney yin and insufficiency of nourishment. This syndrome is usually caused by consumption of kidney yin due to asthenic overstrain and chronic disease; or by consumption of kidney yin at the advanced stage of seasonal febrile disease; or by intemperance of sexual life and hypersexuality which exhausts yin.

Clinical manifestations: Aching and weakness of the loins and knees, dizziness and tinnitus, insomnia and amnesia, seminal emission, scanty menstruation or amenorrhea, or metrorrhagia and metrostaxis, flushed cheeks in the afternoon, bone-steaming tidal fever, night sweating, dry mouth and throat, emaciation, yellowish and scanty urine, reddish tongue with scanty fur and thin and rapid

肿，腰以下肿甚，按之没指；阳虚水停，气机不畅，则腹部胀满；水气凌心，抑遏心阳，则心悸气短；水饮上逆犯肺，肺失宣降，则咳喘痰鸣；肾阳虚衰，温煦失职，阴寒内盛，故畏寒肢冷，腰膝酸冷。舌淡胖，苔白滑，脉沉迟而弱，为肾阳亏虚，水湿内停的征象。

辨证要点：本证以水肿、腰以下为甚，小便短少，以及腰膝酸冷、畏寒肢冷等虚寒的表现为诊断依据。

### （三）肾阴虚证

肾阴虚证是指由于肾阴亏损，失于滋养，虚热内生所表现的证候。本证多由于虚劳久病，耗损肾阴；或温热病后期，消灼肾阴；以及房事不节，情欲妄动，阴枯内损所致。

临床表现：腰膝酸软，眩晕耳鸣，失眠健忘，男子遗精，女子经少或经闭，或见崩漏，午后颧红，骨蒸潮热，盗汗，口燥咽干，形体消瘦，小便黄少，舌红少苔，脉细数。可见于结核、肿瘤等慢性消耗性疾病，

pulse. Such symptoms are seen in some consumptive diseases (such as tuberculosis and tumor), sexual disorder and at the rehabilitative stage of some infectious diseases.

Analysis of the symptoms: Aching and pain in the loins and knees, dizziness and tinnitus as well as amnesia are caused by consumption of kidney yin and malnutrition of cerebral marrow, orifices and bones; seminal emission is caused by yin asthenia and fire exuberance, asthenic fire disturbing sperm house; scanty menstruation and amenorrhea are caused by consumption of blood and insufficiency of blood in the thoroughfare and conception vessels; metrorrhagia and metrostaxis are caused by extravasation of blood due to asthenic fire; restlessness, fever and insomnia are caused by asthenic fire disturbing mind; emaciation, bone-steaming tidal fever, flushed cheeks and night sweating, dry mouth and throat as well as yellow and scanty urine are caused by insufficiency of kidney yin, lack of moistening and nourishment as well as fumigation of asthenic fire; reddish tongue with scanty fur or without fur and thin and rapid pulse are the signs of yin asthenia and endogenous heat.

Key points for syndrome differentiation: This syndrome is marked by aching and pain of the loins and knees, dizziness and tinnitus, seminal emission and irregular menstruation accompanied by yin asthenia and endogenous heat.

### 2.3.5.4 Syndrome of kidney essence insufficiency

Syndrome of kidney essence insufficiency refers to the symptoms of retard growth, decline in reproduction and senilism due to consumption of kidney essence. This syndrome is mainly caused by congenital defect, postnatal malnutrition and insufficiency of primordial qi; or by impairment due to chronic disease, intemperance of sexual

性功能障碍,以及多种感染性疾病的恢复阶段。

证候分析:肾阴亏虚,脑髓、官窍、骨骼失养,则腰膝酸痛,眩晕耳鸣,健忘;阴虚火旺,虚火扰动精室,精关不固,则遗精;阴血亏损,冲任失充,则女子月经量少,经闭;虚火迫血妄行则崩漏;虚火上扰心神,则烦热少寐;肾阴不足,失于滋润,虚火蕴蒸,则形体消瘦,骨蒸潮热,颧红盗汗,口燥咽干,小便黄少。舌红少苔或无苔,脉细数,为阴虚内热的征象。

辨证要点:本证以腰膝酸痛、眩晕耳鸣、男子遗精、女子月经不调等,兼有阴虚内热的表现为诊断依据。

### (四)肾精不足证

肾精不足证是指由于肾精亏损,表现以生长发育迟缓、生殖功能低下、早衰为主症的证候。本证多由于先天禀赋不足,后天失养,元气不充;或久病劳损,房事不节,耗

life and consumption of kidney essence.

Clinical manifestations: Infantile retardation of growth and closure of fontanel, flaccidity of skeleton, retardation of body growth, slowness in action and feeble-mindedness; senilism in adults, aching and weakness of loins and knees, dizziness, tinnitus and deafness, loss of hair and looseness of teeth, flaccidity of feet, amnesia and dull facial expression; sterility due to oligospermia in man, infertility due to amenorrhea in woman and sexual hypoesthesia. Such symptoms are usually seen in infantile malnutrition, rickets, retardation of intelligence, senile dementia, sexual underdevelopment, hypogonadism, sterility in man and infertility in woman.

Analysis of the symptoms: Infantile retardation of growth and closure of fontanel, flaccidity of skeleton, retardation of body growth, slowness in action and feeble-mindedness are caused by asthenia of kidney and its failure in transforming qi and blood as well as malnutrition of the brain and body; senilism in adults, aching and weakness of loins and knees, dizziness, tinnitus and deafness, loss of hair and looseness of teeth, flaccidity of feet, amnesia and dull facial expression are caused by asthenia of kidney essence that fails to control bones and nourish the brain, teeth, hair and spirit; sterility due to oligospermia in man, infertility due to amenorrhea in woman and sexual hypoesthesia are caused by asthenia of kidney essence and insufficiency of the reproductive source.

Key points for syndrome differentiation: This syndrome is marked by retardation of body development in infants, hypogonadism and senilism in adults.

### 2.3.5.5 Syndrome of kidney qi weakness

Syndrome of kidney qi weakness refers to the symptoms due to asthenia of kidney qi and its failure in storage and consolidation. This syndrome is usually caused by

伤肾精所致。

临床表现：小儿生长发育迟缓，囟门迟闭，骨骼痿软，身体矮小，动作迟缓，智力低下；成人早衰，腰膝酸软，眩晕，耳鸣耳聋，发脱齿摇，两足痿软，健忘恍惚，神情呆钝；男子精少不育，女子经闭不孕，性功能低下。可见于小儿营养不良、佝偻病、智能迟缓、老年痴呆、性发育不全、性腺功能低下、不育症、不孕症等。

证候分析：肾精不足，不能化生气血，脑髓、形体失于充养，则小儿生长发育迟缓，囟门迟闭，骨骼痿软，身体矮小，动作迟缓，智力低下。肾精亏虚，不能主骨、充脑、固齿、华发、养神，则成人早衰，腰膝酸软，眩晕，耳鸣耳聋，发脱齿摇，两足痿软，健忘恍惚，神情呆钝。肾精亏虚，生殖无源，则男子精少不育，女子经闭不孕，性功能低下。

辨证要点：本证以小儿发育迟缓、成人生殖功能低下、早衰为诊断依据。

### （五）肾气不固证

肾气不固证是指由于肾气亏虚，封藏固摄功能失职所表现的证候。本证多由于年

weakness in the aged and asthenia of kidney qi; or by congenital defect and insufficiency of kidney qi; or by consumption of kidney qi due to chronic disease and overstrain.

Clinical manifestations: Aching and weakness of loins and knees, dizziness and tinnitus, frequent clear urine, or dripping urination, or enuresis, or frequent nocturnal urination, or incontinence of urine in man, seminal emission, immature ejaculation, dripping menstruation, or thin and profuse leukorrhagia, or excessive movement of fetus and susceptibility to abortion, light-coloured tongue with whitish fur and weak pulse. Such symptoms are usually seen in prostate hyperplasia, hypogonadism, metrostaxis due to dysfunction and habitual abortion, etc.

Analysis of the symptoms: Aching and weakness of loins and knees, dizziness and tinnitus are caused by asthenia of kidney qi and insufficient nutrition; frequent clear urine, or dripping urination, or enuresis, or frequent noctural urination, or incontinence of urine in man are caused by asthenia of kidney qi and dysfunction of bladder; seminal emission and immature ejaculation are caused by asthenia of kidney qi and its failure in storage, dripping menstruation, or thin and profuse leukorrhagia, or excessive movement of fetus and susceptibility to abortion, are caused by insufficiency of kidney qi, dysfunction of the thoroughfare and conception vessels as well as weakness of the belt vessel; light-coloured tongue with whitish fur and weak pulse are the signs of qi asthenia.

Key points for syndrome differentiation: This syndrome is marked by aching and weakness of the loins and knees, frequent and clear urine or dripping urination, seminal emission, immature ejaculation, dripping menstruation, thin and profuse leukorrhagia and weakness of the bladder.

高体弱,肾气亏虚;或先天禀赋不足,肾气不充;以及久病劳损,耗伤肾气所致。

临床表现:腰膝酸软,眩晕耳鸣,小便频数而清,或尿后余沥不尽,或遗尿,或夜尿频多,或小便失禁,男子滑精、早泄,女子月经淋漓不尽,或带下清稀而量多,或胎动易滑,舌淡苔白,脉弱。可见于前列腺增生症、性腺功能低下、功能失调性子宫出血、习惯性流产等。

证候分析:肾气亏虚,失于充养,则腰膝酸软,神疲乏力,耳鸣失聪;肾气亏虚,膀胱失约,则小便频数而清,或尿后余沥不尽,或遗尿,或夜尿频多,或小便失禁;肾气亏虚,封藏失职,精关不固,则男子滑精、早泄;肾气不足,冲任失约,带脉失固,则女子月经淋漓不尽,或带下清稀而量多,或胎动易滑。舌淡,苔白,脉弱,为气虚的征象。

辨证要点:本证以腰膝酸软,小便频数而清或尿后余沥不尽,男子滑精、早泄,女子月经淋漓不尽、带下清稀量多等肾和膀胱不能固摄的临床表现为诊断依据。

## 2.3.5.6 Syndrome of kidney failing to receive qi

Syndrome of kidney failing to receive qi refers to the symptoms of dyspnea and shortness of breath due to asthenia of the kidney qi and its failure to receive qi and direct it to its source. This syndrome is usually caused by consumption of pulmonary qi and impairment of the kidney due to cough in chronic disease; or by consumption of kidney qi due to overstrain; or by congenital deficiency of primordial qi and malnutrition of the kidney; or by asthenia of kidney qi in the aged.

Clinical manifestations: Dyspnea and shortness of breath, more exhalation and less inhalation, aggravation of dyspnea after movement, low and weak voice, spontaneous sweating, lassitude, aching and weakness of loins and knees, light-coloured tongue and weak pulse; or aggravation of dyspnea, profuse cold sweating, cold limbs and cyanotic complexion, floating and large pulse; or shortness of breath and dyspnea, flushed cheeks and dysphoria, vexation, dry mouth and throat, reddish tongue with scanty fluid as well as thin and rapid pulse. Such symptoms are usually seen in chronic obstructive pulmonary emphysema, pulmogenic heart disease, bronchial asthma, lung cancer and failure of respiratory function, etc.

Analysis of the symptoms: Dyspnea and shortness of breath, more exhalation and less inhalation and aggravation of dyspnea after movement are caused by asthenia of kidney qi and its failure in receiving qi and directing qi to its source; low and weak voice, spontaneous sweating, lassitude, aching and weakness of loins and knees, light-coloured tongue and weak pulse are caused by asthenia of lung and kidney qi, declination of thoracic qi and weakness of defensive qi; aggravation of dyspnea, profuse cold

## （六）肾不纳气证

肾不纳气证是指由于肾气虚衰，纳气无权，气不归元，表现以喘息、气短为主症的证候，又称肺肾气虚证。本证多由于久病咳喘，耗伤肺气，损及于肾；或劳伤过度，耗损肾气；或先天元气不足，肾失充养；或老年肾气虚衰所致。

临床表现：喘息气短，呼多吸少，动则喘息尤甚，语声低怯，自汗乏力，腰膝酸软，舌淡脉弱。或喘息加剧，冷汗淋漓，肢冷面青，脉浮大无根；亦可见气短息促，颧红心烦，躁扰不宁，咽干口燥，舌红少津，脉细数。可见于慢性阻塞性肺气肿、肺源性心脏病、支气管哮喘、肺癌、呼吸功能衰竭等。

证候分析：肾气虚，纳气无权，气不归元，则喘息，气短不足以息，呼多吸少，动则喘息尤甚；肺肾气虚，宗气亦微，卫表不固，则语声低怯，自汗乏力，腰膝酸软，舌淡脉弱。若肾阳虚衰欲竭，虚阳外浮，则喘息加剧，冷汗淋漓，肢冷面青，脉浮大无根；若肾气虚

sweating, cold limbs and cyanotic complexion, floating and large pulse are caused by exhaustion of kidney yang and floating of asthenic yang; flushed cheeks and dysphoria, vexation, dry mouth and throat, reddish tongue with scanty fluid as well as thin and rapid pulse are caused by asthenia of kidney qi complicated by consumption of yin fluid and failure of yin to control yang.

Key points for syndrome differentiation: This syndrome is marked by asthmatic cough, shortness of breath, more exhalation and less inhalation, aggravation of dyspnea after movment and accompanied by asthenia of both lung and kidney qi.

## 2.3.6 Syndrome differentiation of stomach disease

Stomach disease mainly reflects the disorders of the stomach and the pathological changes of its functions in receiving food, digesting food and descending. Clinically stomach disease is marked by stomachache, belching, hiccup, nausea and vomiting, etc.

Stomach disease is either asthenic or sthenic. Sthenic stomach disease is usually caused by exogenous pathogenic factors attacking the stomach and improper diet, leading to the formation of stomach cold, stomach heat and retention of food in the stomach. While asthenic stomach disease is usually caused by improper diet, excessive vomiting and diarrhea, impairment of yin by febrile disease, spleen asthenic involving the stomach and other acute and chronic diseases that impair the stomach and lead to asthenic cold in the stomach and consumption of stomach yin.

### 2.3.6.1 Syndrome of stomach cold

Syndrome of stomach cold refers to internal cold

衰兼阴液亏少，阴不制阳，则出现颧红、咽干、心烦、躁扰不宁、舌红少津、脉细数等症。

辨证要点：本证以久病咳喘气短，呼多吸少，动则喘息益甚，兼有肺肾气虚的表现为诊断依据。

## 六、胃病辨证

胃的病变主要反映在胃腑本身以及胃主受纳、腐熟的功能失常，胃气失于和降而上逆等方面，临床以胃脘疼痛、嗳气、呃逆、恶心、呕吐等为常见症状。

胃病的证候有虚实之分，实证多因外邪犯胃，饮食失节，从而形成胃寒、胃热、食滞胃脘等证；虚证多由饮食失调，吐泻过度，热病伤阴，脾虚及胃，以及其他急、慢性疾患损伤胃腑，导致胃气虚寒、胃阴亏虚等。

### （一）胃寒证

胃寒证是指由于寒邪侵

syndrome marked by epigastric and abdominal cold pain due to pathogenic cold attacking on the stomach, or due to weakness of the stomach yang and endogenous yin cold. This syndrome is mainly caused by cold attacking on the epigastrium and abdomen, or excessive intake of cold and uncooked food, or overstrain or asthenic cold of the gastric qi.

Clinical manifestations: Cold pain in the epigastrium which is worsened with cold and alleviated with warmth; or sharp pain which is unpressable or lingering or prefers pressure; nausea and vomiting, relief of pain after vomiting, bland taste in the mouth without thirst, whitish or bluish complexion; or epigastric and abdominal distending pain, gurgling of water in the stomach and regurgitation of clear fluid; or accompanied by dispiritedness and lassitude, cold limbs and preference for warmth and loose stool; light-coloured tongue with whitish slippery fur, sinking, tense or slow pulse. Such symptoms are usually seen in acute gastritis, chronic gastritis, duodenitis, duodenal bulbar ulcer, gastric ulcer, gastric spasm, pylorochesis, gastrointestinal dysfunction, stomach cancer and duodenal cancer, etc.

Analysis of the symptoms: Cold, sharp and unpalpable pain in the stomach is caused by retention of pathogenic cold in the stomach and stagnation of qi; alleviation of pain with warmth and aggravation with cold are due to the fact that cold is a pathogenic factor of yin nature and can only be resolved by yang; cold, lingering, palpable or unpalpable pain in the epigastrium is caused by longer duration of disease, repeated occurrence of stomach, consumption of gastrosplenic yang, or overstrain, asthenic cold of gastric qi and loss of warmth in the stomach; nausea, vomiting and relief of pain after vomiting are due to stagnation of qi and improper descending of gastric qi;

犯胃腑，或胃阳虚弱，阴寒内生，表现以脘腹冷痛为主症的里寒证。本证多由于脘腹受凉，或过食生冷，或劳倦伤中，胃气虚寒所致。

临床表现：胃脘冷痛，得温痛减，遇寒加重，或痛势急剧，拒按，或痛势绵绵喜按，恶心呕吐，吐后痛缓，口淡不渴，面白或青；或脘腹胀满，胃中有振水声，口泛清水；或伴见神疲乏力，肢凉喜暖，大便稀溏。舌淡苔白滑，脉沉紧或迟。可见于急性胃炎、慢性胃炎、十二指肠炎、十二指肠球部溃疡、胃溃疡、胃痉挛、幽门梗阻、胃肠功能紊乱、胃癌、十二指肠癌等。

证候分析：寒邪凝滞胃腑，气机阻滞，则胃脘冷痛，痛势急剧，拒按；寒为阴邪，得阳始化，故疼痛得温则减，遇寒加重；若病程迁延，胃脘疼痛反复发作，中阳耗伤，或劳倦伤中，胃气虚寒，胃腑失于温煦，则胃脘冷痛，痛势绵绵，喜温喜按；寒凝气滞，胃失和降，则恶心呕吐，吐后痛缓；阴盛阳虚，津液未伤，故口淡不渴；阴寒凝滞，则面白或青；寒伤

bland taste in the mouth without thirst is due to the fact that body fluid is not consumed because yin is exuberant and yang is asthenic; whitish or bluish complexion is due to stagnation of yin cold; epigastric and abdominal distension and fullness, gurgling of water in the stomach and regurgitation of clear fluid are due to impairment of gastric yang by cold and upward adverse rise of fluid retention with gastric qi; dispiritedness and lassitude, cold limbs and preference for warmth and loose stool; light-coloured tongue with whitish slippery fur, sinking, tense or slow pulse are the signs of yang asthenia and internal exuberance of yin cold.

Key points for syndrome differentiation: This syndrome is marked by cold pain in the epigastrium, which is alleviated with warmth and aggravated with cold, and internal exuberance of yin cold.

### 2.3.6.2 Syndrome of stomach heat

Syndrome of stomach heat refers to symptoms of sthenic heat due to superabundance of fire and heat in the stomach and failure of gastric qi to descend. This syndrome is usually caused by excessive intake of pungent, warm and dry food which transforms into heat and fire; or by emotional upsets and stagnation of qi which transform into fire and attacks the stomach; or by pathogenic heat attacking the stomach.

Clinical manifestations: Scorching pain in the stomach, gastric discomfort with acid regurgitation, or vomiting right after eating, or preference for cold drinks, or polyorexia, or halitosis, or swelling, pain and ulceration of gum, dental bleeding, constipation, scanty yellowish urine, reddish tongue with yellow fur and slippery and rapid pulse. These symptoms are usually seen in acute and chronic gastritis, digestive ulcer, esophagus cancer and stomach cancer as well as periodontitis and diabetes.

胃阳，水饮不化而随胃气上逆，则脘腹胀满，胃中有振水声，口泛清水。神疲乏力，肢凉喜暖，大便稀溏，舌淡苔白滑，脉沉迟或沉紧，为阳虚阴寒内盛的表现。

辨证要点：本证以胃脘冷痛，得温则减，遇寒加重，以及阴寒内盛的表现为诊断依据。

### （二）胃热证

胃热证是指由于胃中火热炽盛，胃失和降所表现的实热证候。本证多由于过食辛辣温燥之品，化热生火；或情志不遂，气郁化火犯胃；或邪热犯胃等所致。

临床表现：胃脘灼痛，吞酸嘈杂，或食入即吐，或渴喜冷饮，或消谷善饥，或见口臭，或牙龈肿痛溃烂、齿衄，大便秘结，小便短黄，舌红苔黄，脉滑数。可见于急性胃炎、慢性胃炎、消化性溃疡、食管癌、胃癌等消化系统疾病，以及牙周炎、糖尿病等。

Analysis of the symptoms: Scorching and unpalpable pain in the stomach is caused by stagnation of heat in the stomach and obstruction of the gastric qi; gastric discomfort with acid regurgitation or vomiting right after eating is caused by upward adverse rise of liver and gastric qi and fire as well as failure of gastric qi to descend; polyorexia is caused by exuberance of gastric fire and excessive digestion; halitosis is caused by upward adverse rise of gastric heat with turbid qi; preference for cold drinks, constipation and scanty yellow urine are due to consumption of body fluid by pathogenic heat; swelling, pain and ulceration of gum and dental bleeding are caused by fumigation of gastric fire along the meridian, stagnation of qi and blood as well as impairment of the collaterals; reddish tongue with yellow fur and slippery and rapid pulse are the signs of internal exuberance of fire and heat.

Key points for syndrome differentiation: This syndrome is marked by scorching pain in the epigastrium, stomach discomfort with acid regurgitation, polyorexia and internal exuberance of fire and heat.

### 2.3.6.3 Syndrome of food retention in the stomach

Syndrome of food retention in the stomach refers to the symptoms of gastric and abdominal fullness and pain, vomiting, diarrhea, acid regurgitation and halitosis due to retention of food in the stomach. This syndrome is caused by intemperance of food, or congenital weakness of the stomach and spleen as well as dysfunction of the stomach in receiving and digesting food.

Clinical manifestations: Unpalpable gastric and abdominal fullness and pain, eructation with fetid odor, anorexia, or vomiting of fetid food, alleviation of abdominal distension and pain after vomiting, or borborygmus with abdominal pain, unsmooth defecation, foul stool like

证候分析：热郁于胃，胃气壅滞，则胃脘灼痛而拒按；肝胃气火上逆，胃失和降，则吞酸嘈杂，或食入即吐；胃火炽盛，腐熟太过，则消谷善饥；胃热挟浊气上逆，则口臭；热邪伤津，则渴喜冷饮，大便秘结，小便短黄；胃火循经上薰，气滞血壅，血络受损，则牙龈红肿疼痛，甚至化脓溃烂、齿衄。舌红苔黄，脉滑数，为火热内盛的表现。

辨证要点：本证以胃脘灼痛，吞酸嘈杂，消谷善饥，以及火热内盛的表现为诊断依据。

### （三）食滞胃脘证

食滞胃脘证是指由于饮食停滞于胃，以脘腹胀满疼痛，呕泻酸馊腐臭为主症的证候。本证多由于饮食不节，暴饮暴食；或素体脾胃虚弱，运纳失健等因素所引起。

临床表现：脘腹胀满疼痛，拒按，嗳腐吞酸，厌食，或呕吐酸腐食物，吐后胀痛得减，或肠鸣腹痛，泻下不爽，便臭如败卵，舌苔厚腻，脉滑或

decayed eggs, thin and greasy tongue fur, slippery pulse or sinking and sthenic pulse. Such symptoms are usually seen in acute gastritis, acute enteritis, gastric dilatation, chronic gastritis, malabsorption syndrome and Crohn's disease.

Analysis of the symptoms: Unpalpable gastric and abdominal fullness and pain, eructation with fetid odor, anorexia, or vomiting of fetid food, alleviation of abdominal distension and pain after vomiting are caused by retention of food in the stomach, stagnation of qi and upward adverse rise of gastric qi; borborygmus with abdominal pain, unsmooth defecation, foul stool like decayed eggs are caused by retention of food in the intestines, inhibited flow of qi and transportation; thin and greasy tongue fur, slippery pulse or sinking and sthenic pulse are the signs of internal retention of food.

Key points for syndrome differentiation: This syndrome is marked by epigastric and abdominal fullness and pain, vomiting of fetid food, or unsmooth defecation, foul stool like decayed eggs and history of disease due to improper diet.

### 2.3.6.4 Syndrome of asthenic stomach yin

Syndrome of asthenic stomach yin refers to the symptoms due to insufficiency of gastric yin, loss of proper moistening and descending of the stomach as well as internal disturbance of asthenic heat. This syndrome is usually caused by prolonged stomach di-sease; or by consumption of yin fluid at the advanced stage of seasonal febrile disease; or by consumption of body fluid due to excessive vomiting and diarrhea; or by excessive intake of pungent, fragrant and dry foods; or by excessive taking of warm and dry drugs; or by consumption of gastric fluid due to emotional depression and fire transformed from qi stagnation.

沉实。可见于急性胃炎、急性肠炎、胃扩张、慢性胃炎、吸收不良综合征、克罗恩病等。

证候分析：食滞胃脘，气机阻滞，胃气上逆，则脘腹胀满疼痛，拒按，嗳腐吞酸，厌食，或呕吐酸腐食物，吐后胀痛得减。食积于肠，气机不畅，传导不利，则肠鸣腹痛，泻下不爽，便臭如败卵。舌苔厚腻，脉滑或沉实，为食积内阻的表现。

辨证要点：本证以脘腹胀满疼痛，呕吐酸腐食物，或泻下不爽，便臭如败卵，以及有伤食病史为诊断依据。

### （四）胃阴虚证

胃阴虚证是指由于胃阴不足，胃失濡润和降，虚热内扰所表现的证候。本证多由胃病久延；或温热病后期阴液耗伤未复；或吐泻太过，伤津耗液；或过食辛辣、香燥之品；或服用温燥药物太过；或情志郁结，气郁化火，导致胃阴耗伤所形成。

Clinical manifestations: Scorching and dull pain in the epigastrium, hunger without desire to take food, or epigastric fullness and discomfort, or dry vomiting and hiccup, dry mouth and throat, dry feces, scanty urine, reddish tongue with scanty fluid and thin and rapid pulse. Such symptoms are usually seen in acute and atrophic gastritis, malabsorption syndrome, Crohn's disease, esophagus cancer, stomach cancer, liver cirrhosis and liver cancer as well as at the rehabilitative stage of various infectious diseases.

Analysis of the symptoms: Scorching and dull pain in the epigastrium, hunger without desire to take food are caused by insufficiency of gastric fluid, loss of proper moistening in the stomach, internal disturbance of asthenic heat and failure of gastric qi to descend; epigastric fullness and discomfort or dry vomiting and hiccup are caused by loss of proper moistening in the stomach and failure of gastric qi to descend; dry mouth and throat, dry feces and scanty urine are caused by yin asthenia and consumption of body fluid; reddish tongue with scanty fluid and thin and rapid pulse are the signs of yin asthenia and internal heat.

Key points for syndrome differentiation: This syndrome is marked by scorching dull pain in the epigastrium, hunger without desire to take food, or dry vomiting and hiccup as well as dry mouth and throat, reddish tongue with scanty fluid.

## 2.3.7 Syndrome differentiation of gallbladder disease

Syndrome differentiation of gallbladder disease reflects the disorder of the gallbladder proper and the disturbance of its functions in storing and secreting bile to assist digestion and absorption of food as well as in making strategy. The commonly encountered symptoms in clinical

临床表现：胃脘灼热隐痛，饥不欲食，或脘痞不舒，或干呕呃逆，口燥咽干，大便干结，小便短少，舌红少津，脉细而数。可见于慢性萎缩性胃炎、吸收不良综合征、克罗恩病、食道癌、胃癌、肝硬化、肝癌等消化系统疾病，以及各种感染性疾病的恢复阶段等。

证候分析：胃阴不足，胃失濡润，虚热内扰，和降失职，则胃脘灼热隐痛，饥不欲食；胃失濡润，和降失职，则脘痞不舒，或干呕呃逆；阴虚津伤则口燥咽干，大便干结，小便短少。舌红少津，脉细而数，是阴虚内热的征象。

辨证要点：本证以胃脘灼热隐痛，饥不欲食，或干呕呃逆，以及口燥咽干、舌红少津等阴亏失润的表现为诊断依据。

## 七、胆病辨证

胆的病变主要反映在胆腑本身及其贮存和排泄胆汁以助饮食物的消化吸收、主决断的功能失常等方面，临床以胁肋疼痛、口苦、黄疸、惊悸、

practice are hypochondriac pain, bitter taste in the mouth, jaundice, palpitation, timidity and dizziness, etc.

Since the secretion and excretion of bile are closely related to the dispersing function of the liver, the symptoms of gallbladder, such as hypochondriac pain, bitter taste in the mouth and jaundice, usually indicate simultaneous disorder of the liver and gallbladder which will be described in the part of complicated diseases of the viscera. The following mainly describes the syndrome of gallbladder stagnation and phlegm disturbance marked by palpitation, timidity and dizziness.

## Syndrome of gallbladder stagnation and phlegm disturbance

Syndrome of gallbladder stagnation and phlegm disturbance refers to the symptoms of gallbladder failing to disperse due to internal disturbance of phlegm-heat. This syndrome is mainly caused by emotional depression and internal disturbance of the gallbladder by a mixture of phlegm and heat due to fire transformed from qi stagnation which scorches fluid into phlegm.

Clinical manifestations: Timidity and susceptibility to fright, palpitation and restlessness, insomnia and dreaminess, dysphoria, difficulty in making decision, thoracic and hypochondriac oppressin and distension, frequent sigh, dizziness and vertigo, bitter taste in the mouth, vomiting, reddish tongue, yello-wish and greasy fur as well as taut and slippery pulse. Such symptoms are usually seen in neurasthenia, cholecystitis, arrhythmia and climacteric syndrome.

Analysis of the symptoms: Timidity and susceptibility to fright, palpitation and restlessness as well as difficulty in making decision are caused by internal disturbance of phlegm-heat and disorder of gallbladder qi; insomnia and dreaminess and dysphoria are caused by phlegm-heat dis-

胆怯、眩晕等为常见症状。

由于胆汁的分泌、排泄与肝脏的疏泄功能密切相关,故胆病以胁肋疼痛、口苦、黄疸为主症的证候多属于肝胆同病,将在脏腑兼病中介绍。这里主要介绍以惊悸、胆怯、眩晕为主症的胆郁痰扰证。

## 胆郁痰扰证

胆郁痰扰证是指由于痰热内扰,胆失疏泄所表现的证候。本证多由于情志抑郁,气郁化火,灼津为痰,痰热互结,内扰胆腑所致。

临床表现:胆怯易惊,惊悸不宁,失眠多梦,烦躁不安,谋虑不决,胸胁闷胀,善太息,头晕目眩,口苦,呕恶,舌红,苔黄腻,脉弦滑。可见于神经衰弱、胆囊炎、心律失常、更年期综合征等。

证候分析:痰热内扰,胆气不宁,故胆怯易惊,惊悸不安,谋虑不决;痰热内扰心神,故失眠多梦,烦躁不安;胆失疏泄,气机不利,故胸胁闷胀,

turbing mind; thoracic and hypochondriac oppressin and distension as well as frequent sigh are caused by failure of the gallbladder to disperse and inhibited flow of qi; dizziness and vertigo are caused by phlegm-heat attacking the head along the gallbladder meridian; bitter taste in the mouth and vomiting are caused by heat driving gallbladder qi to rise and failure of the stomach to descend; reddish tongue, yellowish and greasy fur as well as taut and slippery pulse are the signs of internal exuberance of phlegm-heat.

Key points for syndrome differentiation: This syndrome is marked by palpitation, insomnia, dizziness, thoracic and hypochondriac oppression and distension, bitter taste in the mouth and yellowish greasy tongue coating.

善太息；痰热循胆经上犯头目，则头晕目眩；热迫胆气上溢，胃失和降，则口苦、呕恶。舌红，苔黄腻，脉弦滑，为痰热内盛的征象。

辨证要点：本证以惊悸，失眠、眩晕，胸胁闷胀，口苦，苔黄腻为诊断依据。

## 2.3.8 Syndrome differentiation of small intestinal disease

## 八、小肠病辨证

Small intestinal disease reflects the disorder of the small intestine and the pathological changes of its functions in receiving and digesting food as well as in separating lucid substance from turbid substance. Clinically the symptoms of small intestinal disease are abdominal distension, borborygmus and loose stool.

小肠的病变主要反映在小肠腑本身及其受盛化物、分别清浊等消化吸收的功能失常方面，临床以腹胀、肠鸣、便溏等为常见症状。

In the theory of viscera and their manifestations, the digestive and absorptive functions of the small intestine are attributed to the spleen. So the disorders of the small intestine are usually included in the disorders of the spleen. The following is a brief description of sthenic heat syndrome of small intestine due to the heart transferring heat to the small intestine.

在藏象学说中，往往把小肠的消化吸收功能归属于脾主运化的范围内，所以小肠虚证的病变一般多归属于脾病的范畴。这里主要介绍心热下移小肠所致的小肠实热证。

### Sthenic heat syndrome of small intestine

### 小肠实热证

Sthenic heat syndrome of small intestine refers to the symptoms due to exuberance of heat in the small intestine. This syndrome is usually caused by the heart trans-

小肠实热证是指小肠里热炽盛所表现的证候。本证多由于心热下移小肠所致。

ferring heat to the small intestine.

Clinical manifestations: Dysphoria and thirst, ulcer in the mouth and on the tongue, scanty and brownish urine, inhibited urination, scorching pain in urination, hematuria, reddish tongue, yellowish tongue fur and rapid pulse. These symptoms are usually seen in Behcet's disease, infection of urinary tract and sicca syndrome.

Analysis of the symptoms: Dysphoria is caused by internal exuberance of heart fire which disturbs mind; thirst is caused by heat scorching body fluid; ulcer in the mouth and on the tongue are caused by hyperactivity of heart fire; scanty and brownish urine, inhibited urination and scorching pain in urination are caused by exuberant heat in the small intestine transferred by the heart because the heart and the small intestine are internally and externally related to each other; hematuria is caused by extravasation of blood due to exuberant heat scorching the yin collaterals; reddish tongue, yellowish tongue fur and rapid pulse are the signs of internal exuberance of heat.

Key points for syndrome differentiation: This syndrome is marked by vexation, thirst, mouth and tongue ulcer as well as scanty urine, inhibited urination and scorching pain in urination.

## 2.3.9 Syndrome differentiation of large intestinal disease

Large intestinal disorder mainly reflects the dysfunction of the large intestine proper and the pathological changes in its functions in transportation and transformation. The clinical symptoms of large intestinal disorder are usually constipation, diarrhea and purulent and bloody dysentery.

Large intestinal disorder is either asthenic or sthenic. The asthenia syndrome of large intestine is usually

临床表现：心烦口渴，口舌生疮，小便短赤，排尿艰涩不畅，尿道灼痛，尿血，舌红，苔黄，脉数。可见于白塞病、尿路感染、干燥综合征等。

证候分析：心火内炽，热扰心神，则心烦；热灼津伤，则口渴；心火上炎，则口舌生疮。小肠有分别清浊的功能，使水液入于膀胱。心与小肠相表里，心热下移小肠，小肠里热炽盛，故小便短赤，排尿艰涩不畅，尿道灼热疼痛；热盛灼伤阴络，迫血妄行，则尿血。舌红，苔黄，脉数，为里热炽盛的征象。

辨证要点：本证以心烦口渴、口舌生疮等心火热炽与小便赤涩、灼痛的表现共见为诊断依据。

## 九、大肠病辨证

大肠的病变主要为大肠腑本身及其传导、变化功能失常等方面，临床以便秘、泄泻、下痢脓血等为常见症状。

大肠病的证候有虚实之分，虚证多因素体阴亏，或热

caused by congenital yin deficiency, or by exuberant heat consuming body fluid, or by excessive vomiting and diarrhea, or by impairment of yin due to chronic disease which lead to consumption of large intestinal fluid; the sthenia syndrome of large intestine is often caused by attack of summer-dampness and heat, or by improper food that lead to retention of damp heat in the large intestine.

### 2.3.9.1 Syndrome of large intestinal fluid consumption

Syndrome of large intestinal fluid consumption refers to the symptoms of retention of dry feces and difficulty in defecation due to consumption of large intestinal fluid and inhibited transportation. This syndrome is usually caused by congenital yin deficiency, or by insufficiency of blood in the aged, or by excessive vomiting and diarrhea, or by consumption of yin due to chronic disease, or by non-restoration of consumed fluid at the advanced stage of febrile disease, or by excessive hemorrhage, etc.

Clinical manifestations: Dry feces and difficulty in defecation, defecation once in several days, dry mouth and throat, or dizziness and halitosis, reddish tongue with scanty fluid, yellow and dry tongue fur, as well as thin and unsmooth pulse. Such symptoms are usually seen in disturbance of intestines, habitual constipation, chronic atrophic gastritis, esophagus cancer, stomach cancer and intestinal cancer as well as the rehabilitative stage of various infectious diseases.

Analysis of the symptoms: Dry feces and difficulty in defecation, defecation once in several days are caused by consumption of large intestinal fluid, loss of moisture in the large intestine and its function in transportation; dry mouth and throat are caused by consumption of fluid and loss of moisture; dizziness and halitosis are caused by stagnation of large intestinal qi and disturbance of lucid

盛伤津,或吐泻太过,或久病伤阴等,导致大肠液亏;实证多因感受暑湿热邪,或饮食不洁,导致大肠湿热蕴结。

### (一)大肠液亏证

大肠液亏证是指由于大肠阴津亏虚,传导不利,表现以大便燥结、排便困难为主症的证候,又称肠燥津亏证。本证多由于素体阴亏,或年老阴血不足,或吐泻太过,或久病伤阴,或热病后期津伤未复,或失血过多等因素所致。

临床表现:大便干燥秘结,难以排出,数日一行,口干咽燥,或头晕口臭,舌红少津,苔黄燥,脉细涩。可见于肠功能紊乱、习惯性便秘、慢性萎缩性胃炎、食道癌、胃癌、肠癌等慢性消耗性疾病,以及各种感染性疾病的恢复阶段。

证候分析:大肠液亏,肠道失却濡润,传导失职,则大便干燥秘结,难以排出,数日一行;津伤失润则口干咽燥;大肠腑气不通,秽浊之气上逆,清阳被扰,则头晕口臭。舌红少津,苔黄燥,脉细涩,为

yang by upward adverse flow of turbid qi; reddish tongue with scanty fluid, yellow and dry tongue fur, as well as thin and unsmooth pulse are the signs of consumption of yin fluid and endogenous dry-heat.

Key points for syndrome differentiation: This syndrome is marked by retention of dry feces and difficulty in defecation as well as manifestations of loss of fluid.

### 2.3.9.2 Syndrome of large intestinal damp-heat

Syndrome of large intestinal damp-heat refers to the symptoms of diarrhea and dysentery due to invasion of damp heat into the intestinal tract and failure of the intestine to transport. This syndrome is mainly caused by invasion of pathogenic damp-heat in summer and autumn into the intestinal tract, or by improper diet, leading to retention of damp-heat and turbid pathogenic factors in the intestinal tract.

Clinical manifestations: Abdominal pain, yellowish and foul fulminant diarrhea, scorching sensation over the anus, or purulent and bloody dysentery, tenesmus, scanty and yellow urine, reddish tongue, yellow and greasy tongue fur as well as slippery and rapid pulse. Such symptoms are usually seen in acute enteritis, dysentery, ulcerative colitis, intestinal tuberculosis and tumor in the intestinal tract.

Analysis of the symptoms: Abdominal pain, yellowish and foul fulminant diarrhea are caused by retention of damp-heat in the large intestine, stagnation of qi in the intestinal tract and failure of the intestine to transport; scorching sensation over the anus is caused by heat invading the large intestine; purulent and bloody dysentery is caused by damp-heat fumigating the large intestinal tract and impairing the collaterals; tenesmus is caused by stagnation of dampness and qi as well as heat fumigating the

阴津亏损、燥热内生的表现。

辨证要点：本证以大便燥结，难以排出，以及津亏失润的表现为诊断依据。

### （二）大肠湿热证

大肠湿热证是指由于湿热侵犯肠道，传导失职，表现以泄泻、下痢为主的证候。本证多由于夏秋之季感受暑湿热邪，侵犯肠道，或饮食不洁，致使湿热秽浊之邪蕴结肠道所致。

临床表现：腹痛，暴注下泻，色黄秽臭，肛门灼热，或下痢脓血，里急后重，小便短黄，舌质红，苔黄腻，脉滑数。可见于急性肠炎、痢疾、溃疡性结肠炎、肠结核、肠道肿瘤等。

证候分析：湿热蕴结大肠，肠道气滞，传导失职，则腹痛，暴注下泻，色黄秽臭；热迫大肠，则肛门灼热；湿热薰蒸肠道，脉络受损，则下痢脓血；湿阻气滞，热蒸肠道，则里急后重。小便短黄，舌质红，苔黄腻，脉滑数，为湿热内阻的表现。

intestinal tract; scanty and yellow urine, reddish tongue, yellow and greasy tongue fur as well as slippery and rapid pulse are the signs of internal stagnation of damp-heat.

Key points for syndrome differentiation: This syndrome is marked by abdominal pain, fulminant diarrhea, or purulent bloody dysentery as well as manifestations of damp-heat.

## 2.3.10 Syndrome differentiation of bladder disease

Bladder disease mainly reflects the disorder of the bladder proper and the pathological changes of its functions in storing and excreting urine. The clinical manifestations are frequent urination, urgency in urination, pain in urination and anuria as well as brownish and turbid urine, hematuria and sandy urine, etc.

Bladder disease is often of sthenic nature due to retention of damp heat in the bladder and inhibited transformation of qi in the bladder. The asthenic disease of the bladder is usually caused by asthenic cold in the lower energizer and unconsolidation of the bladder due to asthenia of kidney yang.

### Syndrome of damp heat in the bladder

Syndrome of damp heat in the bladder refers to symptoms of morbid changes in urine due to retention of damp heat in the bladder and inhibited transformation of qi. This syndrome is frequently caused by invasion of exogenous damp heat in the bladder, or by downward migration of damp heat transformed from improper diet into the bladder.

Clinical manifestations: Frequent and urgent urination, lower abdominal distending pain, scorching pain in urination, scanty and brownish urine, or hematuria, or sandy urine, accompanied by fever, lumbago, reddish tongue, yellowish greasy tongue fur and slippery and rapid pulse. Such symptoms are usually seen in acute pyelitis, cystitis, prostatitis, urethritis and urinary calculus, etc.

Analysis of the symptoms: Frequent and urgent urination, lower abdominal distending pain, scorching pain in urethra are caused by retention of damp heat in the bladder and inhibited transformation of qi; scanty and brownish urine is caused by retention of damp heat and scorching of fluid; hematuria is caused by damp heat impairing yin collaterals; sandy urine is caused by lingering damp heat scorching impurity in the urine into stones; fever and lumbago are caused by fumigation of damp heat involving the kidney; reddish tongue, yellowish greasy tongue fur and slippery and rapid pulse are the signs of internal accumulation of damp heat.

Key points for syndrome differentiation: This syndrome is marked by frequent and urgent urination, burning pain in urethra during urination and yellowish and brownish urine.

## 2.3.11 Syndrome differentiation of accompanying diseases of viscera

Accompanying diseases of viscera refer to simultaneous disease of two or more viscera.

The viscera are different in functions, but they are closely related to each other and form an organic whole. Therefore under pathological conditions, they may affect each other and resulting in accompanying diseases.

The accompanying diseases of viscera are pathologically related to each other and affect each other. For example, accompanying diseases usually occur among the viscera internally and externally related to each other or

数。可见于急性肾盂肾炎、膀胱炎、前列腺炎、尿道炎、尿路结石等。

证候分析：湿热留滞膀胱，气化不利，下迫尿道，则尿频尿急，尿道灼痛；膀胱气滞，则小腹胀痛；湿热内蕴，津液被灼，则小便短赤浑浊；湿热伤及阴络，则尿血；湿热久恋，煎熬尿中杂质成石，则尿有砂石；湿热郁蒸，波及肾府，则发热、腰痛。舌红，苔黄腻，脉滑数，为湿热内蕴的表现。

辨证要点：本证以尿频尿急，排尿灼痛，小便黄赤为诊断依据。

## 十一、脏腑兼病辨证

凡两个或两个以上脏腑相继或同时发病者，称为脏腑兼病。

人体各脏腑虽具有不同的功能，但它们是密切联系的有机整体。因此，在发生病变时，它们可以相互影响而发生脏腑兼病。

脏腑兼病在病理上有着一定内在联系且又相互影响的规律，如具有表里关系的脏腑间，或有生克乘侮关系的脏

promoting, restraining, over-restraining and reverse restraining each other.

The manifestations of accompanying diseases of viscera are not simply the addition of the symptoms of the viscera. Actually the accompanying diseases of viscera have their specific mechanism which results in the corresponding symptoms.

### 2.3.11.1 Asthenia syndrome of heart and lung qi

Asthenia syndrome of heart and lung qi refers to the symptoms of palpitation, cough and dyspnea due to simultaneous asthenia of heart and lung qi. This syndrome is usually caused by consumption of pulmonary qi with the involvement of the heart due to cough and dyspnea in chronic disease; or by weakness in the aged or by overstrain.

Clinical manifestations: Palpitation, shortness of breath, chest oppression, weakness in cough, vomiting of thin and clear sputum, dizziness and dispiritedness, timid and low voice, spontaneous sweating and lassitude, aggravation after movement, pale complexion, light-coloured tongue with whitish fur, or light purplish tongue and lips, sinking and weak or knotted pulse and intermittent pulse. Such symptoms are usually seen in chronic and obstructive pulmonary emphysema, chronic and pulmogenic heart disease, congestive heart failure, pericarditis and mitral valve prolapse syndrome.

Analysis of the symptoms: Palpitation is caused by asthenia of heart qi which fails to propel and nourish the heart; shortness of breath and chest oppression are caused by asthenia of heart and lung qi which lead to insufficient production of thoracic qi and inhibited flow of qi; weakness in cough is caused by asthenia of pulmonary qi, failure of pulmonary qi to depurate and descend as well as upward adverse flow of qi; vomiting of thin and clear

器兼病较为常见。

脏腑兼病的证候表现,并不是病变脏腑证候的简单相加,脏腑兼病特定的病变机理,导致其具有相应的证候表现。

### (一)心肺气虚证

心肺气虚证是指由于心肺两脏气虚,表现以心悸、咳喘为主症的证候。本证多由久病咳喘,耗伤肺气,波及于心;或老年体虚,或劳倦太过所致。

临床表现:心悸,胸闷,气短,咳喘无力,吐痰清稀,头晕神疲,语声低怯,自汗乏力,动则诸症加剧,面色淡白,舌淡苔白,或唇舌淡紫,脉沉弱或结代。可见于慢性阻塞性肺气肿、慢性肺源性心脏病、充血性心力衰竭、心包炎、二尖瓣脱垂综合征等。

证候分析:心气虚,鼓动无力,心失所养,则心悸;心肺气虚,宗气生成不足,气机不畅,则胸闷,气短;肺气虚弱,肃降无权,气机上逆,则咳喘无力;肺气虚,气不布津,水液停聚为痰为饮,则吐痰清稀;气虚功能活动减弱,则头晕神

sputum is caused by asthenia of pulmonary qi which fails to distribute body fluid and leads to accumulation of fluid into phlegm; dizziness and dispiritedness, timid and low voice, spontaneous sweating and lassitude are caused by hypoactivity of the body due to asthenia of qi; aggravation after movement is due to consumption of qi; pale complexion, light-coloured tongue with whitish fur, or light purplish tongue and lips, sinking and weak or knotted pulse and intermittent pulse are the signs of asthenia of heart and lung qi which is weak in transporting blood.

Key points for syndrome differentitation: The major manifestations are both palpitation, cough, asthma and symptoms due to qi deficiency and weakened functional activity.

### 2.3.11.2 Asthenia syndrome of heart and spleen

Asthenia syndrome of heart and spleen refers to the symptoms of malnutrition of the heart, dysfunction of the spleen and weakness of the spleen in controlling blood. This syndrome is usually caused by improper regulation in prolonged disease, or by excessive contemplation, or by intemperance of food and impairment of the spleen and stomach, or by acute and chronic hemorrhage leading to deficiency of heart and spleen qi and blood.

Clinical manifestations: Sallow complexion, lassitude, palpitation, insomnia and dreaminess, dizziness and amnesia, poor appetite, abdominal distension and loose stool, hematemesis, hematochezia, or subcutaneous hemorrhage, or scanty and light-coloured menstruation and dripping menstruation, light-coloured and tender tongue as well as thin and weak pulse. These symptoms are usually seen in arrhythmia, cardiac neurosis, chronic gastritis, digestive ulcer, hemorrhage from upper digestive tract, malabsorption syndrome, iron-deficiency anemia, aplastic

疲,语声低怯,自汗乏力;动则耗气,气虚更甚,故动则诸症加剧。面色淡白,舌淡苔白,唇舌淡紫,脉沉弱或结代,为心肺气虚,运血无力的表现。

辨证要点:本证以心悸,咳喘,与气虚功能活动减弱的表现并见为诊断依据。

### (二) 心脾两虚证

心脾两虚证是指由于心血不足、脾虚气弱而表现的心神失养,脾失健运,统血无权的虚弱证候。本证多由于久病失调,或思虑过度,或饮食失节,损伤脾胃,或急、慢性失血,以致心脾气血亏虚所形成。

临床表现:面色萎黄,倦怠乏力,心悸怔忡,失眠多梦,头晕健忘,食欲不振,腹胀便溏,呕血、便血,或皮下出血,或女子月经量少色淡、淋漓不尽,舌质淡嫩,脉细弱。可见于心律失常、心脏神经官能症、慢性胃炎、消化性溃疡、上消化道出血、吸收不良综合征、缺铁性贫血、再生障碍性

anemia, purpura, leukopenia and dysfunctional uterine bleeding.

Analysis of the symptoms: Insomnia and dreaminess are caused by insufficiency of heart blood, malnutrition of the heart and irritability; dizziness and amnesia are caused by insufficiency of heart blood; poor appetite, abdominal distension and loose stool are caused by spleen asthenia, qi deficiency and dysfunction of transformation; hematemesis, hematochezia, or subcutaneous hemorrhage, or dripping menstruation are caused by failure of the spleen to control blood due to asthenia; sallow complexion, lassitude, light-coloured and tender tongue as well as thin and weak pulse are the signs of qi and blood consumption.

Key point for syndrome differentiation: This syndrome is marked by palpitation, insomnia, abdominal distension, loose stool and manifestations of asthenia of both qi and blood.

### 2.3.11.3 Asthenia syndrome of heart and kidney yang

Asthenia syndrome of heart and kidney yang refers to the symptoms of blood stagnation and retention of fluid due to decline of heart and kidney yangqi. This syndrome is mainly caused by decline of heart yang and prolonged disease involving the kidney; or by retention of fluid attacking on the heart due to deficiency of kidney yang and failure of qi transformation.

Clinical manifestations: Palpitation, cold body and limbs, dispiritedness and lassitude, edema of limbs, dysuria, cyanosis of the lips and nails, light-coloured, dull and purplish tongue, whitish and slippery fur as well as sinking, thin and indistinct pulse. Such symptoms are usually seen in heart and kidney failure due to hypertension, infectious endocarditis, myocarditis, chronic pulmogenic

贫血、紫癜、白细胞减少症、功能失调性子宫出血等。

证候分析：心血不足，心失所养，心神不宁，则心悸怔忡，失眠多梦；气血不足，头目失养则头晕健忘；脾虚气弱，运化失健，则食欲不振，腹胀便溏；脾虚不能摄血，则呕血、便血，或皮下出血，或女子月经淋漓不尽。面色萎黄，倦怠乏力，舌质淡嫩，脉细弱，为气血亏虚的征象。

辨证要点：本证以心悸失眠，食少，腹胀，便溏与气血亏虚的表现共见为诊断依据。

### （三）心肾阳虚证

心肾阳虚证是指由于心肾阳气虚衰，温运无力，致血行瘀滞，水湿内停所表现的虚寒证候。本证多因心阳虚衰，病久及肾；或因肾阳亏虚，气化无权，水气上犯凌心所致。

临床表现：心悸怔忡，形寒肢冷，神疲乏力，肢体浮肿，小便不利，唇甲青紫，舌质淡暗青紫，苔白滑，脉沉细微。可见于高血压病、感染性心内膜炎、心肌病、慢性肺源性心脏病、慢性肾炎、系统性红斑

heart disease, chronic nephritis, systemic lupus erythematosus, diabetes, hypothyroidism and epidemic hemorrhagic fever.

Analysis of the symptoms: Palpitation is caused by asthenia of heart and kidney yang as well as failure of the heart to warm, nourish and propel; edema of limbs and dysuria are caused by asthenia of kidney yang, dysfunction of qi transformation and internal retention of dampness; cyanosis of the lips and nails, light-coloured, dull and purplish tongue are caused by asthenia of heart and kidney yang which fails to transport blood; cold body and limbs, dispiritedness and lassitude, whitish and slippery fur as well as sinking, thin and indistinct pulse are the signs of asthenia of heart and kidney yang as well as internal exuberance of yin cold.

Key points for syndrome differentiation: This syndrome is marked by severe palpitation, edema of limbs, dysuria as well as cold body and limbs, dispiritedness and lassitude.

### 2.3.11.4 Syndrome of disharmony between the heart and kidney

Syndrome of disharmony between the heart and kidney refers to the symptoms of asthenia of heart and kidney yin and hyperactivity of heart and kidney yang due to imbalance between the heart and the kidney. This syndrome is usually caused by excessive contemplation; or by depression which transforms into fire to consume heart and kidney yin; or by overstrain, prolonged disease and intemperance of sexual life.

Clinical manifestations: Restlessness and insomnia, palpitation and dreaminess, dizziness and tinnitus, amnesia, aching and weakness of loins and knees, seminal emission, feverish sensation over the five centers (palms, soles and chest), tidal fever and night sweating, dry

狼疮、糖尿病、甲状腺功能减退症、流行性出血热等多种疾病所导致的心、肾功能衰竭。

证候分析：心肾阳虚，心失温养、鼓动，则心悸怔忡；肾阳亏虚，气化失权，膀胱气化失司，水湿内停，泛溢肌肤，则肢体浮肿，小便不利；心肾阳虚，运血无力，血行不畅，则唇甲青紫，舌质淡暗青紫。形寒肢冷，神疲乏力，脉沉细微，为心肾阳虚，阴寒内盛的表现。

辨证要点：本证以心悸怔忡，肢体浮肿，小便不利，以及形寒肢冷、神疲乏力等虚寒的表现为诊断依据。

### （四）心肾不交证

心肾不交证是指由于心肾水火既济失调所反映的心肾阴虚阳亢证候。本证多由于思虑劳神太过；或情志抑郁，郁而化火，耗伤心肾之阴；或虚劳久病，房事不节所致。

临床表现：心烦少寐，惊悸多梦，头晕耳鸣，健忘，腰膝酸软，遗精，五心烦热，潮热盗汗，口咽干燥，舌红少苔或无苔，脉细数。可见于神经衰

mouth and throat, reddish tongue with scanty fur or without fur and thin and rapid pulse. Such symptoms are usually seen in neurasthenia, arrhythmia, cardiac neurosis, hypertension and hyperthyroidism.

Analysis of the symptoms: Restlessness and insomnia, palpitation and dreaminess are caused by asthenia of heart and kidney yin and relative hyperactivity of yang which disturbs the mind; dizziness and tinnitus, amnesia, aching and weakness of loins and knees are caused by consumption of kidney yin, insufficiency of bone marrow and malnutrition of cerebral marrow and loins; seminal emission is caused by internal exuberance of asthenia fire which disturbs the kidney, feverish sensation over the five centers (palms, soles and chest), tidal fever and night sweating, dry mouth and throat, reddish tongue with scanty fur or without fur and thin and rapid pulse are the signs of yin asthenia and hyperactivity of fire.

Key points for syndrome differentiation: This syndrome is marked by restlessness, insomnia, dreaminess, seminal emission, aching and weakness of loins and knees as well as manifestations of yin asthenia and hyperactivity of fire.

### 2.3.11.5 Syndrome of lung and spleen qi asthenia

Syndrome of lung and spleen qi asthenia refers to the symptoms of asthenia due to asthenia of lung and spleen qi, failure of the lung to disperse and descend as well as failure of the lung to transform. This syndrome is usually caused by cough and consumption of pulmonary qi due to prolonged disease and disorder of the child-organ involving the mother-organ; or by improper diet, impairment of the spleen and stomach involving the lung.

Clinical manifestations: Continuous cough, shortness of breath and dyspnea, profuse thin and clear sputum,

弱、心律失常、心脏神经官能症、高血压、甲状腺功能亢进症等。

证候分析：心肾阴虚，虚阳偏亢，上扰心神，则心烦少寐，惊悸多梦；肾阴亏虚，骨髓不充，脑髓、腰府失养，则头晕耳鸣，健忘，腰膝酸软；虚火内炽，扰动精室，则遗精。五心烦热，潮热盗汗，口咽干燥，舌红少苔或无苔，脉细数，为阴虚火旺的征象。

辨证要点：本证以心烦失眠，多梦遗精，腰膝酸软，以及阴虚火旺的表现为诊断依据。

### （五）肺脾气虚证

肺脾气虚证是指由于肺脾气虚，肺失宣降、脾失健运所表现的虚弱证候。本证多由于久病咳喘，耗伤肺气，子病及母；或饮食不节，脾胃受损，累及于肺而形成。

临床表现：久咳不止，气短而喘，吐痰清稀而多，食欲

poor appetite, abdominal distension and loose stool, low voice and no desire to speak, lack of energy, pale complexion, or edema of limbs, light-coloured tongue with whitish and slippery fur as well as thin and weak pulse. Such symptoms can be seen at the remission stage in chronic bronchitis, chronic bronchial asthma and chronic obstructive pulmonary emphysema as well as in immunological hypofunction due to various factors.

Analysis of the symptoms: Continuous cough, shortness of breath and dyspnea are caused by asthenia of pulmonary qi, failure of the lung to disperse and descend as well as upward adverse flow of qi; poor appetite, abdominal distension and loose stool are caused by asthenia of spleen qi, failure of transformation and transportation; profuse thin and clear sputum is caused by asthenia of qi which fails to distribute fluid and leads to attack of fluid retention on the lung; edema of limbs is caused by failure of the spleen to transform dampness due to asthenia; low voice and no desire to speak, lack of energy, pale complexion, light-coloured tongue with whitish and slippery fur as well as thin and weak pulse are the signs of qi asthenia and hypofunction of the body.

Key points for syndrome differentiation: This syndrome is marked by cough, dyspnea, shortness of breath, poor appetite and loose stool accompanied by qi asthenia and hypofunction of the body.

## 2.3.11.6 Syndrome of spleen and kidney yang asthenia

Syndrome of spleen and kidney yang asthenic refers to asthenic cold symptoms marked by diarrhea or edema due to deficiency of spleen and kidney yang as well as failure of kidney yang to warm and transform. This syndrome is usually caused by consumption of yang due to chronic disease, or by chronic diarrhea or dysentery, or by retention

不振,腹胀便溏,声低懒言,少气乏力,面白无华,或面浮肢肿,舌质淡,苔白滑,脉细弱。可见于慢性支气管炎、慢性支气管哮喘、慢性阻塞性肺气肿等病的缓解期,以及多种因素导致的免疫功能低下症。

证候分析:肺气虚,宣降失职,气逆于上,则久咳不止,气短而喘;脾气虚,运化失健,则食欲不振,腹胀便溏;气虚水津不布,湿聚为痰,上渍于肺,则吐痰清稀而多;脾虚水湿不运,泛溢肌肤,则面肢浮肿。声低懒言,少气乏力,面白无华,舌质淡,苔白滑,脉细弱,为气虚功能衰退的表现。

辨证要点:本证以咳喘气短,食少便溏,兼见气虚功能活动衰退的表现为诊断依据。

## (六)脾肾阳虚证

脾肾阳虚证是指由于脾肾阳气亏虚,温化失权,表现以泄泻或水肿为主症的虚寒证候。本证多由于久病耗气伤阳,或久泄久痢,或水邪久踞,以致肾阳虚衰不能温养脾

of pathogenic dampness, which lead to decline of kidney yang to warm and nourish spleen yang.

Clinical manifestations: Chronic diarrhea and dysentery, morning diarrhea with indigested or thin and cold stool, dropsy of face and body, abdominal distension, dysuria, cold pain in the loins and knees or lower abdomen, bright-white complexion, cold limbs and body, light-coloured and bulgy tongue with whitish slippery fur as well as deep, slow and weak pulse. Such symptoms are usually seen in chronic enteritis, malabsorption syndrome, irritable intestinal syndrome, Crohn's disease, chronic nephritis, purpuric nephritis and chronic failure of the kidney.

Analysis of the symptoms: Chronic diarrhea and dysentery, morning diarrhea with indigested or thin and cold stool are caused by asthenia of spleen and kidney yang, decline of mingmen fire and failure of fire to warm earth; dropsy of face and body, abdominal distension and dysuria are caused by asthenia of spleen and kidney yang leading to failure to warm and transform fluid and internal retention of fluid; cold pain in the loins and knees or lower abdomen are caused by decline of spleen and kidney yang to nourish the body and viscera; bright-white complexion, cold limbs and body, light-coloured and bulgy tongue with whitish slippery fur as well as deep, slow and weak pulse are the signs of internal exuberance of yin cold and internal retention of fluid cold due to yang asthenia.

Key points for syndrome differentiation: This syndrome is marked by morning diarrhea with indigested food, dropsy and cold pain in the loins and abdomen.

## 2.3.11.7 Syndrome of kidney and liver yin asthenia

Syndrome of kidney and liver yin asthenia refers to symptoms of interior disturbance of asthenia-heat due to consumption of liver and kidney yin fluid and failure of yin

阳而形成。

临床表现：久泄久痢不止，五更泄泻，完谷不化，或粪质清冷，面浮身肿，腹胀如鼓，小便不利，腰膝或下腹冷痛，面色㿠白，形寒肢冷，舌质淡胖，舌苔白滑，脉沉迟无力。可见于慢性肠炎、吸收不良综合征、肠易激综合征、克罗恩病、慢性肾炎、紫癜性肾炎、慢性肾功能衰竭等。

证候分析：脾肾阳虚，命门火衰，火不暖土，则久泄久痢不止，或五更泄泻，完谷不化，粪质清冷；脾肾阳虚，无以温化水液，水湿内停，泛溢肌肤，则面浮身肿，腹胀如鼓，小便不利；脾肾阳气虚衰，形体脏腑失于温煦，则面色㿠白，形寒肢冷，腰膝或下腹冷痛。舌质淡胖，舌苔白滑，脉沉迟无力，为阳虚阴寒内盛，水寒之气内停的征象。

辨证要点：本证以五更泄泻，完谷不化，浮肿，以及腰腹冷痛等虚寒表现为诊断依据。

## （七）肝肾阴虚证

肝肾阴虚证是指由于肝肾阴液亏虚，阴不制阳，虚热内扰所表现的证候。本证多

to control yang. This syndrome is marked by consumption of fluid due to chronic disease and improper regulation; or by interior impairment due to emotional disorder and consumption of yin due to hyperactivity of yang; or by consumption of renal essence due to intemperance of sexual life; or by exhaustion of liver and kidney yin fluid due to prolonged duration of febrile disease.

Clinical manifestations: Dizziness, tinnitus and amnesia, dull pain in the hypochondria, aching and weakness of the loins and knees, insomnia and dreaminess, seminal emission, scanty menstruation or amenorrhea, or metrorrhagia and metrostaxis, dry mouth and throat, feverish sensation over the five centers (palms, soles and chest), night sweating and flushed cheeks, reddish tongue with scanty fur, thin and rapid pulse. Such symptoms are usually seen in various consumptive diseases (such as chronic hepatitis, cirrhosis of liver, liver cancer, chronic nephritis, diabetic nephritis, renal tuberculosis, kidney cancer, bladder cancer, systemic lupus erythematosus) and at the rehabilitative stage of various infectious diseases (such as sicca syndrome and sterility).

Analysis of the symptoms: Dizziness, tinnitus and amnesia are caused by consumption of liver and kidney yin; dull pain in the hypochondria, aching and weakness of the loins and knees are caused by asthenia of liver and kidney yin and lack of proper nourishment; insomnia and dreaminess are caused by interior heat disturbing mind due to yin asthenia; seminal emission is caused by asthenia-fire disturbing essence source; scanty menstruation or amenorrhea is caused by asthenia of liver and kidney yin to replenish the thoroughfare and conception vessels; metrorrhagia and metrostaxis are caused by superabundance of fire disturbing the thoroughfare and conception vessels due to yin asthenia; dry mouth and throat, feverish sensa-

由于久病失调,阴液亏虚;或情志内伤,阳亢耗阴;或房事不节,耗损肾之阴精;或温热病日久,肝肾阴液被劫所致。

临床表现:头晕目眩,耳鸣健忘,胁痛隐隐,腰膝酸软,失眠多梦,男子遗精,女子月经量少或经闭,或崩漏,口燥咽干,五心烦热,盗汗颧红,舌红少苔,脉细而数。可见于慢性肝炎、肝硬化、肝癌、慢性肾炎、糖尿病肾病、肾结核、肾癌、膀胱癌、系统性红斑狼疮等慢性消耗性疾病,干燥综合征,不孕症,以及多种感染性疾病的恢复期等。

证候分析:肝肾阴亏,水不涵木,肝阳上扰,则头晕目眩,耳鸣健忘;肝肾阴虚,失于濡养,则胁痛隐隐,腰膝酸软;阴虚内热,扰乱心神,则失眠多梦;虚火扰动精室,则男子遗精;肝肾阴虚,冲任失于充养,则女子月经量少或经闭;阴虚火旺,热扰冲任,则崩漏。口燥咽干,五心烦热,盗汗颧红,舌红少苔,脉细而数,为阴虚失润,虚火内炽的表现。

tion over the five centers (palms, soles and chest), night sweating and flushed cheeks, reddish tongue with scanty fur, thin and rapid pulse are the signs of lack of moistening due to yin asthenia and interior exuberance of asthenia fire.

Key points for syndrome differentiation: This syndrome is marked by aching and weakness of the loins and knees, hypochondriac pain, dizziness, tinnitus and seminal emission as well as interior heat due to yin asthenia.

### 2.3.11.8 Syndrome of liver fire invading lung

Syndrome of liver fire invading lung refers to the symptoms of the lung failing to depurate and clear due to invasion of adverse movement of fire in the liver meridian into the lung. According to the theory of five elements, it is called "wood-fire tormenting metal". This syndrome is usually caused by impairment of liver due to depression and rage and stagnation of qi transforming into fire; or by accumulation of pathogenic heat in the liver meridian attacking the lung.

Clinical manifestations: Scorching pain in the chest and hypochondria, irritability and susceptibility to rage, dizziness and distension of head, flushed cheeks and red eyes, restless fever and bitter taste in the mouth, paroxysmal cough, yellowish thick and sticky sputum, or hemoptysis, dry feces, yellowish and reddish urine, reddish tongue, yellowish thin fur and taut and rapid pulse. Such symptoms are usually seen in bronchiectasis, pulmonary tuberculosis, endobronchial tuberculosis and lung cancer.

Analysis of the symptoms: Scorching pain in the chest and hypochondria, irritability and susceptibility to rage, dizziness and distension of head, flushed cheeks and red eyes are caused by internal stagnation of liver meridian qi and fire; restless fever and bitter taste in the mouth are caused by heat steaming gallbladder qi; paroxysmal

辨证要点：本证以腰膝酸软，胁痛，眩晕耳鸣，遗精，以及阴虚内热的表现为诊断依据。

### （八）肝火犯肺证

肝火犯肺证是指由于肝经气火上逆犯肺，使肺失清肃所表现的证候。按五行理论又称"木火刑金"。本证多由于郁怒伤肝，气郁化火；或邪热蕴结肝经，上犯于肺所致。

临床表现：胸胁灼痛，急躁易怒，头晕头胀，面红目赤，烦热口苦，咳嗽阵作，痰黄稠粘，或咳血，大便干结，小便黄赤，舌质红，苔薄黄，脉弦数。可见于支气管扩张、肺结核、支气管内膜结核、肺癌等。

证候分析：肝经气火内郁，则胸胁灼痛，急躁易怒，头晕头胀，面红目赤；热蒸胆气上逆，则烦热口苦；肝火犯肺，肺失清肃，则咳嗽阵作，痰黄稠粘；火热内盛，灼伤肺络，则

cough, yellowish thick and sticky sputum are caused by liver fire attacking the lung and failure of the lung to clear and depurate; hemoptysis is caused by internal exuberance of fire and heat impairing pulmonary collaterals; dry feces, yellowish and reddish urine are caused by exuberant heat consuming fluid; reddish tongue, yellowish thin fur and taut and rapid pulse are the signs of internal exuberance of sthenia-fire in the liver meridian.

Key points for syndrome differentiation: This syndrome is marked by cough, hemoptysis, scorching pain in the chest and hypochondria, susceptibility to anger and internal exuberance of sthenia-fire.

## 2.3.11.9 Syndrome of imbalance between liver and spleen

Syndrome of imbalance between liver and spleen refers the symptoms of chest and hypochondriac distending pain, abdominal distension and loose stool due to failure of the liver to disperse and convey as well as dysfunction of the spleen. This syndrome is mainly caused by emotional upsets, impairment of the liver due to depression and rage as well as attack of the liver qi on the spleen due to failure of the liver to act freely; or by impairment of the spleen due to improper diet and overstrain as well as the spleen reversely restraining the liver due to dysfunction of the spleen.

Clinical manifestations: Distending pain and wandering pain in the chest and hypochondria, susceptibility to sigh, emotional depression, irritability and susceptibility to rage, anorexia and abdominal distension, loose stool and retention of feces or loose stool and unsmooth defecation, borborygmus and breaking wind, or abdominal pain with desire of diarrhea, alleviation of pain after diarrhea, whitish tongue fur, taut pulse or slow and weak pulse. Such symptoms are usually seen in chronic enteritis, irri-

咳血不止；热盛伤津，则大便干结，小便黄赤。舌质红，苔薄黄，脉弦数，为肝经实火内炽的征象。

辨证要点：本证以咳嗽，咳血，胸胁灼痛，易怒，以及实火内炽的表现为诊断依据。

## （九）肝脾不调证

肝脾不调证是指肝失疏泄，脾失健运而表现以胸胁胀痛、腹胀、便溏为主症的证候。本证多由于情志不遂，郁怒伤肝，肝失条达而横乘脾土；或饮食、劳倦伤脾，脾失健运而反侮于肝所致。

临床表现：胸胁胀痛窜痛，善太息，情志抑郁，急躁易怒，纳呆腹胀，大便溏结不调或便溏不爽，肠鸣矢气，或腹痛欲泻，泻后痛减，舌苔薄白，脉弦或缓弱。可见于慢性肠炎、肠易激综合征、过敏性结肠炎、吸收不良综合征、慢性肝炎等。

table intestinal syndrome, allergic colitis, malabsorption syndrome and chronic hepatitis.

Analysis of the symptoms: Distending pain and wandering pain in the chest and hypochondria, susceptibility to sigh, emotional depression, irritability and susceptibility to rage are caused by failure of the liver to disperse and convey as well as stagnation of qi; anorexia and abdominal distension, loose stool and retention of feces are caused by invasion of adverse liver qi into the spleen and dysfunction of the spleen; loose stool and unsmooth defecation, borborygmus and breaking wind, or abdominal pain with desire of diarrhea are caused by stagnation of qi and retention of dampness; alleviation of pain after diarrhea is due to the fact that stagnation of qi is relieved after defecation; whitish tongue fur, taut pulse or slow and weak pulse are the signs of liver depression and spleen asthenia.

Key points for syndrome differentiation: This syndrome is marked by chest and hypochondriac distension and fullness, anorexia, abdominal pain and borborygmus as well as loose stool and diarrhea.

### 2.3.11.10 Syndrome of incoordination between liver and stomach

Syndrome of incoordination between liver and stomach refers to the symptoms of epigastric and hypochondriac distension and pain due to stagnation of liver qi which invades the stomach and prevents gastric qi from normal descending. This syndrome is mainly caused by emotional upsets, stagnation of liver qi and invasion of liver qi into the stomach.

Clinical manifestations: Hypochondriac and epigastric distending pain or wandering pain, hiccup, belching, acid regurgitation, anorexia, mental depression, irritability and susceptibility to anger and sigh, whitish thin or yellowish thin tongue fur, taut pulse or taut and rapid pulse.

证候分析：肝失疏泄，气机郁滞，则胸胁胀痛窜痛，善太息，情志抑郁，急躁易怒；肝气横逆犯脾，脾失健运，则纳呆腹胀，大便溏结不调；气滞湿阻，则便溏不爽，肠鸣矢气，或腹痛欲泻；排便后气滞得以缓解，故泻后痛减。舌苔薄白，脉弦或缓弱，为肝郁脾虚的征象。

辨证要点：本证以胸胁胀满，纳呆，腹痛肠鸣，大便溏泄为诊断依据。

### （十）肝胃不和证

肝胃不和证是指由于肝气郁滞，横逆犯胃，胃失和降而表现以脘胁胀痛为主症的证候。本证多由于情志不舒，肝气郁结，横逆犯胃所致。

临床表现：胁肋、胃脘胀满疼痛，或窜痛，呃逆，嗳气，吞酸嘈杂，食纳减少，情绪抑郁，烦躁易怒，善太息，舌苔薄白或薄黄，脉弦或弦数。可见

Such symptoms are usually seen in acute gastritis, chronic gastritis, digestive ulcer, reflux esophagitis, cholecystitis and gallstones.

Analysis of the symptoms: Hypochondriac and epigastric distending pain or wandering pain are caused by failure of the liver to disperse and convey, invasion of adverse flowing liver qi into the stomach and failure of gastric qi to descend; hiccup, belching, acid regurgitation and anorexia are caused by stagnation of qi and fire in the stomach and adverse flow of gastric qi; mental depression, irritability and susceptibility to anger and sigh are caused by failure of the liver to act freely, stagnation of qi and transformation of fire from stagnated qi; whitish thin or yellowish thin tongue fur, taut pulse or taut and rapid pulse are the signs of stagnation of liver qi and transformation of fire from stagnated qi.

Key points for syndrome differentiation: This syndrome is marked by distending pain or wandering pain in the chest, hypochondria and stomach as well as hiccup and retching.

### 2.3.11.11 Syndrome of damp-heat in liver and gallbladder

Syndrome of damp-heat in liver and gallbladder refers to the symptoms of dysfunction in dispersion and conveyance due to accumulation of damp-heat in the liver and gallbladder. This syndrome is usually caused by pathogenic damp-heat; or by partiality to greasy and sweet foods which causes internal generation of damp-heat; or by dysfunction of the stomach and spleen which leads to internal production of dampness and the spleen reversely restraining the liver, resulting in accumulation of damp-heat in the liver and gallbladder.

Clinical manifestations: Hypochondriac scorching distending pain, or hypochondriac mass, anorexia and

于急性胃炎、慢性胃炎、消化性溃疡、反流性食管炎、胆囊炎、胆石症等。

证候分析：肝失疏泄，横逆犯胃，胃失和降，则胁肋、胃脘胀满疼痛，或窜痛；气火内郁犯胃，胃气上逆，则呃逆、嗳气，吞酸嘈杂，食纳减少；肝失条达，气机郁滞，气郁化火，则情绪抑郁，烦躁易怒，胸闷善太息。舌苔薄白或薄黄，脉弦或弦数，为肝气郁结，气郁化火的表现。

辨证要点：本证以胸胁、胃脘胀痛，或窜痛，呃逆嗳气为诊断依据。

### （十一）肝胆湿热证

肝胆湿热证是指由于湿热蕴结肝胆，疏泄功能失职所表现的证候。本证多由于感受湿热之邪；或嗜食肥甘，湿热内生；或胃脾纳运失常，湿浊内生，土壅侮木，致使湿热蕴阻肝胆所致。

临床表现：胁肋灼热胀痛，或有痞块，厌食腹胀，口

abdominal distension, bitter taste in the mouth, acid regurgitation and nausea, disorder of defecation, scanty and reddish urine, or alternate chills and fever, yellow coloration of the skin and eyes, or pudendal pruritus, or foul and yellowish leukorrhea, reddish tongue with yellowish and greasy fur, taut and rapid pulse or slippery and rapid pulse. Such symptoms are usually seen in various digestive system diseases (such as viral hepatitis, cirrhosis of liver, jaundice, cholecystitis, pancreatitis, liver cancer, gallbladder cancer and pancreas cancer) as well as orchitis, scrotal eczema, pelvic inflammation and vaginitis.

Analysis of the symptoms: Hypochondriac scorching distending pain, or hypochondriac mass are caused by accumulation of damp-heat, dysfunction of the liver and gallbladder in dispersion and conveyance, stagnation of qi and unsmooth circulation of blood; bitter taste in the mouth is caused by stagnation and steaming of damp-heat; yellow coloration of the skin and eyes is caused by dysfunction of the liver and gallbladder in dispersion and conveyance which leads to extravasation of the bile in the skin and muscles; acid regurgitation and nausea, disorder of defecation, scanty and reddish urine, or alternate chills and fever, anorexia and abdominal distension are caused by stagnation of damp-heat and disorder of the spleen and stomach in ascending and descending; pudendal pruritus, or foul and yellowish leukorrhea are caused by downward migration of damp-heat along the liver meridian; reddish tongue with yellowish and greasy fur, taut and rapid pulse or slippery and rapid pulse are the signs of stagnation of steaming of damp-heat in the liver and gallbladder.

Key points for syndrome differentiation: This syndrome is marked by distending pain in the hypochondria and rib-side, anorexia, abdominal distension, coloration of the skin and eyes and pudendal pruritus.

苦,泛恶欲呕,大便不调,小便短赤,或见寒热往来,身目发黄,或阴部瘙痒,或带下色黄臭秽,舌红苔黄腻,脉弦数或滑数。可见于病毒性肝炎、肝硬化、黄疸、胆囊炎、胆石症、胰腺炎、肝癌、胆囊癌、胰腺癌等消化系统疾病,以及睾丸炎、阴囊湿疹、盆腔炎、阴道炎等。

证候分析:湿热蕴结,肝胆疏泄失职,气机郁滞,血行不畅,故胁肋灼热胀痛,或有痞块;湿热郁蒸,胆气上溢则口苦;湿热蕴结,肝胆疏泄失职,胆汁不循常道而外溢肌肤,则身目发黄;湿热郁阻,脾胃升降失司,运纳失常,故厌食,腹胀,泛恶欲呕,大便不调,小便短赤;邪居少阳,故见寒热往来;肝经湿热下注,可见阴部瘙痒,或带下色黄臭秽。舌红苔黄腻,脉弦数或滑数,为肝胆湿热郁蒸的征象。

辨证要点:本证以胁肋胀痛,厌食腹胀,身目发黄,阴部瘙痒等湿热内蕴的表现为诊断依据。

## 2.4 Other syndrome differentiation methods

### 2.4.1 Introduction to six-meridians syndrome differentiation

Six-meridians syndrome differentiation, a method developed by Zhang Zhongjing, a celebrated doctor in the Han Dynasty, is the principle for syndrome differentiation and treatment in Treatise on Seasonal Febrile Disease and is the basis of syndrome differentiation for the later generations.

Six-meridians syndrome differentiation categorizes the stages of exogenous febrile diseases into six types for selection of treatment according to the main principle of yin and yang, namely taiyang disease, yangming disease, shaoyang disease, taiyin disease, shaoyin disease and jueyin disease.

Six-meridians diseases reflect the pathological changes of the meridians and viscera. Among the six types of diseases, taiyang disease pertains to the external, yangming disease to the internal, shaoyang disease to the semi-external and semi-internal; while the three yin types all pertain to the internal. The three yang types of disease reflect the pathological changes of the six fu organs, while the three yin types of diseases reflect the pathological changes of the five zang organs. So the six-meridians diseases include the pathological changes of both the twelve meridians and viscera. Since the six-meridians syndrome differentiation focuses on the analysis of the pathological changes and transmission rule of diseases caused by exogenous wind-cold, they are not identical with syndrome differentiation of viscera.

第四节 其他辨证方法简介

一、六经辨证概要

六经辨证是汉代张仲景创立的主要用于外感病的一种辨证方法。是《伤寒论》辨证论治的纲领,并为后世各种辨证方法的形成奠定了基础。

六经辨证将外感病发生发展过程中不同阶段所表现的证候,以阴阳为纲,归纳为太阳病、阳明病、少阳病、太阴病、少阴病、厥阴病六类不同证候类型,作为论治的基础。

六经病证是经络、脏腑病理变化的反映。其中,太阳病属表,阳明病属里,少阳病属半表半里,三阴病统属于里。三阳病以六腑病变为基础,三阴病以五脏病变为基础。所以,六经病证基本概括了脏腑和十二经的病变。但由于六经辨证的重点在于分析外感风寒所引起的一系列病理变化及其传变规律,因此不能完全等同于脏腑辨证。

### 2.4.1.1 Taiyang syndrome

Taiyang governs the superficies and controls both nutrient and defensive qi. When wind and cold attacks the human body, it first invades taiyang. Then defensive qi will take action to resist. The struggle between pathogenic factors and healthy qi in the superficies brings about taiyang meridian disease which reflects the primary stage of exogenous febrile disease. If the pathogenic factors are not relieved and enter the fu organs along the meridians, it will cause taiyang fu syndrome.

#### 2.4.1.1.1 Taiyang meridian syndrome

Taiyang meridian syndrome, the disease caused by invasion of pathogenic factors into the superficies, may be divided into taiyang wind-attack syndrome and taiyang cold-attack syndrome according to the constitution of the patients and the nature of pathogenic factors.

**Taiyang wind-attack syndrome**: A syndrome caused by invasion of pathogenic wind into the superficies and disorder of nutrient and defensive qi.

Clinical manifestations: Fever, aversion to wind, sweating, stiffness and pain in the neck and head, whitish thin tongue fur and floating and slow pulse.

Analysis of the symptoms: Fever is caused by invasion of pathogenic wind into the superficies and struggle between defensive qi and pathogenic factors; sweating and aversion to wind are caused by looseness of the muscular interstices and failure of nutrient qi to keep inside because wind tends to open and disperse; stiffness and pain in the neck and head are caused by pathogenic wind attack and disorder of meridian qi because taiyang meridians converge over the head and distribute down to the neck from the head; whitish thin tongue fur is due to the fact that pathogenic factors are still retained in the skin and have penetrated inside; floating and slow pulse is the sign of

### （一）太阳病证

太阳主一身之表，统摄营卫。风寒侵袭人体，太阳首当其冲，卫气奋起抗邪，正邪相争于表，产生太阳经证，是伤寒病的初期阶段。如病邪不解，循经入腑，则出现太阳腑证。

**1. 太阳经证**

太阳经证是指邪气侵袭肌表所致的病证。因患者体质不同，感邪性质各异，又分为太阳中风证和太阳伤寒证。

（1）太阳中风证：太阳中风证是指风邪袭表，营卫失调所表现的证候。

临床表现：发热，恶风，汗出，头项强痛，苔薄白，脉浮缓。

证候分析：风邪袭表，卫阳与邪气相争则发热；风性开泄，腠理疏松，营阴不能内守，则汗出、恶风；太阳经交巅顶、经脑下项，风邪侵袭，经气不舒，则头项强痛；邪在肌表，尚未入里，故苔仍薄白。脉浮缓为表虚的征象。

external asthenia.

**Taiyang cold-attack syndrome**: The disease caused by invasion of pathogenic cold into the superficies, obstruction of defensive qi and stagnation of nutrient qi.

Clinical manifestations: Aversion to cold, fever, no sweating, or dyspnea, stiffness and pain in the neck and head, body pain, whitish thin tongue fur and floating and tense pulse.

Analysis of the symptoms: Aversion to cold is caused by cold attacking the superficies, and stagnation of defensive qi; fever is caused by struggle between defensive qi and healthy qi; no sweating and dyspnea are caused by obstruction of the muscular interstices and failure of the lung to disperse and descend; pain in the head and body is caused by stagnation of nutrient qi and inhibited flow of meridian qi; whitish thin tongue fur, floating and tense pulse are the signs of wind and cold attacking the superficies.

#### 2.4.1.1.2 Taiyang fu syndrome

Taiyang fu syndrome refers to the syndrome due to failure to relieve taiyang meridian syndrome and transmission of pathogenic factors into the bladder along the meridians. It may be divided into taiyang water-accumulation syndrome and taiyang blood-accumulation syndrome according to the pathogenesis.

**Taiyang water-accumulation syndrome**: A syndrome caused by hypofunction of the bladder in transforming qi and accumulation and retention of water due to failure to relieve taiyang meridian syndrome and transmission of pathogenic factors into the bladder.

Clinical manifestations: Fever, aversion to cold, dysuria, lower abdominal distension and fullness, thirst, vomiting after drinking water and floating pulse.

Analysis of the symptoms: Fever, aversion to cold

（2）太阳伤寒证：太阳伤寒证是指寒邪袭表，卫阳被遏，营阴郁滞所表现的证候。

临床表现：恶寒，发热，无汗，或喘，头项强痛，身痛，苔薄白，脉浮紧。

证候分析：寒邪束表，卫阳被遏，则恶寒；卫阳与邪气相争则发热；腠理闭塞，肺失宣降，则无汗而喘；营阴郁滞，经气不利，则头身疼痛。苔薄白，脉浮紧，为风寒束表之象。

2. 太阳腑证

太阳腑证是指太阳经证不解，病邪循经内传下焦膀胱所表现的证候。根据病机之不同，又分为太阳蓄水证和太阳蓄血证。

（1）太阳蓄水证：太阳蓄水证是指太阳经证不解，病邪内传膀胱，致膀胱气化不利，水液停蓄所表现的证候。

临床表现：发热，恶寒，小便不利，小腹胀满，口渴，水入即吐，脉浮。

证候分析：太阳经证不

and floating pulse are caused by failure to relieve taiyang meridian syndrome; dysuria and lower abdominal distension and fullness are caused by transmission of pathogenic heat into the bladder and dysfunction of the bladder in transforming qi; thirst is due to retention of fluid and failure of qi to distribute fluid; vomiting after drinking is due to indigestion and adverse flow of gastric qi.

**Taiyang blood-accumulation syndrome**: This syndrome is caused by internal transmission of pathogenic factors and its mixture with blood in the lower energizer due to failure to relieve taiyang meridian syndrome.

Clinical manifestations: Lower abdominal spasm, fullness or mass, normal urination, mania, deep and unsmooth pulse or deep and knotted pulse.

Analysis of the symptoms: Lower abdominal spasm or even hard mass is due to improper treatment of taiyang meridian syndrome which leads to transmission of pathogenic heat into the internal and its mixture with blood in the lower abdomen; mania is caused by internal stagnation of heat disturbing mind; normal urination is due to the fact that the disease still remains in blood phase and has not affect the function of the bladder in transforming qi; deep and unsmooth or deep and knotted pulse is the sign of obstruction due to stagnation of heat and inhibited flow of blood.

### 2.4.1.2　Yangming syndrome

Yangming syndrome, the syndrome due to invasion of pathogenic factors into yangming meridian, hyperactivity of yang heat and dry-heat in the stomach and intestines, is the critical stage during the course of struggle between pathogenic factors and healthy qi in exogenous febrile disease. Yangming syndrome is usually caused by delayed or improper treatment of taiyang disease which leads to pathogenic factors transmitting inside and transforming into

解,则发热,恶寒,脉浮;邪热内传膀胱,气化功能失职,则小便不利,小腹胀满;水液内停,气不布津,则口渴;水入不消,胃气上逆则吐。

(2)太阳蓄血证:太阳蓄血证是指太阳经证不解,病邪内传,与血相结于下焦所表现的证候。

临床表现:少腹急结或硬满,小便自利,如狂或发狂,脉沉涩或沉结。

证候分析:太阳经证失治,邪热循经内传,与血相结于少腹,故少腹急结,甚则硬满;瘀热内结,上扰心神,故见神志错乱如狂;病在血分,未影响膀胱气化功能,故小便自利。脉沉涩或沉结,是瘀热阻滞,脉道不利之征。

(二)阳明病证

阳明病证是指邪入阳明,阳热亢盛,胃肠燥热所表现的证候。为伤寒病发展过程中邪正斗争的极期阶段。阳明病的发病,多由太阳病失治、误治,病邪内传阳明化热所致;亦有津液素亏而阳气偏盛之人,初感外邪直接引发的。

heat; or by exogenous factors attack on people with frequent deficiency of body fluid and relative superabundance of yangqi. Yangming syndrome can be divided into yangming meridian syndrome and yangming fu syndrome according to the location of disease and the characteristics of syndrome.

#### 2.4.1.2.1 Yangming meridian syndrome

Yangming meridian syndrome refers to the syndrome with no retention of feces in the intestines due to hyperactivity of pathogenic heat.

Clinical manifestations: High fever, no aversion to cold but aversion to heat, profuse sweating, polydipsia, flushed cheeks and dysphoria, reddish tongue with yellowish dry fur and full and large pulse.

Analysis of the symptoms: Fever, flushed cheeks, no aversion to cold but aversion to heat are due to invasion of pathogenic factors into yangming meridian, transformation of heat and dryness, hyperactivity of dryness and heat all over the body; profuse sweating is caused by internal accumulation of heat driving fluid out of the body; polydipsia and yellowish dry tongue fur are caused by excessive heat consuming body fluid; dysphoria is due to heat disturbing mind; full and large pulse is due to superabundance of heat and rapid flow of blood.

#### 2.4.1.2.2 Yangming fu syndrome

Yangming fu syndrome refers to the syndrome with retention of dry feces in the intestines due to mixture of superabundance of pathogenic heat with waste materials in the intestines.

Clinical manifestations: Fever, afternoon tidal fever, continuous sweating over hands and feet, abdominal hardness and fullness with unpressable pain, constipation, restlessness, even delirium, yellowish dry tongue fur or brownish tongue fur, tongue with prickles, deep and pow-

根据病变部位及证候特点的不同，有阳明经证与阳明腑证之分。

**1. 阳明经证**

阳明经证是指邪热亢盛，而肠中无燥屎内结所表现的证候。

临床表现：身大热，不恶寒反恶热，大汗出，大渴引饮，面赤心烦，舌红苔黄燥，脉洪大。

证候分析：邪入阳明，化热化燥，燥热亢盛，弥漫全身，则身热面赤、不恶寒反恶热；热蒸于里，迫津外泄，则大汗出；热盛津伤，则口渴引饮，舌苔黄燥；热扰心神则心烦；热盛血涌则脉洪大。

**2. 阳明腑证**

阳明腑证是指邪热内盛，与肠中糟粕相搏，燥屎内结所表现的证候。

临床表现：身热，日晡潮热，手足濈然汗出，腹满硬痛，拒按，大便秘结，烦躁，甚则神昏谵语，舌苔黄燥或焦黄，舌起芒刺，脉沉实有力。

erful pulse.

Analysis of the symptoms: Fever and sweating are caused by superabundance of heat inside; tidal fever is due to struggle between meridian qi and pathogenic factors because yangming meridian qi is in its peak in the afternoon; constipation and abdominal hardness and fullness with unpressable pain are caused by mixture of dry-heat in the yangming meridian and waste materials in the intestines which leads to retention of dry feces in the intestines; restlessness or even deli-rium is caused by pathogenic heat disturbing the mind; yellowish dry tongue fur or brownish tongue fur, tongue with prickles, deep and powerful pulse are the signs of superabundant heat consuming fluid and internal retention of sthenia-pathogenic factors.

### 2.4.1.3 Shaoyang syndrome

Shaoyang syndrome refers to the syndrome due to pathogenic factors attacking the gallbladder. This syndrome is usually caused by internal invasion of pathogenic factors into the gallbladder when the taiyang disease is not relieved yet. The struggle between healthy qi and pathogenic factors in the external and internal causes shaoyang syndrome. Or it may be caused by direct invasion of pathogenic factors into shaoyang.

Clinical manifestations: Alternate chills and fever, chest and hypochondriac discomfort and fullness, no appetite, vexation and susceptibility to vomiting, bitter taste in the mouth and dry throat, dizziness and taut pulse.

Analysis of the symptoms: Alternate chills and fever is due to struggle between healthy qi and pathogenic factors in the external and internal in which predomination of healthy qi leads to fever and predomination of pathogenic factors results in cold; chest and hypochondriac discomfort and fullness is caused by stagnation of pathogenic factors in shaoyang meridian which circulates along the rib-sides;

证候分析：里热炽盛，蒸腾于外，则身热汗出；日晡正当阳明经气旺时，经气与邪气相争，则发潮热；阳明燥热与肠中糟粕相搏，燥屎内结，腑气不通，则便秘，腹满硬痛，拒按；邪热上扰心神，则烦躁，甚则神昏谵语。苔黄燥或焦黄、舌起芒刺，脉沉实有力，为热盛津伤，实邪内阻的征象。

### （三）少阳病证

少阳病证是指邪犯少阳胆腑，枢机不利所表现的证候。多因太阳病不解，病邪内侵，郁于胆腑，正邪分争于表里之间所致，亦可由病邪直犯少阳而产生。

临床表现：寒热往来，胸胁苦满，默默不欲饮食，心烦喜呕，口苦咽干，目眩，脉弦。

证候分析：邪犯少阳，正邪相争于表里之间，正胜则热，邪胜则寒，正邪互胜，故寒热往来；胆之经脉循于两胁，邪郁少阳，经气不畅，故胸胁苦满；胆热犯胃，胃失和降，则默默不欲饮食，呕吐；热郁则

no appetite and vomiting are caused by gallbladder heat invading the stomach and preventing the stomach qi from normal descent; vexation is due to stagnation of heat; bitter taste in the mouth, dry throat and dizziness are caused by upward migration of gallbladder heat along the meridian; taut pulse is the sign of shaoyang disorder.

### 2.4.1.4　Taiyin syndrome

Taiyin syndrome refers to the syndrome due to decline of spleen yang and internal superabundance of cold-dampness. This syndrome is caused by delayed and wrong treatment of three yang meridian diseases which impairs spleen yang; or by insufficiency of spleen yang and direct attack of pathogenic cold on the spleen.

Clinical manifestations: Abdominal fullness and vomiting, poor appetite, diarrhea, frequent abdominal pain, preference for warmth and pressure, no thirst, light-coloured tongue with white fur and slow and weak pulse.

Analysis of the symptoms: Abdominal fullness, frequent abdominal pain, preference for warmth and pressure and poor appetite are caused by decline of spleen yang, internal exuberance of cold-dampness and stagnation of qi, diarrhea is caused by failure of spleen qi to rise and downward migration of cold-dampness; vomiting is caused by failure of gastric qi to descend; no thirst, light-coloured tongue with white fur and slow and weak pulse are signs of asthenia-cold syndrome.

### 2.4.1.5　Shaoyin syndrome

Shaoyin syndrome refers to the syndrome at the advanced stage of six-meridians pathological changes due to cold-attack. This syndrome is divided into shaoyin cold-transformation syndrome and shaoyin heat-transformation syndrome according to the pathogenic factors and constitution of the patient.

心烦；胆热循经上炎则口苦咽干、目眩。脉弦为病在少阳的征象。

### （四）太阴病证

太阴病证是指脾阳虚衰，寒湿内盛所表现的证候。本证可由三阳病失治、误治，损伤脾阳而成；亦可因中阳不足，寒邪直中太阴而发病。

临床表现：腹满呕吐，食欲不振，腹泻，时腹自痛，喜温喜按，口不渴，舌淡苔白，脉缓弱。

证候分析：脾阳虚衰，寒湿内盛，气机郁滞，则腹满时痛，喜温喜按，食欲不振；脾气不升，寒湿下注则腹泻；胃气不降，浊气上逆则呕吐。口不渴、舌淡苔白、脉缓弱为虚寒证的表现。

### （五）少阴病证

少阴病证是伤寒六经病变发展过程的后期阶段。由于致病因素和体质的不同，有少阴寒化证和少阴热化证两大类型。

### 2.4.1.5.1 Shaoyin cold-transformation syndrome

Shaoyin cold-transformation syndrome refers to the syndrome due to asthenia of heart and kidney yang and pathogenic factors transforming into cold following the nature of yin. This syndrome is usually caused by impairment of heart and kidney yangqi due to delayed and wrong treatment; or by frequent asthenia of the heart and kidney as well as direct attack of pathogenic cold on shaoyin.

Clinical manifestations: Aversion to cold and curled posture in sleep, dispiritedness and sleepiness, cold limbs, diarrhea with indigested food, no thirst or thirst with preference for hot drinks, clear and profuse urine, light-coloured tongue with white fur and deep and indistinct pulse.

Analysis of the symptoms: Aversion to cold and curled posture in sleep, dispiritedness and sleepiness as well as cold limbs are caused by decline of heart and kidney yangqi and lack of warmth; diarrhea with indigested food is caused by decline of kidney yang to warm the spleen to transform food; no thirst is due to internal exuberance of yin cold; thirst with preference for hot drinks is due to failure of kidney to transform qi and produce fluid resulting from asthenia of kidney yang or due to excessive diarrhea consuming body fluid; clear and profuse urine, light-coloured tongue with white fur and deep and indistinct pulse are the signs of decline of yang and exuberance of yin.

### 2.4.1.5.2 Shaoyin heat-transformation syndrome

Shaoyin heat-transformation syndrome refers to the syndrome of asthenia-heat due to asthenia of heart and kidney yin, hyperactivity of heart and kidney yang as well as pathogenic factors transforming into heat from yang.

### 1. 少阴寒化证

少阴寒化证是指心肾阳虚,病邪从阴化寒所表现的虚寒证候。本证多因失治、误治,损伤心肾阳气;或因心、肾素虚,寒邪直中少阴而发病。

临床表现:畏寒蜷卧,精神委靡欲寐,四肢厥冷,下利清谷,口不渴或渴喜热饮,小便清长,舌淡苔白,脉沉微。

证候分析:心肾阳气虚衰,无以温养形体,则畏寒蜷卧、精神委靡欲寐、四肢厥冷;肾阳虚衰,不能温煦脾土以运化水谷,则下利清谷;阴寒内盛,故口不渴;肾阳虚衰,不能化气生津,或下利太甚,损伤津液,则口渴喜热饮,饮量不多。小便清长,舌淡苔白,脉沉微等为阳衰阴盛之象。

### 2. 少阴热化证

少阴热化证是指心肾阴虚阳亢,病邪从阳化热所表现的虚热证候。本证多因邪热不解而耗伤真阴,或素体阴

This syndrome is caused by failure to relieve pathogenic heat and consumption of kidney yin; or by frequent yin asthenia, invasion of pathogenic factors into shaoyin, transformation of pathogenic factors into heat following the nature of yang and consumption of kidney yin scorched by heat.

Clinical manifestations: Vexation and insomnia, dry mouth and throat, reddish tongue tip or deep-red tongue and thin and rapid pulse.

Analysis of the symptoms: Vexation and insomnia are due to deficiency of kidney yin, disharmony between water and fire which leads to hyperactivity of heart fire to disturb the mind; dry mouth and throat, reddish tongue tip or deep-red tongue and thin and rapid pulse are the signs of deficiency of water and superabundance of fire.

### 2.4.1.6 Jueyin syndrome

Jueyin syndrome appears in the advanced stage of six-meridians disorders due to cold-attack, marked by complex changes and mixture of cold and heat in pathogenesis. Upper-heat and lower-cold syndrome is taken as an example to show the characteristics of this syndrome. Jueyin syndrome is usually evolved from the disease lingering in the other meridians.

Clinical manifestations: Thirst, qi rushing up into the heart, pain and feverish sensation in the heart, hunger without appetite, postcibal vomiting of ascaris, cold extremities and diarrhea.

Analysis of the symptoms: Jueyin meridian pertains to the liver and distributes beside the stomach and through the diaphragm. So jueyin disease is marked by dysfunction of the liver and stomach. Complex of heat and cold is due to the fact that jueyin disorder affects dispersion and conveyance which leads to disorder of qi and imbalance between yin and yang; thirst, qi rushing up into the

虚,邪入少阴,从阳化热,热灼真阴所致。

临床表现:心烦不得眠,口燥咽干,舌尖红,或舌绛少苔,脉细数。

证候分析:肾水亏虚,水不济火,致心火独亢,心神被扰,则心烦不得眠;口燥咽干,舌尖红,舌绛少苔,脉细数,为水亏火旺之象。

### (六)厥阴病证

厥阴病证是伤寒六经病变发展过程的较后阶段,病变极为复杂,其病机变化以寒热错杂为基本特点。现以上热下寒证为例说明之。厥阴病多因病在它经不愈发展而成。

临床表现:口渴,气上冲心,心中疼热,饥不欲食,食则吐蛔,厥逆,下利。

证候分析:厥阴之脉属肝挟胃,上贯膈,故厥阴病多出现肝、胃功能失调的症状。厥阴为病,疏泄不利,以致气机逆乱,阴阳失调,故证见寒热错杂。口渴,气上冲心,心中疼热,饥不欲食,强食则吐是

heart, pain and feverish sensation in the heart, hunger without appetite and postcibal vomiting are caused by invasion of adverse flowing liver qi into the stomach as well as heat in the stomach and adverse flow of qi; diarrhea is due to spleen asthenia and cold in the intestines; postcibal vomiting of ascaris is due to upper-heat and lower-cold which drives ascaris to move upward with the rise of gastric qi.

The theory of six-meridians syndrome differentiation holds that the relation between pathogenic factors and viscera, meridians, qi and blood is characterized by transmission, combination of syndromes, complication and direct attack. The change of one meridian disorder into another meridian disorder is called meridian transmission; simultaneous of syndromes involving two or three yang meridians is called combination of syndromes; onset of another meridian disorder before one meridian disorder is relieved is called complication; if pathogenic factors at the primary stage of exogenous febrile disease do not transmit from the yang meridians but directly attack three yin meridians, it is called direct attack.

### 2.4.2 Introduction to syndrome differentiation of defensive qi, qi, nutrient qi and blood

Syndrome differentiation of defensive qi, qi, nutrient qi and blood is a syndrome differentiation method for exogenous epidemic febrile disease developed by Ye Tianshi in the Qing Dynasty. It summarizes the symptoms of exogenous epidemic febrile disease at different stages into four types for the benefit of treatment, namely defensive phase syndrome, qi phase syndrome, nutrient phase syndrome and blood phase syndrome.

Syndrome differentiation of defensive qi, qi, nutrient

肝气横逆犯胃,胃热气逆的表现;下利是脾虚、肠中有寒的表现;上热下寒,蛔虫窜动,随胃气上逆而吐出。

六经辨证理论认为,伤寒病发展过程中,病邪与机体脏腑经络气血之间的力量对比变化,表现为六经病证的传变、合病、并病及直中等多种形式。若某一经病证转变为另一经病证,称为传经。若两个阳经或三个阳经病证同时出现,称为合病。若一经病证未罢,而又出现另一经的病证,称为并病。若伤寒病初起病邪不由阳经传入,而直接侵入三阴经,称为直中。

## 二、卫气营血辨证概要

卫气营血辨证是清代叶天士创立的用于外感温热病的一种辨证方法。它将外感温热病发生发展过程中不同阶段所表现的证候,概括为卫分证、气分证、营分证、血分证四类不同证候类型,作为施治的依据。

卫气营血辨证,是在伤寒

qi and blood was developed on the basis of six-meridians syndrome differentiation due to cold attack, replenishing six-meridians syndrome differentiation and enriching the content of syndrome differentiation for exogenous febrile disease.

### 2.4.2.1 Defensive phase syndrome

Defensive phase syndrome refers to the syndrome due to invasion of pathogenic factors into the lung, disorder of defensive qi and dysfunction of the lung. This syndrome is usually seen at the primary stage of epidemic febrile disease.

Clinical manifestations: Fever, slight aversion to cold and wind, reddish tongue tip, whitish thin or slightly yellow tongue fur, floating and rapid pulse, usually accompanied by headache, cough, dry mouth, slight thirst and swelling pain of the throat.

Analysis of the symptoms: Fever and slight aversion to cold and wind are caused by struggle between pathogenic factors and defensive qi in the superficies; headache is due to febrile pathogenic factors disturbing the head; cough is due to febrile pathogenic factors attacking the lung; slight thirst and dry mouth are due to mild consumption of body fluid at the primary stage of epidemic febrile disease; swelling and painful throat are due to febrile pathogenic factors attacking the lung, scorching the throat and stagnation of qi and blood; reddish tongue tip, whitish thin or slightly yellow tongue fur, floating and rapid pulse are the signs of febrile pathogenic factors invading the superficies.

### 2.4.2.2 Qi phase syndrome

Qi phase syndrome refers to internal sthenia-heat syndrome due to febrile pathogenic factors penetrating inside and attacking the viscera, marked by superabundance of healthy qi and sthenia of pathogenic factors. The manifestations of this syndrome are different due to different

六经辨证的基础上发展起来的,其弥补了六经辨证的不足,从而极大地丰富了中医学辨治外感热病的内容。

### (一)卫分证

卫分证是指温热病邪侵犯肺卫,卫气功能失调,肺失宣降所表现的证候。本证多见于温热病的初期阶段。

临床表现:发热,微恶风寒,舌边尖红,苔薄白或微黄,脉浮数,常伴头痛,咳嗽,口干微渴,咽喉肿痛。

证候分析:温热病邪侵犯肌表,卫气与之相争则发热,微恶风寒;温热之邪上扰清空则头痛;温邪犯肺,肺失宣降,则咳嗽;温病初起伤津不甚,则口干微渴;温热袭肺,上灼咽喉,气血壅滞,则咽喉肿痛。舌边尖红,苔薄白或微黄,脉浮数,为温热犯表的征象。

### (二)气分证

气分证是指温热病邪入里,侵犯脏腑,表现为正盛邪实,阳热亢盛的里实热证。本证多见于温热病的极期阶段。由于邪热侵犯脏腑、部位不同,

location of pathogenic febrile factors in invading the viscera.

Clinical manifestations: Fever, aversion not to cold but to heat, vexation and thirst, sweating, reddish urine, reddish tongue, yellowish tongue fur and rapid pulse, or accompanied by cough, chest pain, expectoration of yellowish thick sputum; or accompanied by vexation, heartburn and restlessness; or high fever, profuse sweating, polydipsia and preference for cold drinks as well as full and large pulse; or afternoon tidal fever, unpressable abdominal hardness and pain, constipation or watery diarrhea, yellowish dry tongue fur, or even dry blackish tongue fur with prickles, deep and sthenia pulse; or alternate chills and fever like malaria, pain in the rib-side and bitter taste in the mouth, vexation and retching as well as taut and rapid pulse.

Analysis of the symptoms: Fever, aversion not to cold but to heat, vexation, thirst and reddish tongue with yellowish tongue fur are caused by internal exuberance of heat and severe struggle between pathogenic factors and healthy qi; cough, chest pain and expectoration of yellowish thick sputum are caused by accumulation of pathogenic heat in the lung and dysfunction of the lung in depuration and descending; vexation and heartburn are due to dysphoria resulting from disturbance of diaphragm by heat; high fever, profuse sweating and serious thirst are due to superabundance of gastric heat and steaming of internal heat; hectic fever, abdominal fullness, distension and pain as well as constipation are due to retention of heat in the intestines and stagnation of intestinal qi; alternate chills and fever like malaria, pain in the rib-side and bitter taste in the mouth are due to retention of pathogenic factors in the gallbladder.

### 2.4.2.3 Nutrient phase syndrome

Nutrient phase syndrome refers to the syndrome due to internal transmission of pathogenic febrile factors,

气分证的表现也不尽相同。

临床表现：发热，不恶寒反恶热，心烦口渴，汗出，尿赤，舌红，苔黄，脉数。或兼咳喘，胸痛，咯痰黄稠；或兼心烦懊憹，坐卧不安；或壮热，大汗出，大渴喜冷饮，脉洪大；或日晡潮热，腹满硬痛，拒按，大便秘结或下利稀水，苔黄燥，甚则焦黑起刺，脉沉实；或寒热如疟，胁痛口苦，心烦干呕，脉弦数。

证候分析：里热炽盛，邪正剧争，故出现身热、不恶寒反恶热，心烦口渴，舌红苔黄等里实热证的表现。邪热壅肺，肺失清肃，则咳喘胸痛，咯痰黄稠；热扰胸膈，心神不宁，则心烦懊憹；胃热亢盛，里热蒸腾，则壮热、大汗、大渴；热结肠道，腑气不通，则出现潮热、腹满胀痛、便秘等症；邪郁胆腑，枢机不利，则出现寒热如疟、胁痛口苦等症。

### (三) 营分证

营分证是指温热病邪内陷，劫灼营阴，心神被扰所表

consumption of nutrient yin and disturbance of the mind. This syndrome appears at the serious stage of epidemic febrile disease.

Clinical manifestations: Severe fever in the night, mild thirst, vexation and insomnia, or even delirium, appearance of macules and eruption, deep-red tongue with scanty fur and thin and rapid pulse.

Analysis of the symptoms: Severe fever in the night is due to invasion of pathogenic febrile factors into nutrient phase and scorching nutrient yin; vexation and insomnia, or even delirium are due to invasion of pathogenic heat into nutrient phase and disturbing the mind; mild thirst is due to pathogenic heat steaming nutrient yin to rise up; appearance of macules and eruption are due to heat invading blood collaterals; deep-red tongue with scanty fur and thin and rapid pulse are the signs of heat scorching yin.

#### 2.4.2.4 Blood phase syndrome

Blood phase syndrome is caused by invasion of pathogenic febrile factors into yin blood and leading to disturbance of blood, generation of wind and consumption of yin. This syndrome appears at the critical stage of epidemic febrile disease.

Clinical manifestations: Worsened fever in the night, restlessness, or even delirium, mania, appearance of purplish or blackish macules and eruptions, or hematemesis, epistaxis, hematochezia, hematuria, deep-red tongue, and rapid pulse; or convulsion, stiffness of neck, episthotonos, upward staring of eyes, lockjaw and taut and rapid pulse; or continuous low fever, evening fever with alleviation in the morning, feverish sensation over the five centers (palms, soles and chest), emaciation and dispiritedness, deafness and thin pulse; or tremor of hands and feet and flaccidity.

现的证候。本证是温热病过程中较为深重的阶段。

临床表现：身热夜甚，口不甚渴，心烦不寐，甚或神昏谵语，斑疹隐现，舌红绛少苔，脉细数。

证候分析：温热病邪深入营分，燔灼营阴，则身热夜甚；邪热入营，心神被扰，则心烦不寐，甚或神昏谵语；邪热蒸腾营阴上承，则口不甚渴；热迫血络，则斑疹隐现。舌红绛少苔，脉细数，为热灼阴伤的征象。

#### （四）血分证

血分证是指温热病邪深入阴血，导致动血、动风、耗阴所表现的一类证候。本证是温热病过程中最深重的阶段。

临床表现：身热夜甚，躁扰不宁，甚或神昏谵语，躁狂，斑疹显露，色紫或黑，或吐血、衄血、便血、尿血，舌色深绛，脉数；或见抽搐，颈项强直，角弓反张，目睛上视，牙关紧闭，脉弦数；或见持续低热、暮热早凉、五心烦热，形瘦神疲，耳聋，脉细；或见手足蠕动，瘛疭。

Analysis of the symptoms: Worsened fever in the night is due to exuberant heat in blood phase scorching blood; restlessness, delirium and mania are due to heat disturbing the mind; appearance of purplish or blackish macules and eruptions and various bleeding are caused by heat scorching collaterals and causing extravasation of blood; deep-red tongue, and rapid pulse are signs of exuberance of heat in blood phase; convulsion, stiffness of neck and episthotonos are due to exuberant heat in blood phase to scorch vessels and tendons; low fever, evening fever with alleviation in the morning, feverish sensation over the five centers (palms, soles and chest) are due to retention of pathogenic heat consuming liver and kidney yin and internal disturbance of asthenia-heat due to yin asthenia; emaciation and dispiritedness and thin pulse are due to deficiency of yin essence and malnutrition of the body; dispiritedness is due to malnutrition of spirit; deafness is due to consumption of kidney yin and malnutrition of ears; tremor of hands and feet and flaccidity are signs of endogenous asthenia-wind due to consumption of liver yin and malnutrition of tendons.

Exogenous epidemic febrile disease usually starts from defensive phase, gradually developing into qi phase, nutrient phase and blood phase as the pathological conditions are gradually getting worsened. Such a progress is called due transmission. If pathogenic factors enter defensive phase and directly penetrates into blood phase without passing through qi phase, coma and delirium will be caused. Such a progress is known as adverse transmission. Besides, there are still some other ways of transmission, such as "simultaneous involvement of defensive phase and qi phase", "heat in both qi phase and nutrient phase" and "heat in both qi phase and blood phase".

证候分析：热炽血分，营血受邪热燔灼，则身热夜甚；热扰心神，故躁扰不宁，甚则神昏谵语，躁狂；热灼络伤，迫血妄行，则见斑疹显露，以及各种出血。舌质深绛，脉数，为血热炽盛的征象。血分热炽，燔灼筋脉，则出现项强、抽搐等动风表现。邪热久羁，劫灼肝肾之阴，阴虚而虚热内扰，则出现低热、暮热早凉、五心烦热等症；阴精亏损，形体失于充养，则形瘦、脉细；神失所养，则神疲；肾阴亏耗，耳窍失养，则耳聋。肝阴亏损，筋失所养，则出现手足蠕动、瘛疭等虚风内动的表现。

外感温热病多起于卫分，渐次转入气分、营分、血分，病情逐渐加重，此为顺传。若邪入卫分不经过气分阶段，而直接深入营血分，出现神昏谵语等症，则为逆传。此外，尚有"卫气同病"、"气营两燔"和"气血两燔"等。

# Postscript

The Compilation of *A Newly Compiled English-Chinese Library of TCM* was started in 2000 and published in 2002. In order to demonstrate the academic theory and clinical practice of TCM and to meet the requirements of compilation, the compilers and translators have made great efforts to revise and polish the Chinese manuscript and English translation so as to make it systematic, accurate, scientific, standard and easy to understand. Shanghai University of TCM is in charge of the translation. Many scholars and universities have participated in the compilation and translation of the Library, i. e. Professor Shao Xundao from Xi'an Medical University (former Dean of English Department and Training Center of the Health Ministry), Professor Ou Ming from Guangzhou University of TCM (celebrated translator and chief professor), Henan College of TCM, Guangzhou University of TCM, Nanjing University of TCM, Shaanxi College of TCM, Liaoning College of TCM and Shandong University of TCM.

The compilation of this Library is also supported by the State Administrative Bureau and experts from other universities and colleges of TCM. The experts on the Compilation Committee and Approval Committee have directed the compilation and translation. Professor She

# 后 记

《(英汉对照)新编实用中医文库》(以下简称《文库》)从2000年中文稿的动笔,到2002年全书的付梓,完成了世纪的跨越。为了使本套《文库》尽可能展示传统中医学术理论和临床实践的精华,达到全面、系统、准确、科学、规范、通俗的编写要求,全体编译人员耗费了大量的心血,付出了艰辛的劳动。特别是上海中医药大学承担了英语翻译的主持工作,得到了著名医学英语翻译家、原西安医科大学英语系主任和卫生部外语培训中心主任邵循道教授,著名中医英语翻译家、广州中医药大学欧明首席教授的热心指导,河南中医学院、广州中医药大学、南京中医药大学、陕西中医学院、辽宁中医学院、山东中医药大学等中医院校英语专家的全力参与,确保了本套《文库》具有较高的英译水平。

在《文库》的编撰过程中,我们始终得到国家主管部门领导和各中医院校专家们的关心和帮助。编纂委员会的国内外学者及审定委员会的

Jing, Head of the State Administrative Bureau and Vice Minister of the Health Ministry, has showed much concern for the Library. Professor Zhu Bangxian, head of the Publishing House of Shanghai University of TCM, Zhou Dunhua, former head of the Publishing House of Shanghai University of TCM, and Pan Zhaoxi, former editor-in-chief of the Publishing House of Shanghai University of TCM, have given full support to the compilation and translation of the Library.

With the coming of the new century, we have presented this Library to the readers all over the world, sincerely hoping to receive suggestions and criticism from the readers so as to make it perfect in the following revision.

Zuo Yanfu
Pingju Village, Nanjing
Spring 2002

专家对编写工作提出了指导性的意见和建议。尤其是卫生部副部长、国家中医药管理局局长佘靖教授对本书的编写给予了极大的关注，多次垂询编撰过程，并及时进行指导。上海中医药大学出版社社长兼总编辑朱邦贤教授，以及原社长周敦华先生、原总编辑潘朝曦先生及全体编辑对本书的编辑出版工作给予了全面的支持，使《文库》得以顺利面世。在此，一并致以诚挚的谢意。

在新世纪之初，我们将这套《文库》奉献给国内外中医界及广大中医爱好者，恳切希望有识之士对《文库》存在的不足之处给予批评、指教，以便在修订时更臻完善。

左言富
于金陵萍聚村
2002年初春